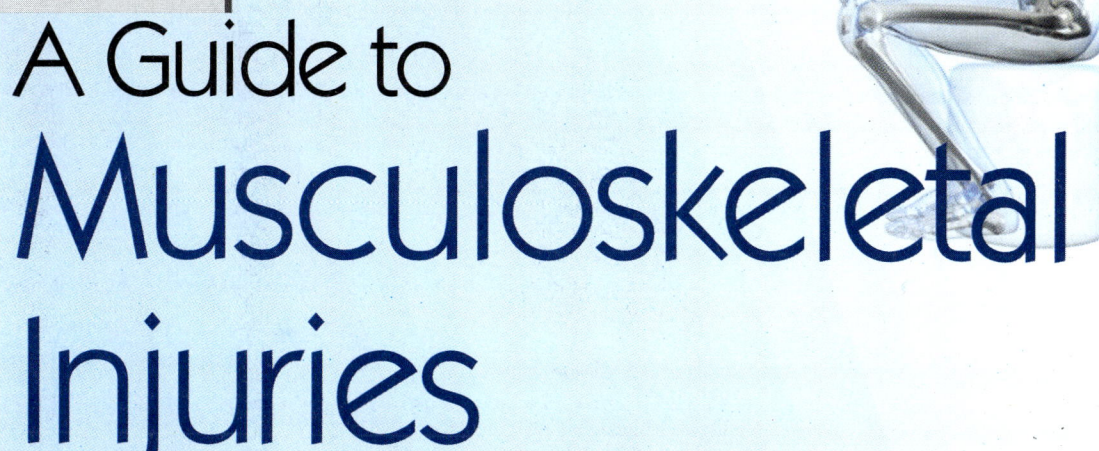

A Guide to
Musculoskeletal
Injuries

A Guide to Musculoskeletal Injuries

B Seetharama Rao MBBS, MS (Ortho), MCh (Ortho)
Senior Orthopaedic Consultant
Former
Head of Department Orthopaedics
Kasturba Medical College, Mangalore and
Melaka Manipal Medical College, Melaka in Malaysia

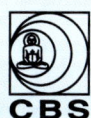

CBS

CBS Publishers & Distributors Pvt Ltd

New Delhi • Bengaluru • Chennai • Kochi • Kolkata • Mumbai
Hyderabad • Jharkhand • Nagpur • Patna • Pune • Uttarakhand

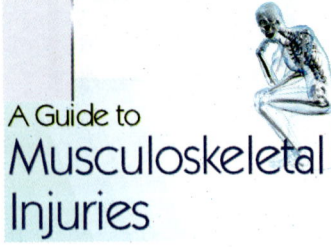

A Guide to
Musculoskeletal
Injuries

ISBN: 978-93-54660-70-2

First Edition: 2022

Published by Satish Kumar Jain and produced by Varun Jain for

CBS Publishers & Distributors Pvt Ltd

4819/XI Prahlad Street, 24 Ansari Road, Daryaganj, New Delhi 110 002, India.
Ph: 011-23289259, 23266861, 23266867   Website: www.cbspd.com
Fax: 011-23243014   e-mail: delhi@cbspd.com; cbspubs@airtelmail.in.

Corporate Office: 204 FIE, Industrial Area, Patparganj, Delhi 110 092
Ph: 011-4934 4934   Fax: 011-4934 4935   e-mail: publishing@cbspd.com; publicity@cbspd.com

Branches

• **Bengaluru:** Seema House 2975, 17th Cross, K.R. Road, Banasankari 2nd Stage, Bengaluru 560 070, Karnataka
  Ph: +91-80-26771678/79   Fax: +91-80-26771680   e-mail: bangalore@cbspd.com
• **Chennai:** 7, Subbaraya Street, Shenoy Nagar, Chennai 600 030, Tamil Nadu
  Ph: +91-44-26680620, 26681266   Fax: +91-44-42032115   e-mail: chennai@cbspd.com
• **Kochi:** 42/1325, 1326, Power House Road, Opp KSEB, Ernakulum, Kochi 682 018, Kerala, India
  Ph: +91-484-4059061-65,67   Fax: +91-484-4059065   e-mail: kochi@cbspd.com
• **Kolkata:** 6/B, Ground Floor, Rameswar Shaw Road, Kolkata-700014 (West Bengal), India
  Ph: +91-33-2289-1126, 2289-1127, 2289-1128   e-mail: kolkata@cbspd.com
• **Mumbai:** PWD Shed, Gala no 25/26, Ramchandra Bhatt Marg, Next to JJ Hospital Gate no. 2, Opp. Union Bank of India, Noorbaug Mumbai-400009, Maharashtra
  Ph: +91-22-66661880/89   e-mail: mumbai@cbspd.com

Representatives

• Hyderabad   0-9885175004   • Jharkhand   0-9811541605   • Nagpur   0-9421945513
• Patna   0-9334159340   • Pune   0-9623451994   • Uttarakhand 0-9716462459

Printed at Goyal Offset Works Pvt. Ltd., Haryana (INDIA)

to

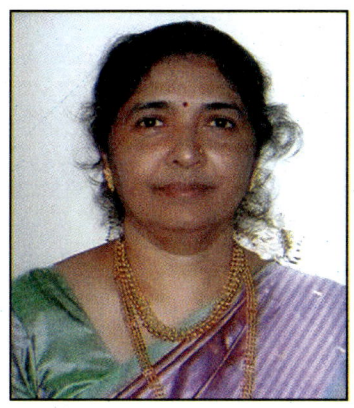

(1958–2020)

*my beloved wife, **Mrs. GEETHA B***
who has been the pillar of my life and
has been a great source of inspiration...

Foreword

It gives me great pleasure to pen a few lines as foreword to a book *A Guide to Musculoskeletal Injuries* written by my good friend Dr B Seetharama Rao, former HOD and Professor of Orthopaedics at KMC Hospital, Attavar. I know him from 1976 when I joined KMC Manipal for first MBBS when he was 1 year my senior and a role model for juniors even then. Thereafter all through his innings as UG and PG in orthopaedics in Kasturba Medical College Mangalore, he has a number of academic achievements which enabled him to get trained in United Kingdom after which he came back and headed the department as its youngest HOD from 1997 to 2002 during which time department rose to great heights under his leadership.

A gentleman to the core he is an excellent teacher, gifted surgeon and a great mentor to his students. His case presentations to Clinical Society are a class apart—outstanding and looked forwards to.

I am very sure the book he has written will blaze a new trail for his students to travel upon and follow his footsteps to reach their academic destination.

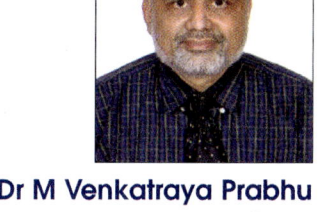

Dr M Venkatraya Prabhu
Dean
Kasturba Medical College
Mangalore

Foreword

"It is the supreme art of the teacher to awaken joy in creative expression and knowledge"
—Albert Einstein

I feel proud to write a brief foreword to a book *A guide to Musculoskeletal injuries*— written by my senior colleague Dr B Seetharama Rao, Professor of Orthopaedics and former Head of Department Orthopaedics, KMC, Mangalore. I had known him for last two decades and witnessed his teaching and professionalism in the department. This book is going to be companion for orthopaedics undergraduates and postgraduates as well as practicing orthopaedic surgeons. Also it is aimed to benefit trainees in Emergency medicine and physiotherapy students.

I am sure that this book is going to awaken creative expression and knowledge in orthopaedic trainees and other readers.

Prof Dr Surendra Umesh Kamath
Dip (Ortho), DNB (Ortho), FRCS (Edinburg), FRCS (Glasgow)
Professor and HOD
Department of Orthopaedics
Kasturba Medical College, Mangalore

Preface

Musculoskeletal injuries are on the rise and hence the need to have a good knowledge related to them, especially their management. The concerned medical person, be it a student or a staff, has to know the basics with quick references. Keeping this in mind, this book is written in such a style that common injuries are described with line diagrams, clinical pictures, simple tables and algorithms. Particular attention is given to highlight the incidence, mechanism of injury, various classification systems, relevant investigations, management protocol and the complications.

At the end of each chapter, references are given, related to important articles in literature. In addition, to gain a visual impact, website references, including short video clippings, are stated for better understanding.

Any suggestions, remarks or feedback are most welcome by the reader(s) for future amendments in bringing out new addition of this book.

B Seetharama Rao
belpusrao@gmail.com

Contents

Orthopaedic Case Notes

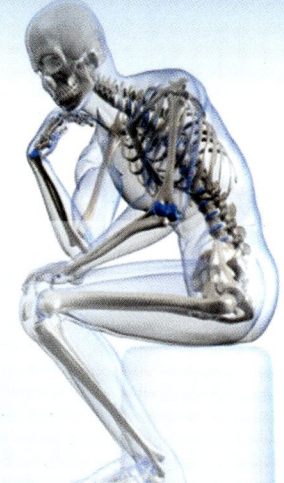

Unlike in other fields of medicine, the following facts have to be borne in mind while taking patient's history:
- Age of the patient
- Occupation of the patient
- Dexterity
- Disability
- Ambulatory status of the patient (in lower limb/spinal pathology)

In orthopaedics, the treatment option depends on the above factors and the decision-making is crucial which varies from case to case basis. For appendicitis, appendicectomy or for tonsillitis, tonsillectomy is the easy and standard solution, irrespective of the profession of the patient. But for correction of a deformity or treatment of a fracture, the choices are many. The treating surgeon should be aware of all the possible options in treating his patient and select the best line with specific advantages and benefits. No similar case may be treated in a similar fashion. The choice of treatment depends on several factors like patient's age, clinical stage or radiological findings, quality of bone, patient's socio-economic status and many others.

Detailed treatment history for the present ailment should be noted down. Significant major medical problems or hospitalization should be recorded. In children, a detail of the birth history along with developmental milestones is very important. Socioeconomic status and living atmosphere play significant role in the etiology and treatment of many orthopaedic disorders.

The common symptoms in orthopaedics are:
- Pain
- Swelling
- Deformity
- Stiffness of a joint
- Loss of function
- Disability
- Limb length discrepancy
- Weakness of limb(s) or part of a limb
- Numbness or coldness of a limb
- Sinus/wound/ulcer
- Constitutional symptoms

History of present illness should elaborate on the type of onset of the ailment, its duration, nature, aggravating and relieving factors, and so on. Chronological order of the onset of symptoms has to be followed. Details of the treatment history need to be noted. Significant family history and major medical illnesses or hospitalizations in the past are of great significance. Various personal habits might contribute to the etiopathogenesis of a given orthopaedic disease.

It is a good idea to write down a diagnosis or set of differential diagnosis at this level before proceeding to examination of the patient.

General examination of the patient should revolve around the underlying orthopaedic

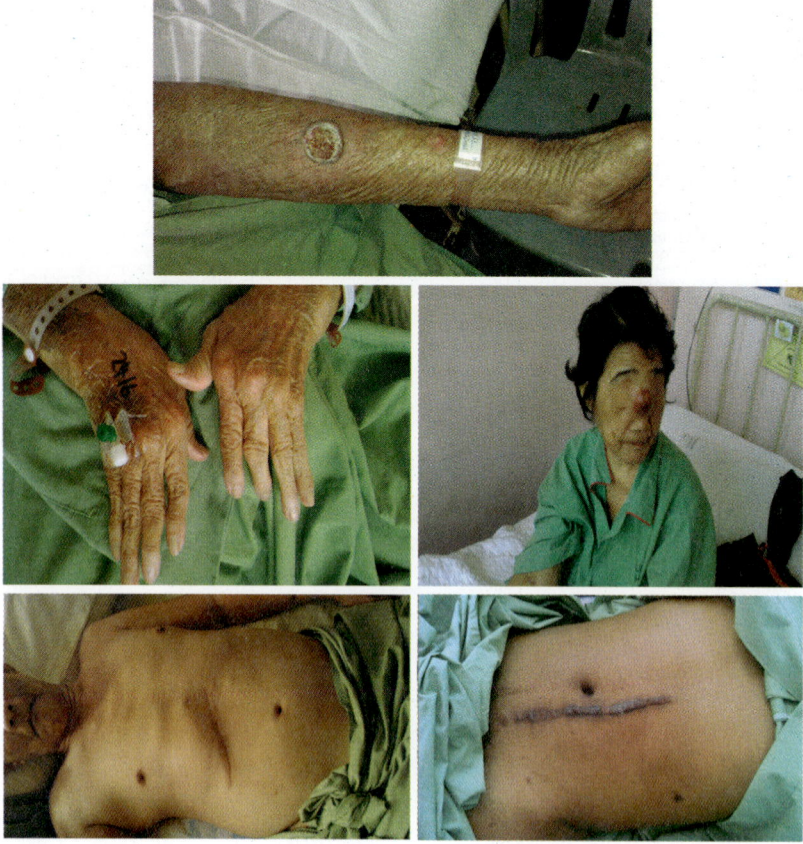

Fig. 1.1: An abdominal scar or a scar over iliac crest may give some clue to the surgical procedure undertaken in the past

pathology (e.g. lungs for primary focus of TB; primary tumours in case of bony secondaries; hypermobile joints in recurrent dislocation of a joint, etc.).

Though it is essential to examine the patient from head-to-toe, if there are no significant findings, it may be summarized in 4–5 sentences as follows:

"On general examination, patient is conscious and co-operative. He is averagely built and well nourished. He has no pallor or generalized lymphadenopathy. His vital signs are stable. There are no significant systemic abnormalities detected".

Local examination in orthopaedics should be systematic:

• Look (inspection)
• Feel (palpation)
• Move (movements)
• Measure (measurements)
• Special tests
• Distal neurovascular status
• Local lymph nodes
• Neighbouring joints

At the end of clinical examination, a provisional diagnosis or a set of differential diagnosis has to be offered with valid reasons.

The diagnosis has to be confirmed before offering treatment. Thus, management of the patient includes investigations, followed by treatment.

The important investigations include: Haemogram, bone profile screening, X-rays, various types of scans and biopsy of the lesion in some cases.

A given orthopaedic injury or disease may be treated by non-operative (conservative) or operative method. The best method of treatment has to be selected on individual case-to-case basis, with clear-cut indications.

To summarise, following is the method of writing up a case note in orthopaedics:

- Name of the patient
- Age
- Sex
- Occupation
- Chief complaints (in chronological order)
- History of presenting illness (HOPI)
- Past medical history (PMH)
- Family history (FH)
- Social (personal) history (SH)
- Diagnosis at history level
- General examination
- Local examination:
  - Inspection
  - Palpation
  - Movements (active and passive)
  - Measurements (limb length and muscle bulk)
  - Special tests, if any
  - One joint proximal and one joint distal
  - Distal neurovascular status
- Clinical diagnosis/differential diagnosis
- Investigations ordered and their results
- Management planned
- Treatment offered
- Progress in hospital, including complications
- End-result

Orthopaedic surgery includes study of injuries and diseases of the musculoskeletal system.

The injuries include those of bones (fractures), joints (dislocations) and soft tissues like nerves, muscles, tendons, vessels, capsule, synovium, bursae and others.

Orthopaedic disorders may be classified into the following (Table 1.1): Congenital (hereditary or non-hereditary), or acquired:

- Traumatic
- Developmental
- Metabolic
- Inflammatory
- Infective
- Neoplastic
- Degenerative

Table 1.1: Classification of orthopaedic disorders

Condition	Examples
Congenital	Developmental dysplasia of the hip (DDH) Congenital talipes equinovarus (CTEV) Spina bifida
Traumatic	Fractures, dislocations, tendon/nerve injury, sprains and strains
Developmental	Spondylolysis, bone dysplasias
Metabolic	Rickets, osteomalacia, Paget's disease, osteoporosis
Inflammatory	Various arthritides (rheumatoid, gouty, sero-negative arthritis)
Infective	Osteomyelitis, pyogenic arthritis, tuberculous arthritis
Neoplastic	Various soft tissue sarcomas and bone tumours (benign and malignant)
Degenerative	Osteoarthritis, cervical and lumbar spondylosis

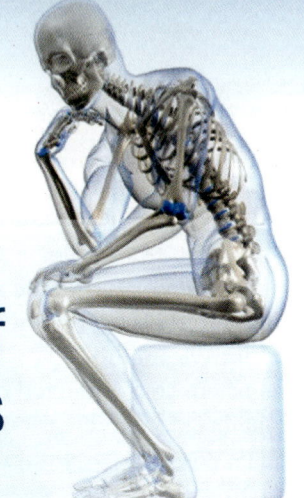

The Foundations of Modern Orthopaedics

It was not until the 12th century that Europe began to gradually awake from its Dark Ages. Universities and hospitals were beginning to be established, human dissection resumed and the great Greek texts were being translated from Arabic to Latin. However, until the 16th century, all developments remained within the shadow cast by Hippocrates.

AMBROISE PARÉ (1510–1590)

Ambroise Paré is regarded as the most famous surgical figure of the 16th century and "the father of French surgery". He was born in Bourg Herent in France. In 1532, he became an apprentice to a Parisian barber-surgeon, then worked for four years at Hotel Dieu in Paris. In 1541, he became a master barber-surgeon and did some work as an army surgeon. In 1564, he published a monumental work on surgery, the *"Dix Livres de la Chirurgie"*. The first part contained anatomy and physiology and the second, surgery. In this, many surgical techniques were described, one of the most significant being the use of ligature for large vessels in amputations. He also used a tourniquet in his amputations, to hold the muscles retracted with the skin, prohibit the flux of blood and to dull the senses. He designed a wide variety of forceps, instruments and braces of all kinds. With the help of armourers, he made a variety of artificial limbs from iron. The majorities were cosmetic, although Pare did design a scoliosis corset and a clubfoot boot.

NICOLAS ANDRY (1658–1742)

Andry was the professor of medicine at the University of Paris and Dean of the faculty of

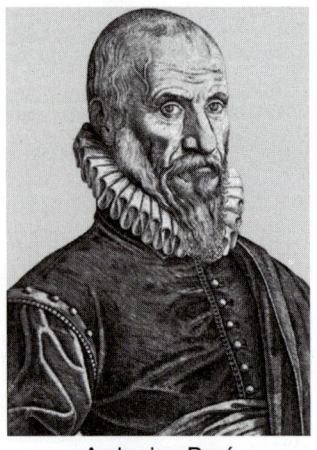

Ambroise Paré

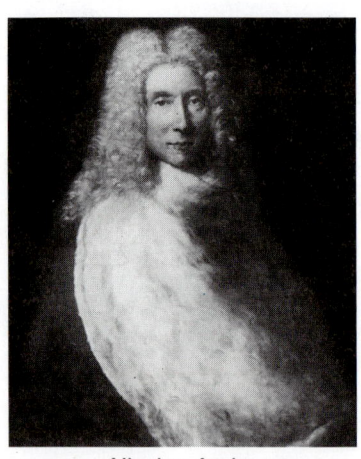

Nicolas Andry

Physick. In 1741, at the age of 81, he published a famous book called "*Orthopaedia* or the art of correcting and preventing deformities in children. By such means that may easily be put into correcting and preventing deformities in children. By such means that may easily be put into practice by parents themselves and all such as are employed in educating children". In this book, Andry presents the work orthopaedic, which derives from the Greek words "straight" and "child". Andry was interested in postural defects and this has been reflected by his famous illustration, which is known as "the tree of Andry". Andry believed that skeletal deformities were due to faults of posture and shortness of muscles. Some regard Andry as the father of orthopaedics, by many strongly disagree, believing that his work was un-scientific and that his only contribution was the use of the word orthopaedics.

THOMAS SYDENHAM (1624–1689)

Sydenham is likened to Hippocrates because his writings cover a large field and are characterized by good observation. Likewise, he is also known as "the father of English medicine". He was born at Winford Eagle, and studied at Oxford and Montpellier. He himself suffered from gout and wrote an excellent description of the disease, detailing the attack, the changes in urine and the link with renal stones. He described acute rheumatism,

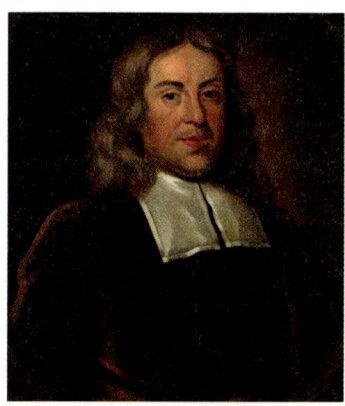

Thomas Sydenham

chorea, and the articular manifestations of scurvy and dysentery.

PERCIVALL POTT (1714–1788)

Pott was from London and worked in St. Bartholomew's Hospital, where he received the diploma of the Barber-Surgeons' company in 1763. He is best known for the fracture that bears his name "Pott's fracture", as he gave a good description of this ankle fracture. In 1756, he received a fracture of his own. It was an oblique compound fracture of the lower third of the tibia, which was acquired after falling from his horse. He refused to be moved until he had purchased a door to be carried on, as he believed that the jolting of a carriage would have exacerbated the injury. Immediate amputation was usually conducted on such injuries, but at the last moment, amputation was stopped and the limb was saved. Pott's most famous work is on the paraplegia of spinal tuberculosis, where he stressed that the condition was not related to spinal cord compression, but associated with "strumous disorders" in the lungs. This is known as Pott's paraplegia.

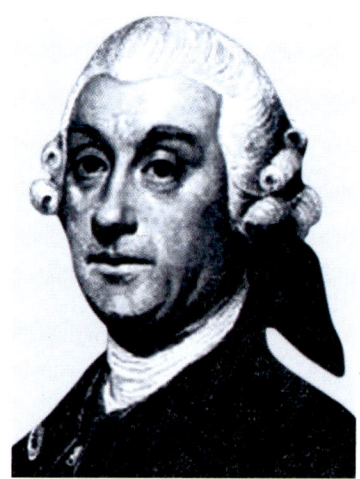

Percivall Pott

WILLIAM HEBERDEN (1710–1801)

Heberden was born in London where he also built up a busy practice. He is known for initiating the medical transactions in 1766, but even more so for his description of Heberden's nodes.

JOHN HUNTER (1728–1793)

Hunter worked on a lowland farm until he was 20 years of age. Until he was 32, he was a pupil and house surgeon at St. George's Hospital in London and also worked in his brother's dissecting room in Covent Garden. In the seven years' war, he served as a military surgeon. He set up a research centre in London's golden square and taught and lectured at Leicester square until angina eventually lead to his death. Hunter's contribution was immense and even stemmed through the pupils he taught (e.g. Abernethy, Chessher, Jenner and Philip Syng Physick). Hunter himself was a pupil of Percivall Pott. Although he received little formal education (unlike his brother William, an obstetrician in London), Hunter put the practice of surgery on a scientific foundation and laid the framework for the twentieth century developments. His saying "don't think, try the experiment" has inspired generations of modern surgeons.

Much of Hunter's knowledge may be attributed to his military experience and his experiments on animals. He described how to assess muscle power in a weak muscle. With joint injury and disease, he states that voluntary movement should not be permitted until inflammation has settled, otherwise contracture is promoted. He believed that healing depended on the body's innate power, and that the surgeon's task was to aid this. He studied loose bodies in joints, pseudoarthroses and fracture healing, where he described the transformation from fracture haematoma to fibrocartilaginous callus to the deposition of new bone, trabeculation, re-establishment of the medullary canal and the resorption of excess bony tissue. Hunter wrote "a treatise on the blood, inflammation and gunshot wounds" in 1794, and also made attempts at tissue grafting.

His collection of specimens (initially over 14,000 POT's; half destroyed in the bombing of London) is in the College of Surgeons, London. They describe the development of the various systems from the simplest (insects) to the most complex. It is a humbling and inspiring experience to visit the museum and see one man's monumental contribution to surgery.

JEAN-ANDRÉ VENEL (1740–1791)

Jean-André Venel was a Genevese physician who studied dissection at Montpellier at the age of 39, and in 1780, established the first orthopaedic institute in the world at Orbe, in Canton Waadt.

This was the first true hospital that dealt specifically with the treatment for crippled children's skeletal deformities. Venel recorded and published all his methods and for this he was known as the first true orthopaedist. He is also regarded as the father of orthopaedics, as his institute acted as a model for hospitals throughout Europe. Venel stressed the importance of sunlight and made various braces and appliances at the workshops within the institute.

WILLIAM HEY (1736–1819)

William Hey was born in Pudsey near Leeds. At the age of 14, he was apprenticed to a surgeon and apothecary and nearly died of an overdose of opium whilst studying its effects. He was the founder of surgery at Leeds and trained at St. George's Hospital. Hey wrote a

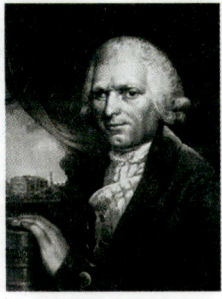

William Hey

book on surgery which contained several chapters on orthopaedics. Subacute osteomyelitis of the tibia was described and he advocated deroofing of the lesion. In 1773, Hey banged his knee getting out of the bath, and many attribute his subsequent interest in the knee to this. He coned the phrase "internal derangement of the knee", and described meniscal injuries. Hey described loose bodies and introduced tarsometatarsal amputation.

GIOVANNI BATTISTA MONTEGGIA (1762–1815)

Monteggia was born at Lake Maggiore and was a Milanese pathologist who acquired syphilis by cutting himself at autopsy and became a surgeon and professor at Milan. He is particularly remembered for his description in 1814 of the fracture that bears his name, Monteggia's fracture.

ABRAHAM COLLES (1773–1843)

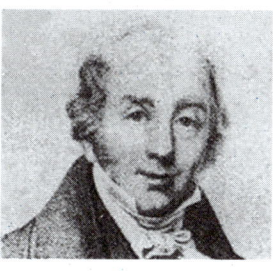

Abraham Colles

Colles was born in Kilkenny, Ireland of humble origins. Nevertheless, he became professor of surgery at the College of Surgeons in Dublin from the age of 29. He was the first to tie the subclavian artery, but is best known for his description of Colles' fracture, in 1814 (the same year as Monteggia).

BARON GUILLAUME DUPUYTREN (1777–1835)

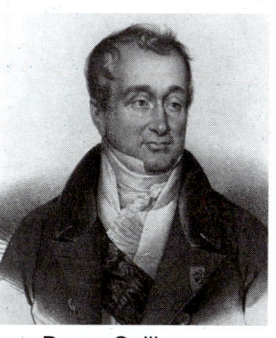

Baron Guillaume Dupuytren

Dupuytren was born in central France. He was kidnapped as a boy by a rich woman from Toulouse on account of his good looks. He was taken to Paris and educated, but endured great poverty throughout his studies. Dupuytren became surgeon in chief at the Hotel Dieu and worked tremendously hard and became very rich. He was described as an unpleasant person to met, yet his work was delightful to read. He was characterized as "first among surgeons, last among men". He was an accurate clinical observer with a great interest in pathology. Dupuytren's name is most associated with the contracture of palmar fascia and a particular ankle fracture that he described. He wrote on many subjects, including congenital dislocation of the hip, the nature of callus formation, subungal exostosis, the Trendelenburg sign, tenotomy in torticollis and he differentiated osteosarcoma from "spina ventosa".

JAMES SYME (1799–1870)

Syme was born in Edinburgh. As a student at Edinburgh University, he found a way of dissolving rubber. Syme opened a school of anatomy and later opened a very successful private clinic. In 1833, he became professor of surgery in Edinburg and held that position until his death. (He had actually made an agreement with his predecessor to pay him a pension, if he resigned.) Syme is known for introducing conservative alternatives to the major amputations that were carried out at the time. In 1831, he released a booklet, which detailed cases where joint excision could be used instead of amputation for grossly diseased joint, as in tuberculosis, and injured joints. In 1842, Syme described an amputation at the ankle. This amputation bears his name,

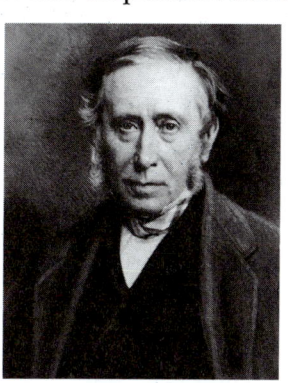

James Syme

as it replaced a portion of below knee amputations, which were ordinary practice at that time.

SIR BENJAMIN COLLINS BRODIE (1783–1862)

Brodie was a national figure. He was a surgeon at St. George's Hospital and a friend of the Thomas family (that of Hugh Owen Thomas). He first published his book, "on the diseases of joints" in 1819, which proved to be a popular reference for many years. In 1832, he described the chronic bone abscess that has been named after him. The patient was a man of 24 who had recurring symptoms in the lower extremity of his right tibia. On examination, Brodie found a pus filled cavity, for which he believed that amputation could be avoided by trephination of that cavity. He recognized the association of arthritis with gonorrhoea and that all children's hip disorders were associated with infection. In 1843, he introduced the fellowship examination of the Royal College of Surgeons in order to improve the education and standing of surgeons.

JOHN RHEA BARTON (1794–1871)

Barton was born in Lancaster, Pennsylvania, USA. He studied at the Pennsylvania Hospital and later worked for Physick (the father of American surgery) who in turn was a student of Hunter. It was said that Barton was ambidextrous and that once he had positioned himself for an operation, he did not move about. In 1826, he performed a subtrochanteric

osteotomy of the femur for a severe flexion-adduction deformity of the hip. Barton is best known for his innovative corrective osteotomies for ankylosed joints. In 1834, Barton wired a fractured patella and in 1835, he described "Barton's fracture".

ROBERT WILLIAM SMITH (1807–1873)

Smith was born in Dublin, he studied and worked there. He became professor of surgery at Trinity College in Dublin. Smith founded the Dublin Pathological Society with Colles, Graves, Corrigan and Stokes. In 1847, Smith wrote a classic book called "a treatise on fractures in the vicinity of joints, and on certain forms of accidents and congenital dislocations". Here he describes the eponymous "Smith's fracture", and Madelung's deformity before Madelung described it. In 1849, he published "a treatise on the pathology, diagnosis and treatment of neuroma". This book was said to be so large that it was larger than an ordinary sized dinning room table when opened up. Smith wrote on neurofibromatosis in great detail, much before von Recklinghausen did.

ANTONIUS MATHIJSEN (1805–1878)

Mathysen was a Dutch military surgeon who in 1851 invented the plaster of Paris (POP) bandage which was to become so important to orthopaedic practice.

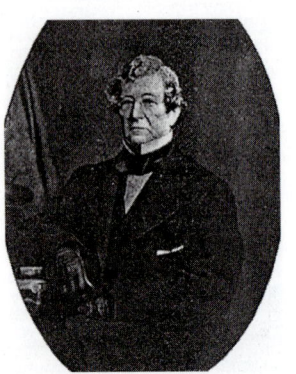

John Rhea Barton

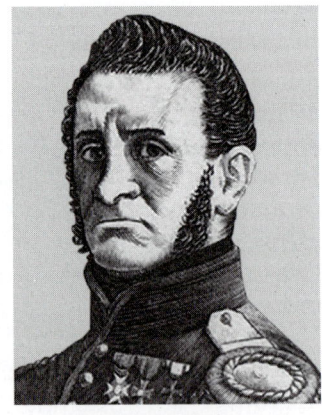

Antonius Mathijsen

To this day, a POP cast is the mainstay of fracture immobilization.

WILLIAM JOHN LITTLE (1810–1894)

Little was educated at the Jesuit seminary at St. Omer. He himself had a paralytic clubfoot. The treatment in London was amputation, however, he found a cure in Germany by tenotomy. Little was a founder of the Royal Orthopaedic Hospital. He published a detail report, in 1862, of the then ill-understood group of deformed and partly retarded children and young adults. This type of spastic paralysis with paraplegia of the lower limbs was then called Little's disease for many years.

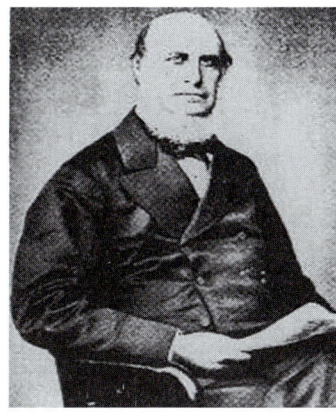

William John Little

JOSEPH LISTER (1827–1912)

Lister studied at the University College Hospital in London, although he did his famous work in Scotland, first at Glasgow (where he first instituted antiseptic surgery), and then as professor of surgery at Edinburgh (where he was at the Royal Infirmary). In 1853, he became Syme's house surgeon at the Royal Infirmary. He there married Syme's daughter. In 1854, he became assistant surgeon to the Royal Infirmary, and in later life came to London as professor of surgery at Kings College Hospital. Lister is known for the introduction of antisepsis. He first applied carbolic acid to a compound fracture in 1965. It was soon clear that the practices had had a dramatic effect in reducing in particular abscesses, pyaemia, hospital gangrene, erysipelas and amputation mortality. Lister was made a baronet in 1883, and later in his life was thought to have trialed the application of the Penicillium mould directly to wounds.

JEAN-MARTIN CHARCOT (1825–1893)

Charcot was from Salpetriere in Paris and is known worldwide as the first Professor of Neurology. He wrote a thesis distinguishing gout, rheumatoid arthritis and osteoarthritis. Charcot also first described the arthropathy that bears his name, Charcot's joints. He was first to write about amyotrophic lateral sclerosis, intermittent claudication, disseminated sclerosis, intermittent hepatic fever and herpes zoster.

EMIL THEODOR KOCHER (1841–1917)

Kocher was born in Berne and studied in Berlin, London, Paris and Vienna. In 1872, he became professor of surgery in Berne. Kocher had a great interest in anatomy and in 1870, he described his eponymous method of reducing a dislocated shoulder. Kocher wrote a remarkable book in which he detailed many useful surgical incisions that he had developed,

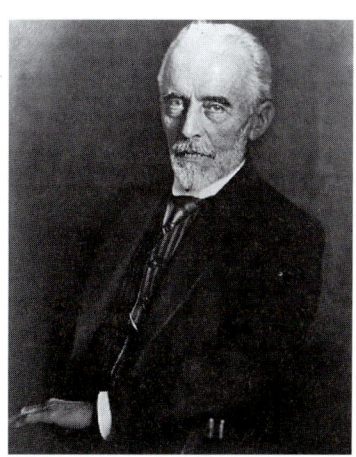

Emil Theodor Kocher

such as his posterolateral exposure of the hip. He also developed several surgical instruments, but his main interest was in thyroid disease.

SIR JAMES PAGET (1814–1899)

Paget was a graduate of St. Bartholomew's Hospital in London, where he remained for the rest of his career. It was in 1877 that Paget gave the first description of what he called "osteitis deformans", but what is now commonly called Paget's disease. He noted the increased incidence of osteosarcoma, the increasing head size and deformities. (One of Paget's original drawings is shown.) Paget was also a remarkable lecturer with a great interest in bone pathology. His name is also associated with other pathological processes.

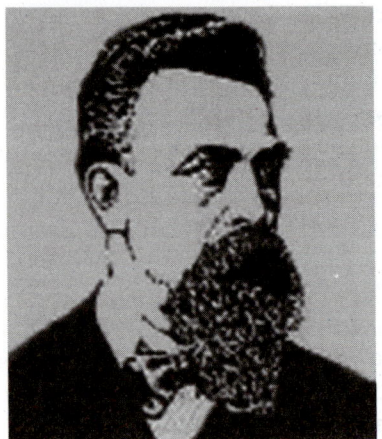
Sir William Macewen

of his grafts were performed on people who had had portions of their bones excised, but who had otherwise normal function. Macewen was also a pioneering neurosurgeon and cardiothoracic surgeon. He worked on cerebral tumours and abscesses and also performed the first pneumonectomy.

RICHARD VON VOLKMANN (1830–1889)

Volkmann was from Halle, Saxony. He was the first in Germany to Institute Lister's antiseptic methods. In 1881, Volkmann published his famous paper on ischaemic muscular paralyses and contractures. Here he attributed the cause of the contractures to direct changes

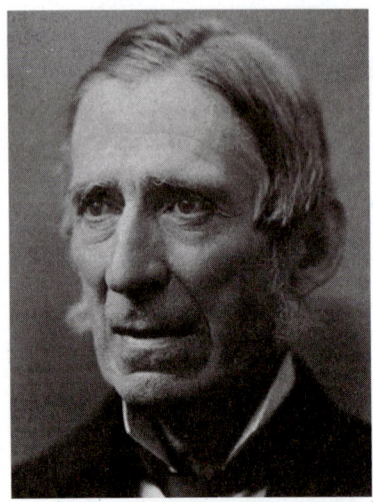
Sir James Paget

SIR WILLIAM MACEWEN (1848–1924)

Macewen studied in Glasgow and had Syme and Lister as teachers. The new era of antisepsis enabled him to make many contributions to surgery. In terms of his orthopaedic contributions, he performed many osteotomies and developed a one-piece osteotome. Macewen's main research interest was in bone growth and in 1879 he performed the first of his pioneering bone grafts. Many

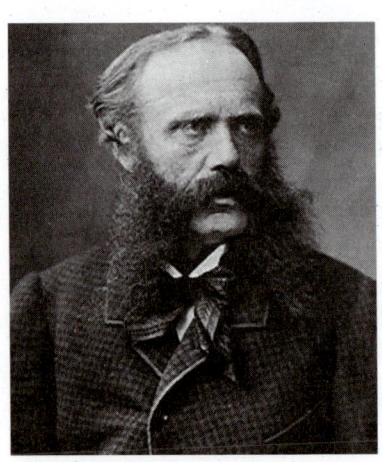
Richard von Volkmann

in the muscles produced by arterial occlusion and emphasized the early warning of preliminary weakness. These contractures are otherwise known as Volkmann's ischaemic contractures. It is interesting to note that Volkmann wrote popular poems and fairy stories and also founded a surgical journal.

EDUARD ALBERT (1841–1900)

Albert was born in Bohemia and studied in Vienna. He is best known for producing "artificial ankyloses" in paralysed limbs and wrote a paper on this in 1881. Albert performed tarsal and shoulder arthrodesis for paralysis and recurrent dislocation, and was the first to use the term "arthrodesis". Albert also described synovectomy, the transplantation of nerves, sciatic scoliosis and Achilles bursitis.

EDWARD HALLARAN BENNETT (1837–1907)

Bennett studied at Trinity College, Dublin. He collected specimens of bone pathology and with these wrote a paper on fractures of the metacarpal bones in 1882. In this paper, Bennett described his eponymous fracture dislocation of the base of the thumb metacarpal. Bennett is said to have introduced antisepsis to Dublin and to have performed many osteotomies for rickets. He became President of the Royal College of Surgeons of Ireland.

HUGH OWEN THOMAS (1834–1891)

If you could only read about one person in the history of orthopaedics, then you would have to read about Hugh Owen Thomas, "the father of British orthopaedics". Hugh Owen Thomas was the eldest of five sons born to a well-known bonesetter at that time. All studied medicine. Thomas was a thin and nervous child who was somewhat delicate. His peculiar temperament in adulthood led many to ignore him and his immense contributions to orthopaedic surgery during his lifetime. Hugh Owen Thomas could not even work with his father and never held a

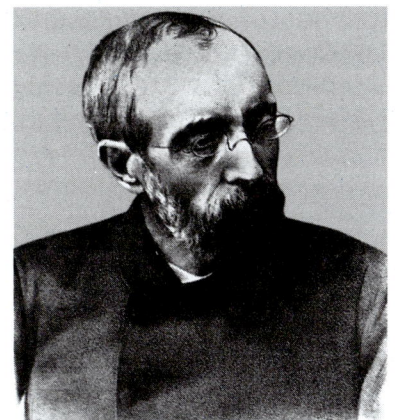

Hugh Owen Thomas

hospital appointment. He treated all his patients at his home. His practice was so busy that he started his rounds at five or six in the morning and never left his home for other than professional purposes. Thomas would designate Sunday as his "free day" and hundreds of patients from the country would surround his house in order to be treated.

The people of Liverpool knew Thomas as a short and quick man. A man who always wore a black coat buttoned up to the neck and a sailor's cap pulled over a damaged eye. A

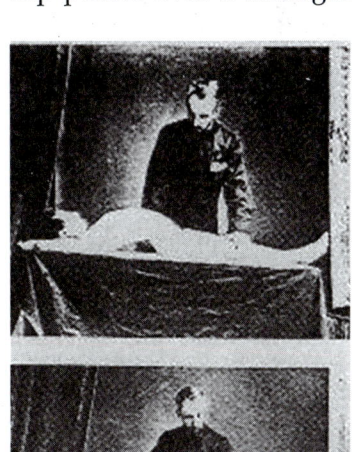

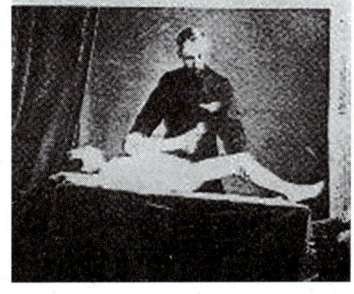

cigarette was also seen constantly in his mouth. Despite Thomas's busy schedule, Thomas wrote prolifically in the night and developed many new techniques and surgical instruments. He believed in enforced, prolonged and uninterrupted rest for the treatment of tuberculous joints. Thomas developed a great number of splints in order to achieve this. These include, the cervical collar, metatarsal bar, heel wedge and knee splint. Many of these are still in use, such as the Thomas splint. Thomas was also able to recognize early cases of hip disease. He was the first to demonstrate concealed flexion of the hip joint and a way of unmasking this by performing the "Thomas test".

It should be remembered that Hugh Owen Thomas had studied medicine and was interested in litholopaxy and the management of acute abdomen as well as orthopaedics. It has been said that the medical profession might not have practiced the "black art" of bone setting, if Hugh Owen Thomas had not graduated from a medical school.

SIR WILLIAM ARBUTHNOT LANE (1856–1943)

Lane was a Scot from Inverness who trained and later worked at Guy's Hospital in London. Lane is known for his attempts at improving alignment of fractures by using internal fixation. He started off using silver wire, then he used steel screws and this was followed by the use of plates and screws. Lane was said to have been eccentric, regarding humans as machines and performed total colectomies as a cure for "autointoxication". He also initiated the programmes of health education that are present today. Lane wrote columns in the news papers, held public lectures and improved the distribution of fruits and vegetables.

FRITZ DE QUERVAIN (1868–1940)

De Quervain was born at Sion in the Valais Canton of Switzerland. He studied at Berne and succeeded Kocher as Professor of Surgery

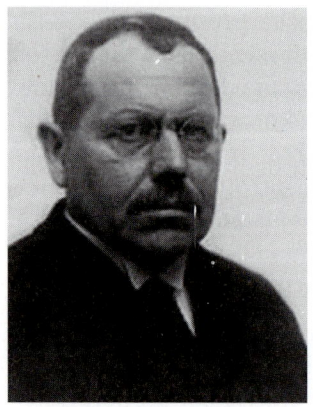
Fritz de Quervain

there. In 1895, de Quervain described a form of chronic tenovaginitis, which is now known as de Quervain's stenosing tenovaginitis. Like Kocher, he studied thyroid disease and is responsible for the introduction of iodized table salt.

FRIEDRICH TRENDELENBURG (1844–1924)

Trendelenburg was born in Berlin. He studied Medicine in Glasgow and in Berlin. Trendelenburg's name is associated with the Trendelenburg sign and the Trendelenburg gait, which he described in association with coxo-femoral incompetence in 1895. Trendelenburg also devised pulmonary embolectomy, but it was one of his pupils, Kirshner who first met success with the procedure many years later in 1924.

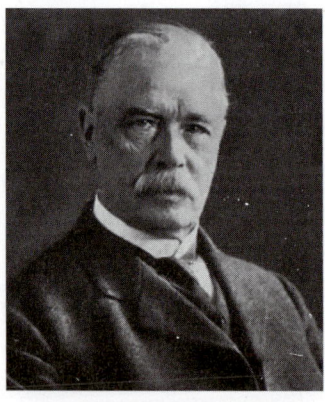
Friedrich Trendelenburg

PIERRE MARIE (1853–1940)

Marie was born in Paris, he worked for Charcot and eventually succeeded him as Professor of Neurology at Salpetriere. Marie described peroneal muscular trophy (Charot-Marie-Tooth disease). He was the first to associate acromegaly with a pituitary tumour in 1886. In 1980, he described hypertrophic pulmonary osteoarthropathy. In 1898, he gave the first account of craniocleidal dystosis and noted the partial aplasia of the clavicles, the increased skull diameter, the disordered dentition and the failure of ossification at the fontanelles. Also in 1898, he published a classic paper on ankylosing spondylitis, which he referred to as "spondylosis rhizomelique". Marie believed that poliomyelitis was infectious.

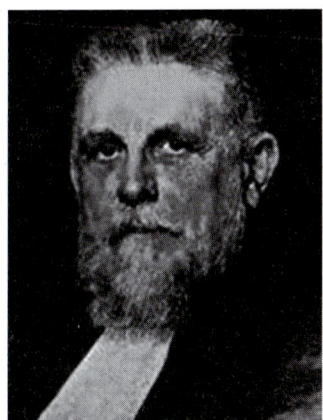

Pierre Marie

LOUIS XAVIER ÉDOUARD LÉOPOLD OLLIER (1830–1900)

Ollier was born in Vans in Ardeche and studied at Lyons and Ontpellier. Ollier, lie Macewen, performed pioneering bone grafts. Although both were successful, their methods and the theory behind them were in fierce opposition. In 1877, Ollier suggested that bone growth may be inhibited in order to correct certain deformities by resecting the epiphyseal plate. In 1899, Ollier first described dyschondroplasia or "Ollier's disease". Ollier researched bone growth to an enormous extent and believed that it might be

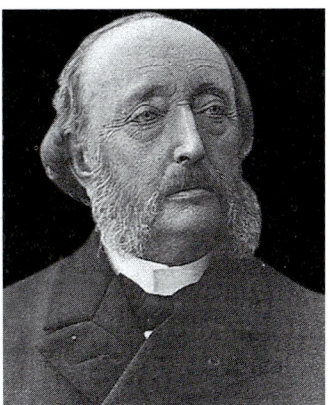

Louis Xavier Édouard Léopold Ollier

possible one day to treat patients by stimulating their cartilage to ossify.

WILHELM CONRAD RÖNTGEN (1845–1923)

Although Röntgen was a Professor of Physics at Wurzburg, his discovery of X-rays (Rontgen rays) and their use has provided an enormous contribution to orthopaedics and is still of great value to orthopaedic practice. The first radiography that Röntgen took was of his wife's hand on the 22nd of December, 1895. This was allegedly her Christmas present. Rontgen received the Nobel Prize for his discovery in 1901.

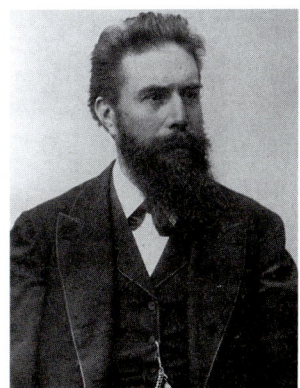

Wilhelm Conrad Röntgen

HISTORY OF ORTHOPAEDICS

Royal Whitman (1896) defined orthopaedic surgery as a division of surgery, which treats disabilities and diseases of the locomotor apparatus and involves prevention and treatment of the deformities of the framework of the body.

Orthopaedics may be defined as a special branch of surgery, which deals with injuries, and diseases of the musculoskeletal system. Thus, it is a vast subject, which includes study of not only conditions of bones and joints, but also disorders of the soft tissues surrounding the skeleton.

Orthopaedic surgery has developed through a necessity to correct deformity, restore function and alleviate pain.

Nicolas Andry was a Professor of Medicine at University of Paris, and in 1741, at the age of 81 years, he published a famous book called "Orthopaedia" or the art of correcting and preventing deformities in children.

The term 'Orthopaedics' was coined in the year 1751 by Nicolas Andry using two Greek words: *Ortho* = straight and *Paedia* = child. In ancient times, a lot of children were disabled with metabolic bone disorders and ended up with grotesque deformities of the spine. It was a challenge for the then orthopaedic surgeon to make these children straight. In the modern era, not only children but also elderly with severe osteoporotic back need to be promptly treated by the orthopaedic surgeon. Its emblem is a crooked tree tied by a rope to a supporting post. The analogy is the knowledge to correct deformity. Nicolas Andry is considered as the father of orthopaedics.

Evolution of Orthopaedics

The history of orthopaedic surgery is one of the progressive evolutions. Progress is difficult to forecast. The past is our foundation for future developments.

Like in other fields of medicine, Hippocrates has contributed a lot in the history of orthopaedics. He defined for the first time the position and role of a doctor in society. Hippocratic oath will always remain central to our practices. He had a thorough understanding of fractures and dislocations. In the management of fractures, he stressed that the following concepts to be followed: Antisepsis, bandaging, reduction, splinting, and traction. He stated that these concepts would supplement/reinforce the "healing power of nature".

Between 1st and 15th century, superstition prevented studies of gross anatomy and pathology and thus there was no progress in orthopaedics.

It was Galen, "father of sports medicine", who observed that when an abscess bursts open and starts pouring pus, the inflammatory signs subside. Therefore, he thought that presence of pus in a wound is a good sign and coined the term "laudable pus".

In the 16th century, Ambroise Paré, "father of French surgery", designed a wide variety of instruments and braces and also tourniquet. He was a "barber surgeon" and one of the greatest surgeons of all times. He made a famous statement: "I dressed him, God cured him".

Thomas Sydenham is considered as "father of English medicine", who himself suffered from gout in early 17th century and described this condition in detail.

In 1756, Percivall Pott from London sustained an oblique compound fracture of lower third of tibia from a horse fall and thus gave a good description of ankle fractures. He also wrote his famous work on paraplegia of spinal tuberculosis.

The first successful internal fixation of a fracture was reported in 1775 when a fracture shaft or humerus was fixed using circlage wires made of brass.

The 19th and 20th centuries were the main age of revolutions in Orthopaedics. Orthopaedic surgery became a recognized part of operative surgery in the mid-19th century at about the same time as ophthalmology.

Hugh Owen Thomas of the 19th century is considered as "father of British orthopaedics". He was born to a family of well-known bonesetters in Liverpool. He had a busy practice all days and nights. He wrote prolifically in the nights.

Sir Robert Jones is the greatest orthopaedic surgeon that the world had ever seen. He was the nephew of Hugh Owen Thomas. He worked closely with his uncle and documented the fundamental concepts of principles in orthopaedics. It was said that when he operated, time stood still. In World War I, he headed the orthopaedic section of the British forces.

Thomas Porter McMurray worked for Robert Jones and was the first to perform a displacement osteotomy for un-united fracture of neck of femur.

Many achievements and discoveries are related to Wars.

In 1843, Malgaigne applied an external fixator for fracture patella.

Various indigenous splints were in use to treat fractures, which were made of resins, gums, waxes, lime and egg white.

Sir William Mcewen from Glasgow became the pioneer in bone grafting surgery in the late 19th century.

In 1852, Mathijsen, a Dutch military surgeon, introduced plaster of Paris in the form of cotton bandages impregnated with gypsum powder.

In 1865, Joseph Lister of London first applied carbolic acid to a compound fracture. Wilhelm Conrad Roentgen of Wurzburg discovered X-rays in 1895.

Fritz Steinmann, a Swiss Surgeon, devised a pin in 1908, which has been named after him and is used for applying skeletal traction.

Martin Kirschner of Germany devised Kirschner wire in the year 1909. Subsequently, Lambotte, Hay Groves and Rush introduced various intramedullary nails. The major breakthrough in the management of fractures of femur and tibia was made by Gerhard Kuntscher, a German Surgeon, during the World War II. He designed Kuntscher nail and laid down the principles of intramedullary nailing.

Lane, Sherman, and Eggers devised several bone plates for the internal fixation of fractures. But the results were poor, as these plates did not have any compression effect at the fracture site.

In 1940, Sir Reginald Watson Jones from Liverpool published his book on fractures and joint injuries. He was a leading teacher in fracture treatment therapy.

In 1958, about 10–12 Swiss surgeons reviewed the whole situation of plate osteosynthesis and formed an association called AO (Association for Osteosynthesis), also known as ASIF (Association of Surgeons for Internal Fixation). A new plate, dynamic compression plate (DCP), was introduced which exhibited compression effect at the fracture site, thus producing better results.

Major advances in the 20th century deal with arthroplasty of hip and knee, arthroscopic surgery and orthopaedic trauma.

In the 1950s, Gavril A Ilizarov developed ring external fixator in Soviet Union for wide use in bony injuries and deformities.

In the 1960s, Sir John Charnley of Manchester pioneered modern total hip arthroplasty and spent the next two decades refining all aspects of the procedure. He wrote a classic book on non-operative approach to fractures, "the closed treatment of common fractures". He also developed bone cement.

From 1970s onwards, fragmentation into regional subspecialties in orthopaedics became obvious.

Evolution of Orthopaedics in India

"Great teachers don't teach; they inspire"

Sushrutha (400 BC) is the "father of Indian medicine". He studied, practiced and taught the art of surgery on the banks of the river Ganges in India. He wrote a book called *Sushrutha Samhita* and defined health as not only the absence of diseases, but also a state of equilibrium of body, mind, soul and sense organs. Sushrutha is held in great esteem in ayurvedic medicine. He divided 1120 diseases into natural and supernatural diseases. Sushrutha stated that surgery is the first and the highest division of the healing art, pure in itself, perpetual in its applicability, a working product of heaven and sure of fame on earth. He was the pioneer of most teaching techniques in experimental and clinical surgery. He is rightly considered as the "father of surgery" and "patron of a surgeon in training". Sushrutha described the anatomy, physiology, pathology of all diseases, and also described 125 instruments.

Sushrutha, Charaka and Vagbhata formed a great triad of ancient times. The encyclopedic works of Charaka and Sushrutha are the products of a fully evolved system which resembles those of Hippocrates, and Galen in some respects; and which in others had developed beyond them.

Julius Jolly has stated that Medicine can now be regarded as the oldest of the Indian Sciences, and have been proved to be the Science in which Indians specialized first.

Dr MG Kini (like HO Thomas) is the fore-runner of orthopaedic surgery in India. Dr NS Narasimha Aiyar of Madras and Dr SR Chandra of Calcutta were the pioneers in this field and toiled very hard. In 1952, Dr Mukhopadhaya suggested the formation of Indian Orthopaedic Association. Dr AK Talwalkar started the Johnson and Johnson and Smith and Nephew Fellowships. The Kini Memorial Oration started in the year 1958 and Sir Harry Platt was the first Orator. The first issue of Indian Journal of Orthopaedics started in 1967 as Prof Prakash Chandra as the editor. In 1980, CME programmes were introduced at the Bombay Silver Jubilee Conference and 16 regional chapters were also included. Dr Duraisamy, Dr Dholakia, Dr TK Shanmugasundaram, Dr Natarajan, Dr Mohandas, Dr Devadoss, Dr BN Sinha, Dr Verghese Chacko, Dr Massalawalla, Dr Venkataswamy, Dr Srinivasan, Dr Natarajan, Dr Maini, Dr Sanchethi, Dr Babulkar and Dr Shantharam Shetty are just a few legendary figures to mention in the history of Indian Orthopaedics chapter.

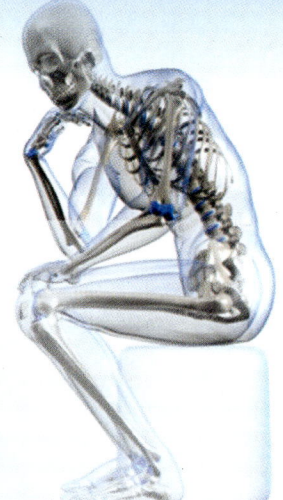

Common Orthopaedic Terminologies

Orthopaedics: Defined as a branch of general surgery which deals with injuries and diseases of the musculoskeletal system (bones, joints and their soft tissues like muscles, tendons, nerves, vessels, capsule, synovium, ligaments, bursae, etc.).

Ortho = straight, *paedics* = children

The term orthopaedics is coined by Nicholas Andry, a French physician and writer, with the aim of preventing and correcting deformities in children.

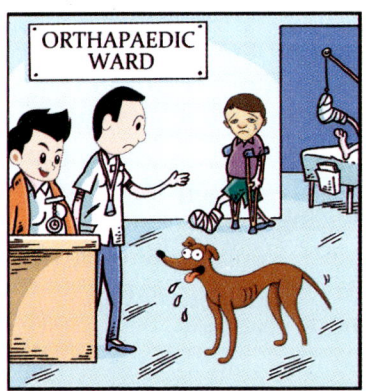

"He's started hanging around ever since he found out orthopaedic means bones!"

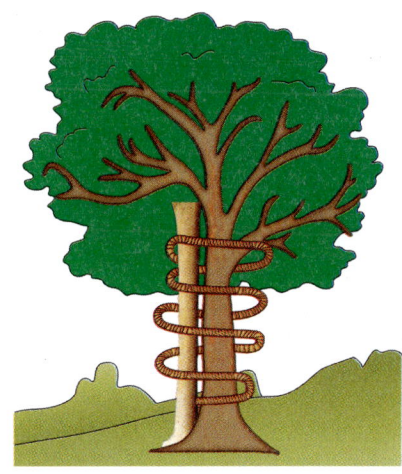

The logo/emblem used to represent orthopaedics (a bent tree is supported for straight growth).

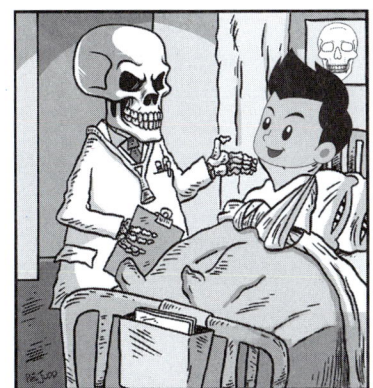

"Hello Mr Jones, I'm the Bone Specialist."

- *Fracture:* A break in the continuity of bone, which may be incomplete or complete.
- *Dislocation:* A complete loss of contact of bones forming a joint.
- *Subluxation:* A partial discontinuity of bones forming a joint.
- *Strain:* Injury to a muscle.
- *Sprain:* Injury to a ligament.
- *ORIF:* Open reduction and internal fixation.
- *MUA/CR:* Manipulation under anaesthesia/closed reduction.

- *Osteosynthesis:* A novel method of treating fractures surgically, wherein bone fragments are retained (and not excised) to achieve union.
- *Traction:* A force or pull applied to a part of the body (usually the limbs), either through skin or bone.
- *Splint/brace/orthosis:* A device used to support a weak part of the body with various functions.
- *Prosthesis:* A device which will replace a missing part of the bone (internal) or a part of the limb (external).
- *Arthralgia:* Pain in a joint.
- *Arthritis:* Inflammation of a joint.
- *Ankylosis:* Marked stiffness of a joint typically observed with end-stage arthritis.
- *Arthrotomy:* Surgical exposure of a joint.
- *Arthrocentesis:* Aspiration of a joint.
- *Arthroscopy:* Endoscopic examination of a joint for diagnostic or therapeutic cause or for both.
- *Arthrodesis:* Surgical fusion of a joint.
- *Arthroplasty:* Surgical reconstruction/ resurfacing of a diseased joint.
- *Arthrolysis:* Facilitating free range of movement of a stiff joint by closed or open method.
- *Osteotomy:* Surgical division of a bone.
- *Osteoclasis:* Breaking of a bone manually either by closed or open method.
- *Neurolysis:* Surgical release of fibrous adhesions surrounding a peripheral nerve.
- *Neurorrhaphy:* Surgical repair of a severed peripheral nerve.
- *Nerve grafting:* Surgical reconstruction of a peripheral nerve wherein the underlying gap is reconstituted with a donor nerve.
- *Neurotisation:* The implantation of a nerve into a paralyzed muscle.
- *Bone grafting:* A surgical procedure wherein bone healing is promoted using bone grafts.
- *Tenotomy:* Surgical release/division of a tendon.
- *Tenodesis:* Stabilisation procedure on a joint by attaching a tendon across it.
- *Tendon grafting:* A surgical procedure wherein a gap present in the tendon is rectified using a donor tendon.
- Tendon transfer: A surgical procedure performed to augment a weak tendon by transferring another tendon onto it.
- *Implant:* Internal fixation device used to stabilize a fractured bone.
- *Instrument:* Device used to perform surgery.

Polytrauma

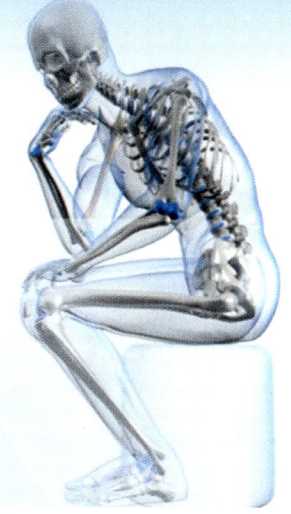

Polytrauma is a major cause of morbidity and mortality in developed and developing countries. Polytrauma refers to injuries that affect two or more body systems or organs, with one of the injuries usually being a traumatic brain injury (TBI), and at least one of the injuries being potentially life-threatening in severity. These injuries can lead to impairments in physical, cognitive, psychological, or psychosocial functioning.

The definition and use of the term "polytrauma" is inconsistent and lacks validation. According to the international consensus opinion, both anatomical and physiological parameters should be included in the definition of polytrauma. Polytrauma (multitrauma) is a short verbal equivalent used for severely injured patients usually with associated injury (i.e. two or more severe injuries in at least two areas of the body), less often with a multiple injury (i.e. two or more severe injuries in one body area).

'Polytrauma' is a medical term which is defined as a clinical state following injury to the body leading to profound physiometabolic changes involving multisystem. It is also defined as:

- Two major system injury + One major limb injury
- One major system injury + Two major limb injury
- One major system injury + One open grade III skeletal injury

- Unstable pelvic fracture with associated visceral injury

The term "polytrauma" has been frequently defined in terms of a high injury severity score (ISS) and has been generally used interchangeably with terms such as "severely injured" or "multiple trauma". Every patient having multiple trauma, which is equal with multiple critical injuries on different anatomical areas of the body, or having injury severity score (ISS) >15, is considered to be polytrauma patient. ISS is an international scale of describing, categorizing and estimating the severity of polytrauma patient's injuries. Such scale is revised trauma score (RTS) too. At least one out of two or more injuries or the sum total of all injuries endangers the life of the injured person with polytrauma. Polytrauma is generally used to describe trauma patients whose injuries involve multiple body regions, compromise the patient's physiology and potentially cause dysfunction of uninjured organs.

Polytrauma may be defined as injury to at least two body regions with abbreviated injury scale ≥3 and with the presence of systemic inflammatory response syndrome on at least 1 day during the first 72 hours. It remains the leading cause of death and disability in children and young adults. The most common causes are road traffic accidents, fall from heights, bullet injuries, etc. The majority of mortality occurs within the 1st hour following trauma, often defined as "the golden hour".

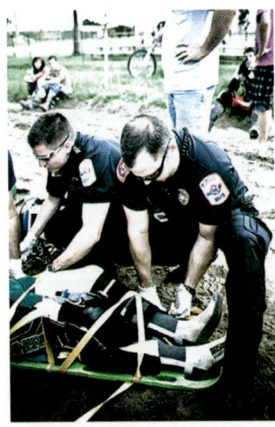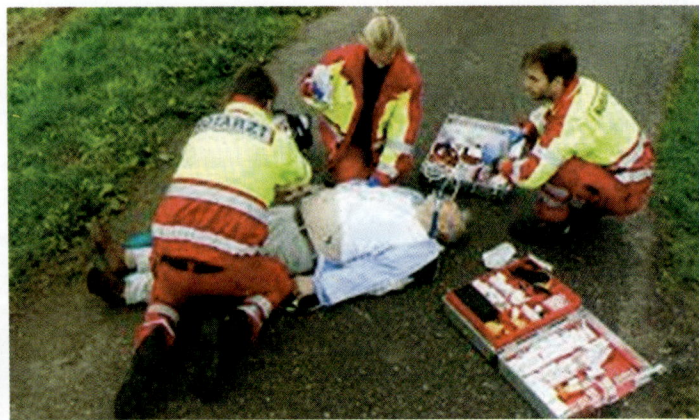

Fig. 4.1: Polytrauma—roadside assistance

Polytrauma patients are expected to have a higher risk of mortality than that obtained by the summation of expected mortality owing to their individual injuries. Polytrauma patients had significantly higher odds for worse haemodynamic measures and the requirement of procedures at the ED than non-polytrauma patients.

Definition of polytraumatized patients	
Arterial $paCO_2$	>50 mm Hg
Haemoglobin	<9.5 g/dl
pH value	<7.2
Lactate level	>4 mmol/l
Base excess	≤6 mmol/l
Shock index	>1
Horowitz index	<300

Polytrauma patients have nearly twofold higher odds of mortality than non-polytrauma patients.

Abrassart et al. defined haemodynamic instability as a combination of haemorrhagic shock, estimated blood loss above 1,500 ml, tachycardia, hypotension (not more than 90 mm Hg systolic blood pressure), and delayed capillary refill for at least two seconds.

Treatment algorithms are highly regimented and follow advanced trauma life support (ATLS) protocols. ATLS is a periodically updated, evidence- and consensus-based training course taught by the American College of Surgeons to physicians who care for trauma patients.

ADVANCED TRAUMA LIFE SUPPORT (ATLS)

The principles of treating the multiply injured can be divided into four phases: Primary survey (ABCDE) and resuscitation, re-evaluation, secondary survey (full head-to-toe examination) and transfer to definitive care (Fig. 4.1). Using these principles, problems are identified and addressed in a stepwise manner in a sequence that allows all injuries to be identified. Should the patient's condition deteriorate at any stage, the attending team must restart the primary survey at A (airway) once again.

Polytrauma remains the leading cause of death and disability in children and young adults. Systematic organized team effort is essential for improving the survival in trauma victims. Initial assessment includes preparation, triage, rapid primary survey and resuscitation, secondary survey and definitive

Philosophy

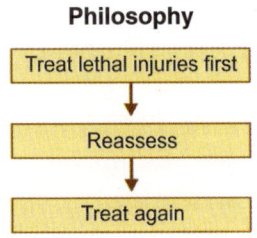

The treatment of seriously injured patients requires rapid assessment of injuries and initiation of life-preserving therapy. Because time is precious, systematic approach that can be easily reviewed and practiced is essential. This process is known as initial assessment and includes:

1. Preparation
2. Triage
3. Rapid primary survey (ABCDE)
4. Resuscitation
5. Adjuncts to primary survey
6. Consideration of need for patient transfer
7. Secondary survey (head-to-toe evaluation and patient history)
8. Adjuncts to secondary survey
9. Continued post-resuscitation monitoring and re-evaluation
10. Definitive therapy.

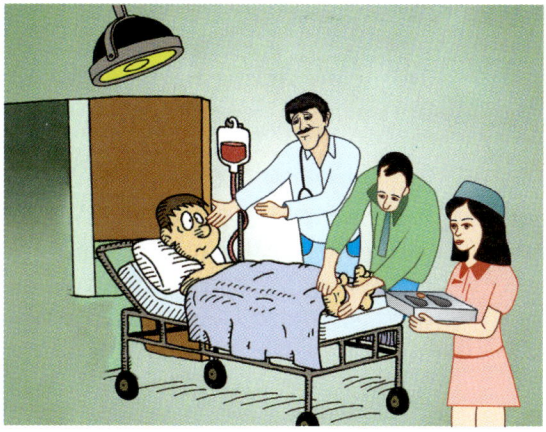

Fig. 4.2: Assessment of polytrauma patient

care (Fig. 4.2). ABCDE of primary survey includes airway maintenance with cervical spine control, breathing and ventilation. Circulation and haemorrhage control, disability and exposure with prevention of hypothermia. Secondary survey includes head-to-toe examination of the trauma patient including a complete history and physical examination and reassessment of all vital signs. Definitive care may involve shifting the patient to radiology/operating room/intensive care unit.

Aggressive resuscitation with crystalloids and blood products is of paramount importance in treating polytrauma victims (Fig. 4.3).

Triage involves sorting of patients based on their need for treatment and the resources available for that treatment. It also pertains to the sorting of patient in the field and the decision regarding to which medical facility they should be transported.

PRIMARY SURVEY AND RESUSCITATION

The examination and associated interventions are divided into primary and secondary surveys, with the primary survey following the mnemonic ABCDE, which stands for airway, breathing, circulation, disability, and exposure.

A: Open the **airway**; address any obstruction by suction of secretions, foreign body removal, protective oral or nasal airway placement, and oral, nasal, or surgical airway management.

B: Stabilize **breathing** through provision of oxygen, managing life-threatening chest trauma such as a pneumothorax or haemothorax with a chest tube, and management of mechanical ventilation.

C: Establish **circulation** through intravenous, intraosseous, or central venous access;

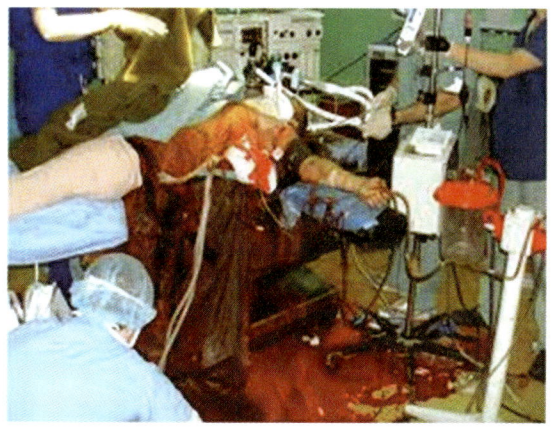

Fig. 4.3: Resuscitation of polytrauma patient

administer crystalloid fluid and blood products, as well as any medications that may support the patient's circulation.

D: Assess **disability** from neurological injury such as paralysis and altered mental status.

E: Expose the patient by removing his or her clothes and evaluating for immediate life-threatening injuries such as femur fractures, penetrating wounds, and arterial bleeding.

Should a life-threatening injury or problem be identified at any level of ABCDE, it is addressed before moving on. Parts or all of the primary ABCDE evaluation may be repeated frequently during the management of the trauma patient.

Circulation and Haemorrhage Control

Haemorrhage is the most important cause of preventable death after injury. Hypotension after injury must be considered hypovolemic unless proved otherwise. Haemorrhage can be classified into four classes based upon the extent of blood loss as given in Table 4.1.

Table 4.1: Classification of haemorrhage based on extent of blood loss

Parameter	Class I	Class II	Class III	Class IV
Blood loss (ml)	>750	750–1500	1500–2000	>2000
Blood loss (%)	<15	15–30	30–40	>40
Pulse rate (beats/min)	<100	100–120	>120	>140
BP	Normal	Decreased	Decreased	Decreased
Respiratory rate	14–20	29–30	30–40	>40
Urine output (ml/h)	>30	20–30	5–15	Negligible
CNS symptoms	Normal	Anxious	Confused	Lethargic

CNS: Central nervous system, BP: Blood pressure

Glasgow Coma Scale (GCS)

Assessment area	Score
Eye opening (E)	
Spontaneous	4
To speech	3
To pain	2
None	1
Best motor response (M)	
Obeys to commands	6
Localized response to pain	5
Withdrawal response	4
Abnormal flexion (decorticate)	3
Abnormal extension (decerebrate)	2
Nil	1
Verbal response (V)	
Oriented	5
Confused conversation	4
Inappropriate words	3
Incomprehensible sounds	2
Nil	1

GCS score: E + M + V. Best possible score: 15, Worst possible score: 3

SECONDARY SURVEY

The secondary survey does not begin until primary survey (ABCDE) is completed, resuscitation efforts are underway, and normalization of vital functions has been demonstrated. The secondary survey is a head-to-toe evaluation of the trauma patient that is a complete history and physical examination, including reassessment of all vital signs.

History

"AMPLE" is a useful mnemonic:
- A: Allergies
- M: Medications currently used
- P: Past illness/past pregnancy
- L: Last meal
- E: Events/environment related to injury.

The secondary survey is a thorough head-to-toe examination that identifies and documents evidence of traumatic injury. Adjunctive survey measures are conducted, such as ultrasonography for a focused assessment with sonography for trauma (FAST) examination, and chest and pelvic X-rays. Many additional procedures (surgical interventions, laceration repairs, splinting, etc.), evaluations (expert evaluations, laboratory studies, CT scans, etc.), and interventions (medications, vent management, etc.) can be conducted after this initial evaluation and management.

Within 24 hours, a tertiary survey—a repeat of the primary and secondary surveys—is performed by the trauma service to identify injuries missed during sometimes—chaotic initial surveys and management.

Re-Evaluation

Trauma patients must be re-evaluated constantly to ensure that new findings are not overlooked and to discover deterioration in previously noted findings (Fig. 4.4).

Damage control focuses on control of haemorrhage management of soft tissue injury

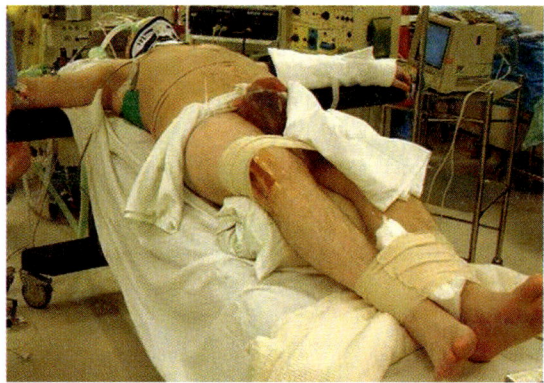

Fig. 4.4: Polytrauma patient

ATLS—Component steps
Primary survey
Identify what is killing the patient
Resuscitation
Treat what is killing the patient
Secondary survey
Proceed to identify other injuries
Definitive care
Develop a definitive management plan

and achievement of provisional fracture stability. The goals are: Fast resuscitation, bleeding control, pain relief, and minimize the second hit. Early total surgery is indicated in stable or borderline stabilized patient. It should be performed within 24 hours after trauma and always in trauma centres with adequate human and material resources. Open reduction and internal fixation will be made according to the principles of osteosynthesis for each type of fracture.

AIMS IN MANAGEMENT

To restore the patient back to his preinjury status, having following priorities:
- Life salvage
- Limb salvage
- Salvage of total function, if possible

The initial management of a patient with polytrauma is of vital importance in minimizing both patient morbidity and mortality. The main principle behind trauma management is an organized team approach, i.e. polytrauma victims are best managed by a team. The delay from any member of the team may lead to death of the patient. Accordingly, standard operating procedure is suggested in managing polytrauma patients of a tertiary care institute.

1. There should be a polytrauma management team consisting of general surgeon, anaesthetist, orthopaedic surgeon, neurosurgeon, cardiothoracic surgeon, ENT surgeon, nurses and other paramedical staff.

2. A proper system for triage should be formed at the reception of the patient as per the prefixed criteria. Triage of patients can be done on the basis of the following injury scale:

Level of	AIS score	Colour code
1	Minor	Green
2	Moderate	Yellow
3	Critical	Red

3. Coloured bands on the wrist of the patient and coloured stamp on the OPD card of the polytrauma patient can be used to differentiate them from other patients depending on the type of injury.

4. After triaging, the general surgeon as team manager should attend the patient and decide the treatment plan accordingly.

5. All the communication regarding treatment should be done through the team manager to avoid confusion. Proper record maintenance by the team manager is a must.

Management of the skeletal injuries in the polytrauma patient is a dynamic process that should be carried out according to the physiological situation of the patient. We must consider the impact that the treatment of the fractures can have on the patient (second hit). What we must do is clear: Stabilize immediately the fractures. How we can do it depends on patient situation. We have two options: Damage control surgery or early definitive surgery. Stable polytrauma patients with associated head injury require special consideration. In contrast, trauma patients with thoracic trauma, if they are stable, can be subjected to early nailing of long bone fractures without increasing the risk of respiratory distress. Spinal injury associated with multiple trauma has special characteristics. It may be undiagnosed. Furthermore, a poor handle of the patient or incorrect immobilization can trigger a neurological damage that previously did not exist. A complete and adequate exploration of the spine, including CT scan and MRI as possible, should be carried out in all trauma patients. Open fractures in multiple injured patients follow the same principles of management for fractures with soft tissue damage. In most cases, damage control surgery by external fixation is the best option.

Trauma Deaths

First peak
- Within minutes of injury
- Major neurological or vascular injury
- Medical treatment will rarely improve outcome

Second peak
- Occurs during the gold hour
- Due to intracranial haematoma, major thoracic or abdominal injury

Third peak
- Days or weeks later
- Sepsis, multiple organ failure

BIBLIOGRAPHY

- https://journalofethics.ama-assn.org
- https://www.jotr.in/article.asp?issn
- https://ota.org/
- https://regionalmedicalsanjose.com
- https://emedicine.medscape.com
- https://link.springer.com
- https://www.youtube.com/watch?v=2PUAbexHl_s

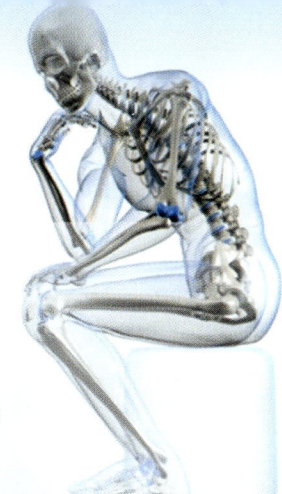

Fractures of Clavicle

Fracture union usually progresses regardless of the treatment initiated. Historically, clavicle fractures have been considered best treated non-operatively, with good outcomes. Controversy remains concerning operative versus non-operative treatment of middle and distal clavicle fractures.

ANATOMICAL CONSIDERATIONS (Fig. 5.1)

The clavicle is the first bone in the body to ossify, beginning at the fifth week of gestation. Through age 5 years, the growth is primarily through intramembranous ossification. The junction of the middle and distal thirds of the clavicle is a common site of fracture because

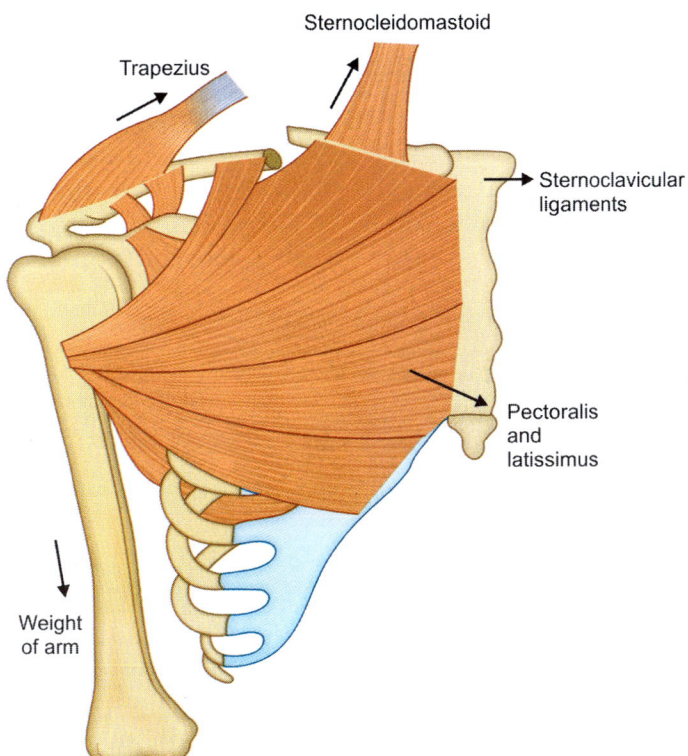

Fig. 5.1: Muscular attachments around clavicle

this is the thinnest part of the bone, and there is relatively little protection by muscular attachments. Three muscles originate from (sternohyoid, pectoralis major and deltoid) and three muscles insert on (sternocleido-mastoid, subclavius and trapezius) the clavicle.

Incidence: Accounts for 10–16% of all fractures in children and 2.6 to 5% in adults. 70–82% of the fractures involve the middle third of clavicle. Male:female—2.5:1.

Clavicle fractures may be caused by direct or indirect trauma. The most common mechanism is an indirect one, involving a fall directly onto the lateral shoulder. A less common mechanism for clavicle fractures is a fall onto an outstretched hand (i.e. a FOOSH injury).

An anteroposterior (AP) view and a 40–45° cephalic tilt view are standard for the initial radiographic evaluation (Fig. 5.2).

CLAVICLE FRACTURE CLASSIFICATIONS

Allman (Fig. 5.3)

- Group I fractures: Middle third injuries
- Group II fractures: Distal third injuries
- Group III fractures: Medial (proximal) third injuries

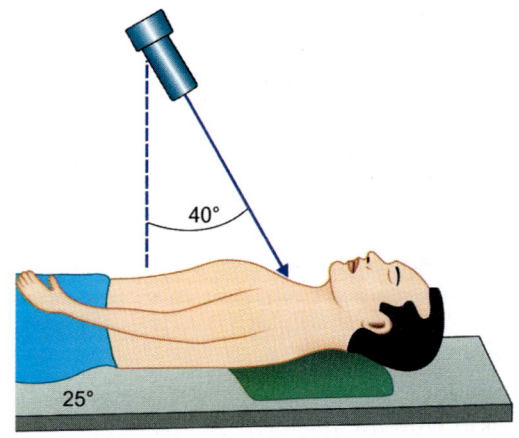

Fig. 5.2: AP view X-ray

Associated Injuries

Pulmonary injury, injury to brachial plexus, subclavian artery, fracture of scapula or ribs, closed head injuries, open fractures.

TREATMENT

The vast majority heal with non-operative management, which includes use of a simple shoulder sling. The focus of treatment of middle third fractures remains non-operative. Such treatment can be divided into the following two categories:

- *Simple support of the extremity:* As in a sling or a sling and swath

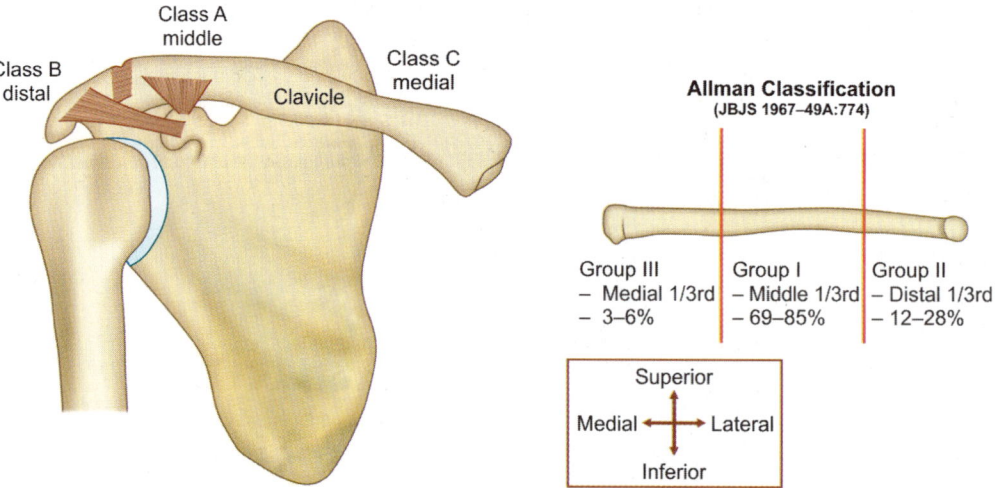

Fig. 5.3: Allman grading

- *Reduction and immobilization:* Typically with figure-of-eight brace (Fig. 5.4a and b)
  Labourers may return to light lifting after 6 weeks and full duty at 12 weeks. Athletes may return to contact sports after 3 months.
  Younger children generally require shorter periods of immobilization (2–4 weeks) than do adolescents and adults (4–8 weeks).

Surgical indications include the following:
- Complete fracture displacement
- Severe displacement causing tenting of the skin with the risk of puncture
- Fractures with 2 cm of shortening
- Comminuted fractures with a displaced transverse "zed" (or Z-shaped) fragment
- Neurovascular compromise: Distal third fractures (high risk of non-union)
- Displaced medial clavicular fractures with mediastinal structures at risk
- Polytrauma (with multiple fractures): To expedite rehabilitation
- Open fractures
- An inability to tolerate closed treatment
- Fractures with interposed muscle

- Established, symptomatic non-union
- Concomitant glenoid neck fracture (floating shoulder)

Implants commonly used: An intramedullary device or fixation with a plate and screws. Obtaining purchase in 6 cortices on either side of the fracture is recommended when plate is used. LC-DCP or reconstruction plate is used. Lag screw fixation is also appropriate when the fracture pattern allows. Cancellous bone grafting is indicated in cases of comminution and/or bone loss (Fig. 5.5).

Complications

- Neurovascular injuries include damage of brachial plexus, subclavian artery and vein, internal jugular vein and axillary artery.
- Intrathoracic injuries involving lungs, pleura, subclavian vessels and axillary artery.
- Malunion, in which the fracture heals with significant angulation and shortening with disfigurement. Mild malunion is common after clavicle fractures, but it is not usually clinically significant. Corrective osteotomy is indicated in selective cases only.

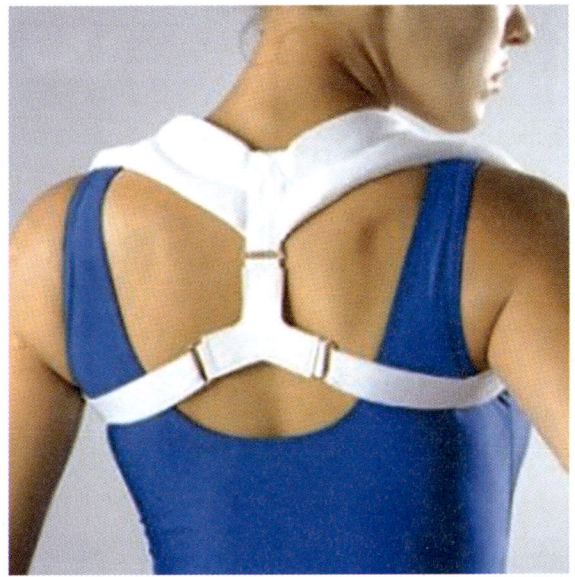
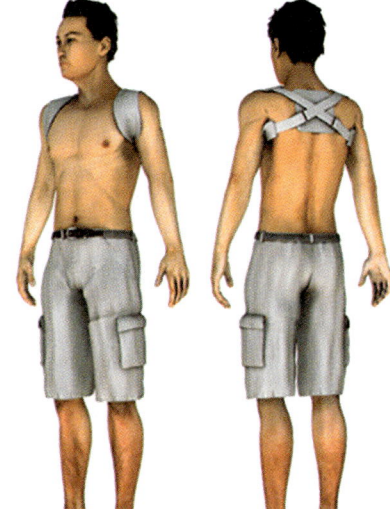

Fig. 5.4a: Figure of eight brace

Classification of fracture of lateral third of clavicle is given in Table 5.2.

Table 5.2: Neer classification of lateral third (10–15%)		
Type I	• Fracture occurs lateral to coracoclavicular ligaments (trapezoid, conoid) or interligamentous • Usually minimally displaced • Stable because conoid and trapezoid ligaments remain intact	Non-operative
Type IIA	• Fracture occurs medial to intact conoid and trapezoid ligament • Medial clavicle unstable • Up to 56% non-union rate with non-operative management	Operative
Type IIB	• Fracture occurs either between ruptured conoid and intact trapezoid ligament or lateral to both ligaments torn • Medial clavicle unstable • Up to 30–45% non-union rate with non-operative management	Operative
Type III	• Intra-articular fracture extending into AC joint • Conoid and trapezoid intact, therefore, stable injury • Patients may develop post-traumatic AC arthritis	Non-operative
Type IV	• A physeal fracture that occurs in the skeletally immature • Displacement of lateral clavicle occurs superiorly through a tear in the thick periosteum • Clavicle pulls out of periosteal sleeve • Conoid and trapezoid ligaments remain attached to periosteum and overall the fracture pattern is stable	Non-operative
Type V	• Comminuted fracture • Conoid and trapezoid ligaments remain attached to comminuted fragment • Medial clavicle unstable	Operative

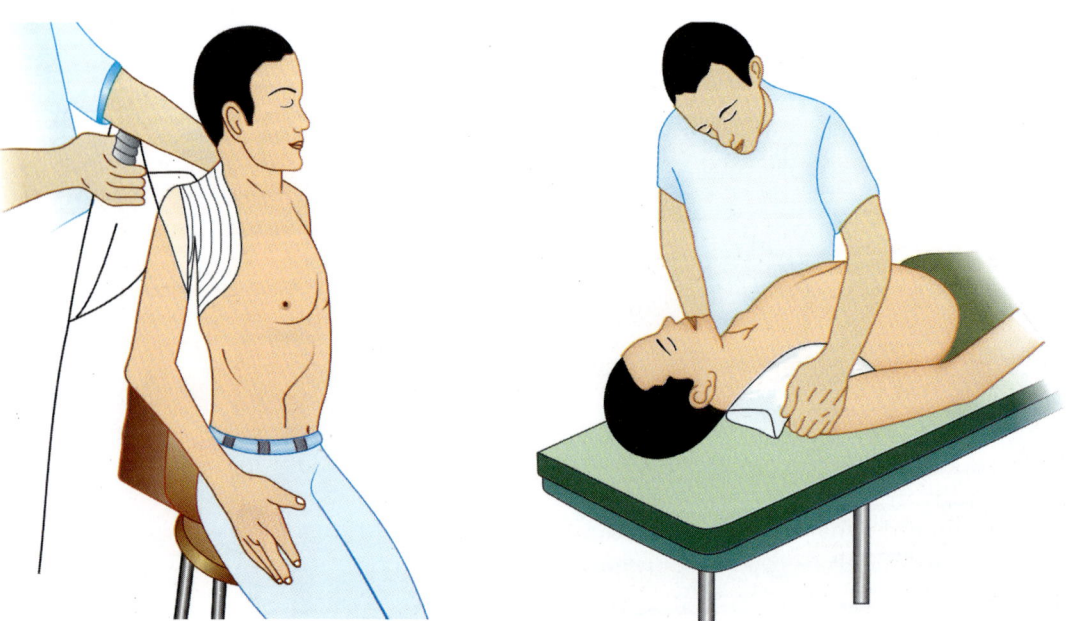

Fig. 5.4b: Closed reduction techniques

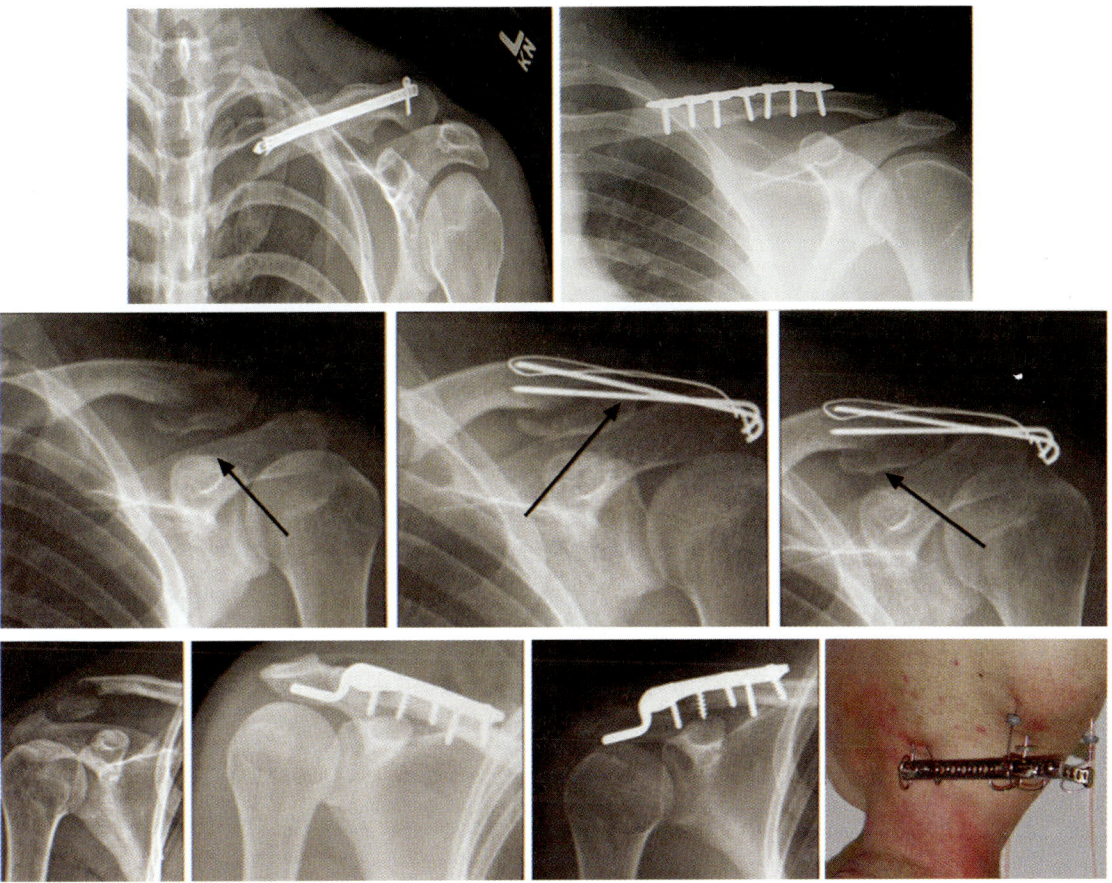

Fig. 5.5: Implants used to fix fracture clavicle

- Non-union is rare (about 6%), where the fracture fails to heal even after 4–6 months. Many non-unions are asymptomatic and require no treatment. Cessation of smoking needs to be included in the treatment of diaphysial clavicle fractures because smoking is one of the risk factors for non-union.

FRACTURE LATERAL THIRD OF CLAVICLE

Displaced lateral-end fractures have a higher risk of non-union after non-operative treatment than do shaft fractures. However, non-union is difficult to predict and may be asymptomatic in elderly individuals. The results of operative treatment are more unpredictable than they are for shaft fractures. Surgical reconstruction should be considered for patients with persistent discomfort associated with a non-union or acromio-clavicular osteoarthritis six months or more after the injury.

The most effective method of treatment for younger individuals (less than 35 years of age) is yet to be determined.

Surgical options include the use of the following implants: Dorsal locking plate, hook plate (Fig. 5.6), and endobutton.

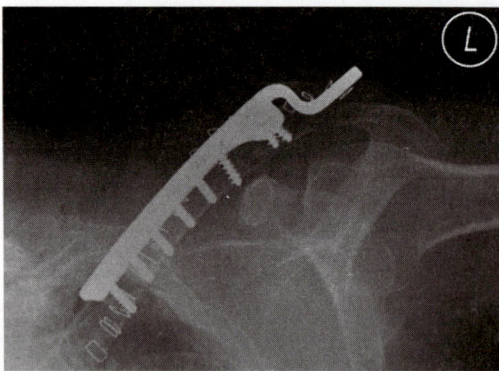

Fig. 5.6: Hook plate

Points to Remember

- Clavicle fractures are most common in children and young adults, typically occurring in persons younger than 25 years.

- Most clavicle fractures occur in the midshaft and can be treated non-operatively. A prominent callus is common in children, and parents may require reassurance.
- Surgery is an option in fractures that have high potential for non-union.
- Non-union is defined as absence of radiographic healing by 4 months.

BIBLIOGRAPHY

- www.orthofracs.com/adult/trauma/shoulder/fractures-clavicle.html
- www.slideshare.net/lenhan68/fractures-of-the-clavicle
- www.morphoedics.wikidot.com
- www.nabilebraheim.mp4
- www.orthobullets.com/trauma/1011/clavicle-fractures

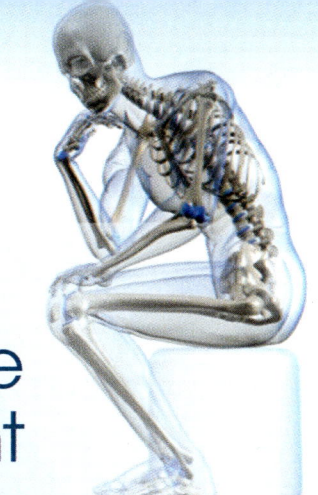

Injuries of the Acromioclavicular Joint

The acromioclavicular (AC) joint is a link between the arm and the trunk and is the only joint between the shoulder blade and the rest of the body (Fig. 6.1).

The most common mechanism for an acromioclavicular joint injury is a fall directly onto the acromion, with the arm adducted up against the body. A fall onto an outstretched hand (FOOSH injury) and a downward force on the upper extremity have also been implicated in acromioclavicular joint injuries. Athletes participating in contact sports (e.g. football, rugby, hockey, martial arts) are at increased risk of acromioclavicular joint

injuries. Males are more commonly affected than females, with a male-to-female ratio of approximately 5:1.

Allman and Tossy initially proposed a 3-grade classification that Rockwood expanded to 6 types of injury (Fig. 6.2). Type I-III acromioclavicular injuries are the most common injuries.

Treatment of acromioclavicular separations has been a subject of debate. In general, types I and II injuries are treated non-operatively in the acute setting, and types IV, V, and VI injuries generally require surgical repair. Conservative treatment involves application

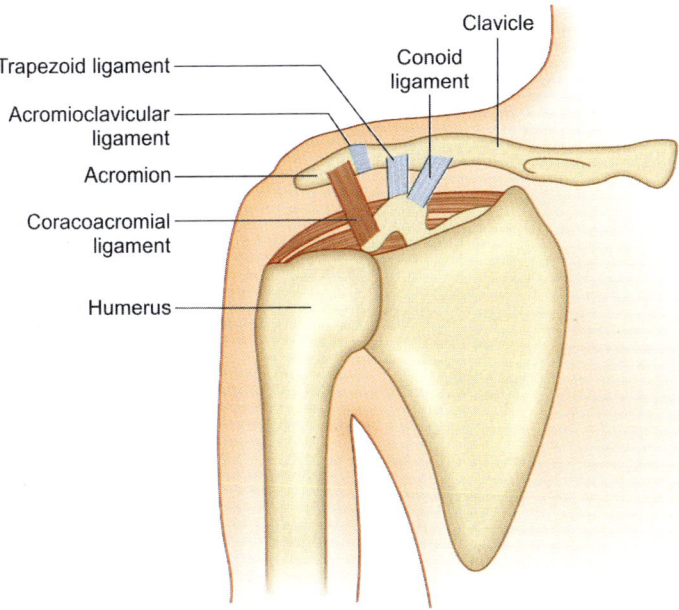

Fig. 6.1: Anatomy of AC joint

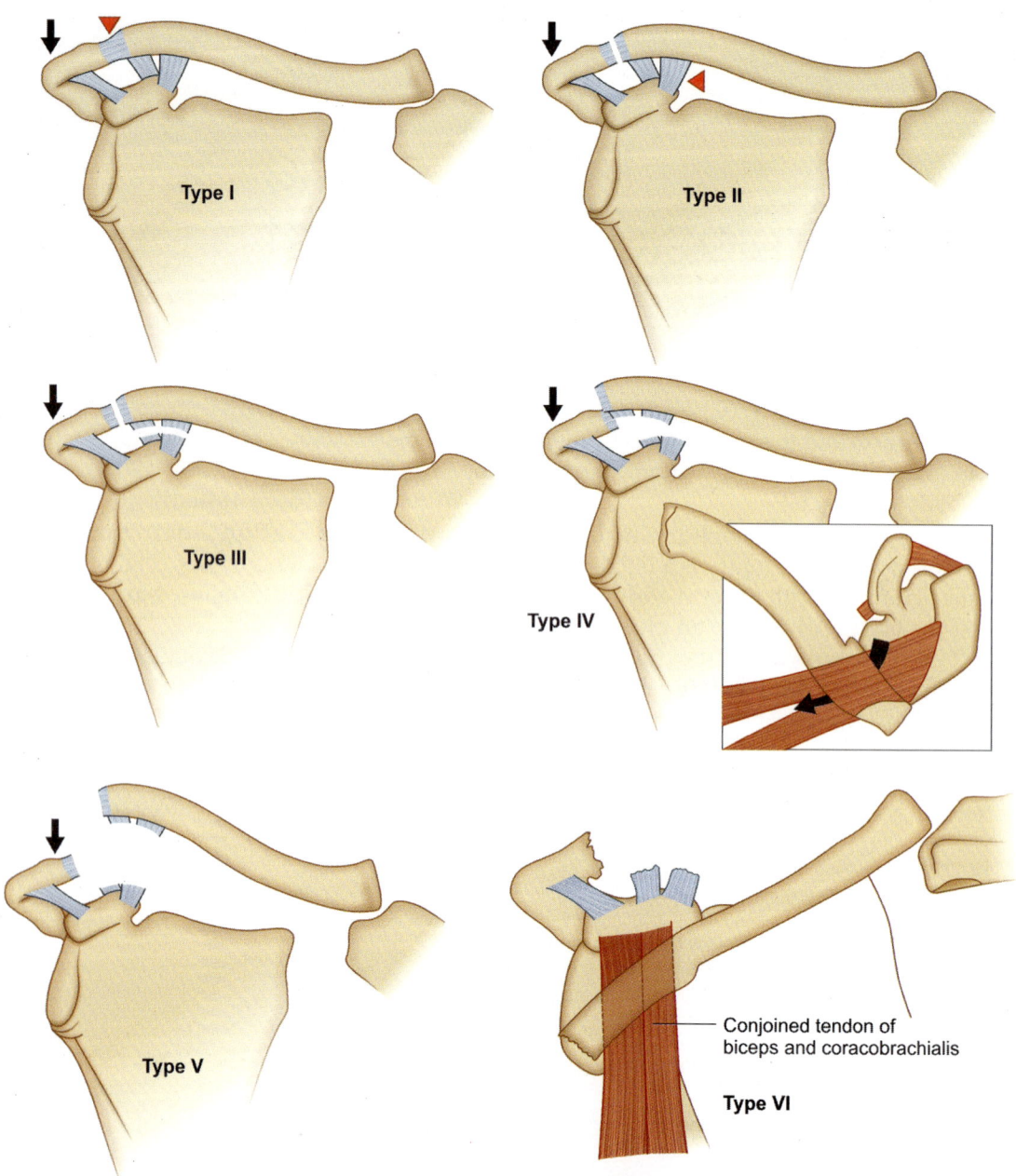

Fig. 6.2: Rockwood classification

of a sling for comfort and activity modification, ice, and analgesic agents until the symptoms subside and the range of motion is reasonably comfortable (Fig. 6.3).

However, reaching a consensus regarding the optimal management of acute type III injuries has been difficult. Types IV, V, and VI injuries generally do well with surgical repair. Published studies of patients undergoing both arthroscopic and open resection have reported good or excellent results in approximately 60–100% of cases of acromioclavicular joint injuries.

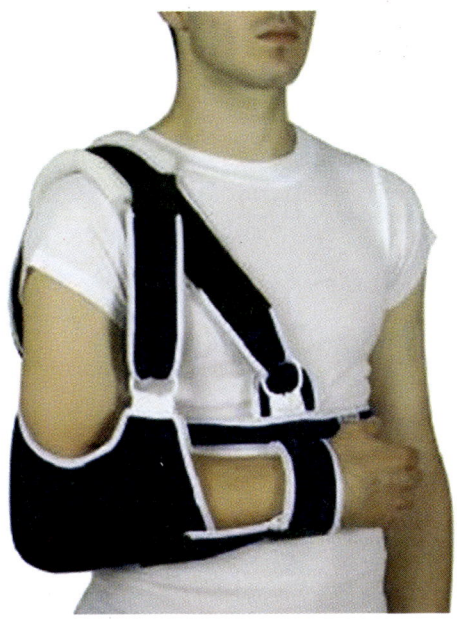

Fig. 6.3: Acromioclavicular support

In general, surgical management should be offered acutely only to those who require high-level upper extremity function and late to those with significant shoulder pain and/or dysfunction refractory to non-operative treatment.

Surgical repair can be divided into anatomical or non-anatomical, or historically into four types:

- Acromioclavicular repairs (intra-articular repair with wires/pins, percutaneous pins, hook plates)
- Coracoclavicular repairs (Bosworth screws, Cerclage, Copeland and Kessel repair)

- Distal clavicular excision
- Dynamic muscle transfers

For sequelae of untreated types IV–VI, or painful types II and III injuries, the Weaver Dunn technique is advocated. This involves removing the lateral 2 cm of the clavicle and reattaching the acromial end of the coracoacromial ligament to the cut end of the clavicle, thus reducing the clavicle to a more anatomical position.

Complications

- Degenerative arthritis of AC joint
- Shoulder impingement syndrome
- Cosmetic deformity
- Osteolysis of lateral end of clavicle

Points to Remember

The management of these injuries is non-operative in the majority of cases. Types I and II injuries are treated symptomatically. The current trend in uncomplicated type III injuries is a non-operative approach. In athletes involved in heavylifting or prolonged overhead activities, surgery may be considered acutely. Types IV–VI injuries are generally treated operatively.

BIBLIOGRAPHY

- https://www.youtube.com/watch?v=lLaTxKhOahU
- https://www.youtube.com/watch?v=OfcSvG-dgbY
- https://www.youtube.com/watch?v=oJz76hYa4jI
- https://www.youtube.com/watch?v=LerMY0XpKE4

Fractures of the Scapula

The first investigator to publish on the topic of scapula fractures was Desault in 1805 (Fig. 7.1).

Scapular fractures occur infrequently and account for approximately 1% of all fractures and fewer than 5% of shoulder girdle injuries. Many of them can be treated without surgery. Scapular fractures are usually the result of significant blunt trauma. Scapular fractures are often associated with other injuries:

- Clavicle fracture
- Rib fracture
- Sternal fracture
- Spinal fracture
- Pneumothorax and/or pulmonary contusion
- Brachial plexus injury.

One or more parts of the scapula may be fractured (Fig. 7.2).
- Scapular body (50 to 60% of patients)
- Scapular neck (25% of patients)
- Glenoid
- Acromion
- Coracoid

An anteroposterior shoulder view along with a lateral scapular view demonstrates the

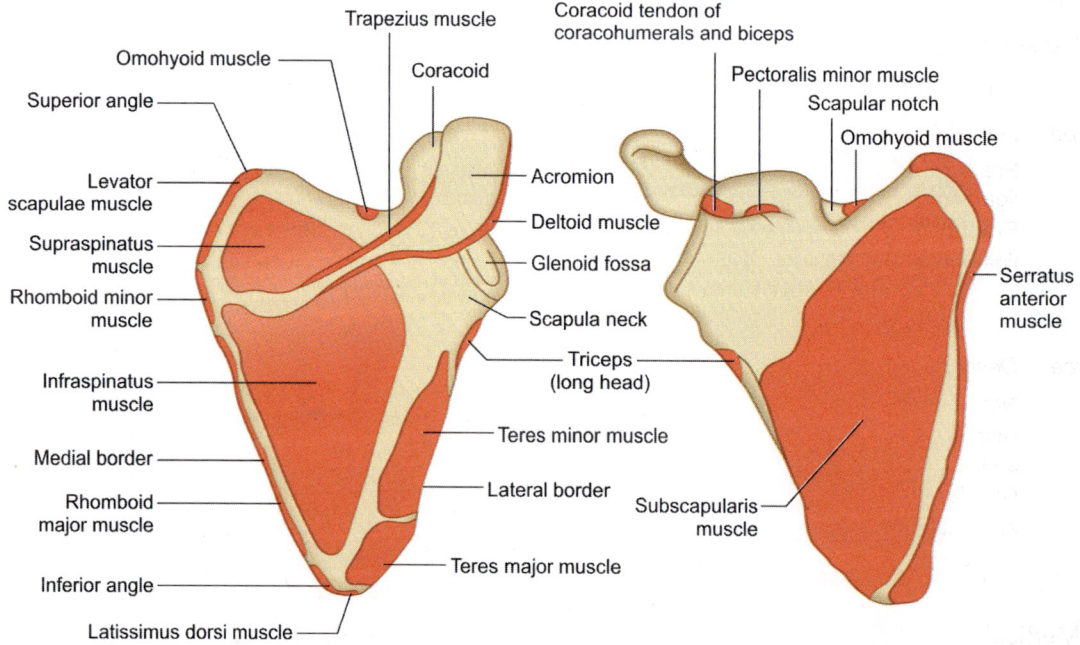

Fig. 7.1: Muscular attachments of scapula

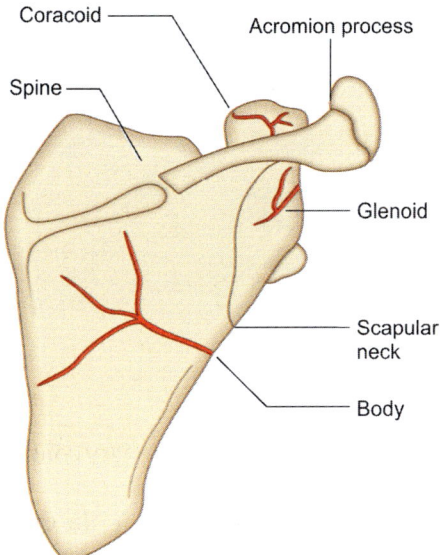

Fig. 7.2: Anatomy of scapula

vast majority of scapular fractures. A lateral axillary view isolates the coracoid process and helps to delineate associated shoulder dislocations.

Tangential oblique views aid in the evaluation of small or subtle scapular body fractures.

Table 7.1: Classification of fracture of scapula

Coracoid process fractures	
Type	Description
I	Fracture proximal to the coracoclavicular ligament
II	Fracture distal to the coracoclavicular ligament

Acromion fractures	
Type	Description
I	Non- or minimally-displaced
II	Displaced but not affecting the subacromial space
III	Displacement compromising the subacromial space.

Glenoid fractures

Medical therapy for patients with scapula fractures generally is the same as that for any trauma patient. Perform fluid resuscitation, stabilize the cardiopulmonary system, and treat life-threatening injuries prior to operative fixation of scapula fractures.

Non-displaced fractures of the acromion usually can be treated with sling immobilization, ice, and analgesics and early motion. Most fractures will heal by 6 weeks.

Displaced fractures and those associated with rotator cuff injuries often require surgical intervention.

Operative

Open reduction internal fixation
Indications
- Glenohumeral instability
  - >25% glenoid involvement with subluxation of humerus
  - >5 mm of glenoid articular surface step off or major gap
  - Excessive medialization of glenoid
    - Displaced scapula neck fractures: With >40° angulation or 1 cm translation
    - Open fracture
    - Loss of rotator cuff function
    - Coracoid fractures with >1 cm of displacement
  - *Outcomes:* 70% good to excellent results with operative treatment

Implants used
- 3.5 mm cortex screws or 4.0 mm cancellous screws as lag screws
- 1/3rd tubular plate may be applied below glenoid to lateral border of scapula as a buttress.

Recognizing the exact indications for operative treatment of scapula fractures is a major issue for the future.

BIBLIOGRAPHY
- https://www.youtube.com/watch?v=0R9YsbE6K-o
- https://www.youtube.com/watch?v=9z0j_jgPA3w

Shoulder Dislocation

The shoulder is the most commonly dislocated joint in the body. The main stabilizers of the shoulder joint are the ligaments and the capsule complex. Multiple ligaments are present, but the inferior glenohumeral ligament is the most important and the one most commonly injured during an anterior shoulder dislocation. Approximately 95% of shoulder dislocations result from a major traumatic event, and 5% result from atraumatic causes. Anterior shoulder dislocation is by far the commonest type of dislocation and usually results from forced abduction, external rotation and extension.

An anteroposterior (AP) view of the shoulder and an axillary lateral view are done. If an axillary lateral radiography cannot be obtained, then a scapular Y view may be taken in its place (Fig. 8.1).

Anterior dislocations can be further divided according to where the humeral head comes to lie (Fig. 8.2):

- Subcoracoid—most common
- Subglenoid
- Subclavicular
- Intrathoracic—very rare

In most of those, the head of the humerus comes to rest under the coracoid process, referred to as subcoracoid dislocation. Subglenoid, subclavicular, and, very rarely, intrathoracic dislocations may also occur. Inferior dislocation is the least likely, occurring in less than 1%. This condition is also called

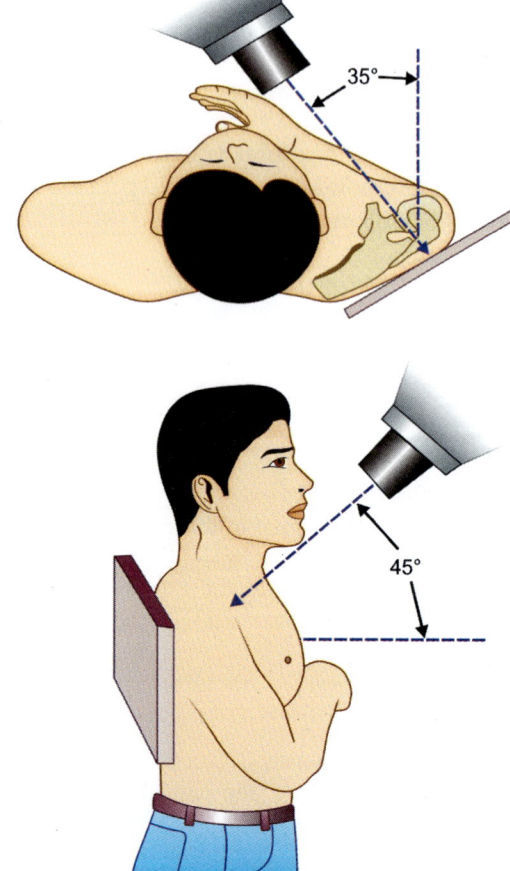

Fig. 8.1: Positioning for X-rays of shoulder

luxatio erecta because the arm appears to be permanently held upward or behind the head.

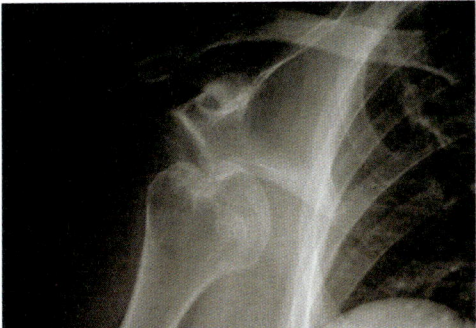
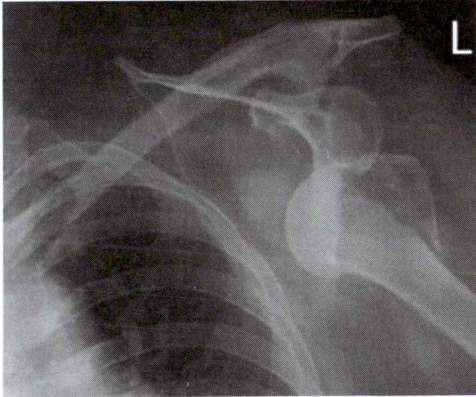
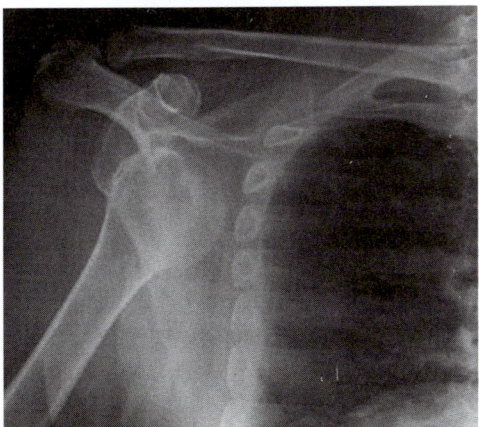

Fig. 8.2: X-rays showing anterior dislocation of shoulder

Approximately 25% of shoulder dislocations have associated fractures.

CLOCKWISE APPROACH TO LABRAL PATHOLOGY
(Figs 8.3 and 8.4)

A clockwise approach to the labrum is the easiest way to diagnose labral tears and

to differentiate them from normal labral variants.

There are two types of labral tears: SLAP tears and Bankart lesions.

- SLAP is an acronym that stands for superior labral tear from anterior to posterior.
- SLAP tears start at the 12 o'clock position where the biceps anchor is located, which tears the labrum off the glenoid.
- SLAP tears typically extend from the 10 to the 2 o'clock position, but can extend more posteriorly or anteriorly and even extend into the biceps tendon.
- Bankart lesions are typically located in the 3–6 o'clock position because that's where the humeral head dislocates.

Hill-Sachs Lesion

On MRI scan, a Hill-Sachs defect is seen at or above the level of the coracoid process.

- Hill-Sachs is a posterolateral depression of the humeral head.
- It is above or at the level of the coracoid in the first 18 mm of the proximal humeral head.
- It is seen in 75–100% of patients with anterior instability.

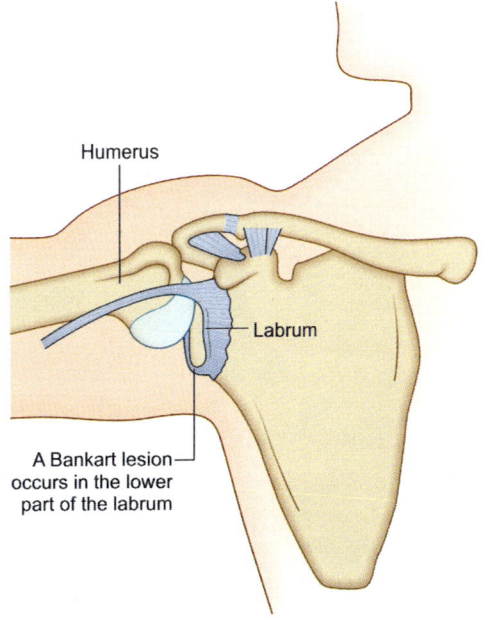

Fig. 8.3a: Bankart lesion

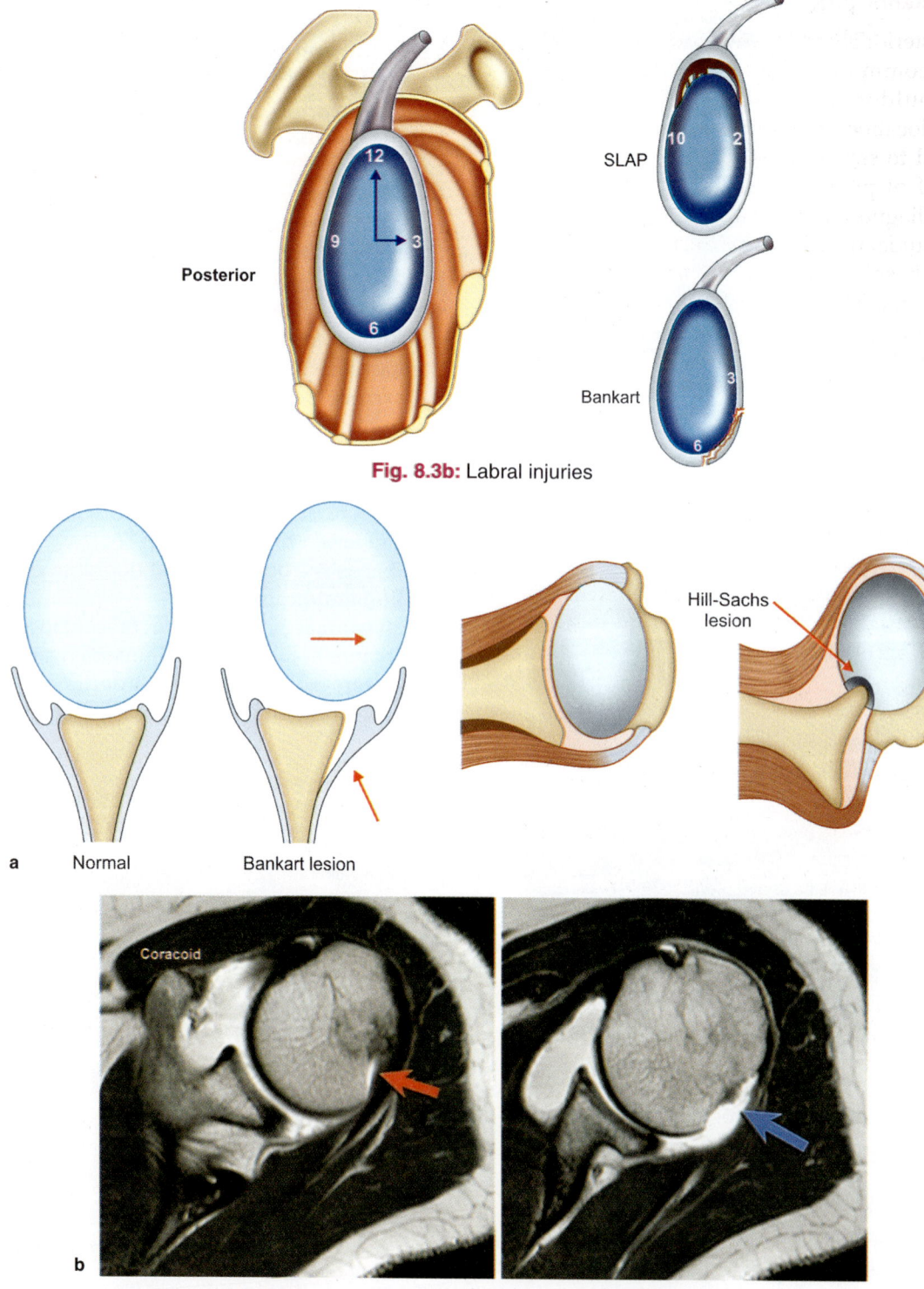

Fig. 8.3b: Labral injuries

a   Normal   Bankart lesion

Hill-Sachs lesion

b

Fig. 8.4a and b: (a) Labral pathology; (b) MRI of shoulder

Posterior Dislocation

Posterior shoulder dislocations are relatively uncommon, comprising only 2–4% of all shoulder dislocations. Thus, posterior dislocations often go undiagnosed, and can lead to severe consequences. Approximately half of posterior shoulder dislocations go undiagnosed on initial presentation. Posterior shoulder dislocations are classically associated with seizures, electrocution and severe trauma. The highest incidence of posterior dislocation is in males between the ages of 35 and 55. Typically the arm is held in internal rotation and adduction. The most significant finding on examination is a limited range of active and passive external rotation of the effected arm as the head of the humerus is caught to the glenoid rim. Palpation of the humeral head in a posterior position is the only other clear diagnostic feature on examination. Other physical signs such as increased prominence of the coracoid process and acromion anteriorly, and the head of humerus posteriorly may be present but are less significant.

The AP view of the normal shoulder demonstrates the normal asymmetry of the humeral head in anatomic position. The larger portion is on the medial side, seated in the glenoid fossa. With internal rotation in the setting of a posterior dislocation, this larger portion rotates out of view producing the rounder and symmetric "light bulb sign" of the humeral head. Other signs include the rim sign (>6 mm gap between the medial humeral head and anterior glenoid rim), the trough sign/reverse Hill-Sachs lesion (compression fracture of anteromedial humeral head), or fracture of the lesser tuberosity.

Several radiological signs have been described on AP view, these include:

- *Light bulb sign:* The head of the humerus in the same axis as the shaft producing a light bulb shape (Fig. 8.5).
- Internal rotation of the humerus

- The 'rim sign'—widening of the glenohumeral space
- The vacant glenoid sign—where the anterior glenoid fossa looks empty.
- The 'trough' sign—a vertical line made by the impression fracture of the anterior humeral head.

Treatment of Anterior Shoulder Dislocation

Traditional reduction techniques such as Hippocrates' and Kocher's are rarely used anymore.

Various manoeuvres described include:

- Hippocratic method—in which the surgeon puts his foot in the armpit of the patient and applies traction with his hands (Fig. 8.6).
- Kocher's method—in which the surgeon first applies traction to the limb followed by external rotation, then adduction and lastly internal rotation. The dislocation should reduce at the point of adduction and then only should the limb be internally rotated. If this is not followed, then fracture of the humerus can occur.
- Stimson's method—in which the patient is made to lie on his belly and the dislocated

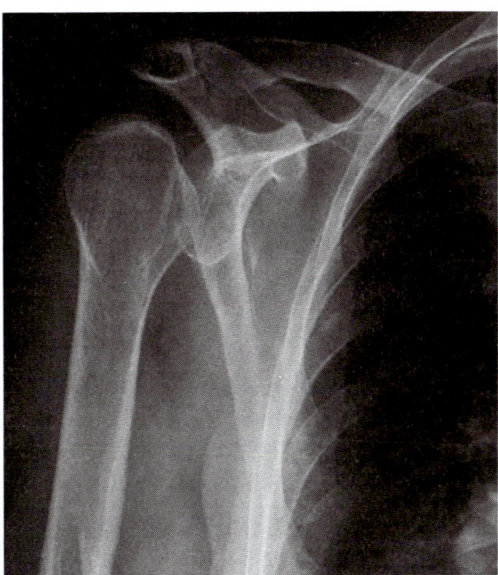

Fig. 8.5: Light bulb sign

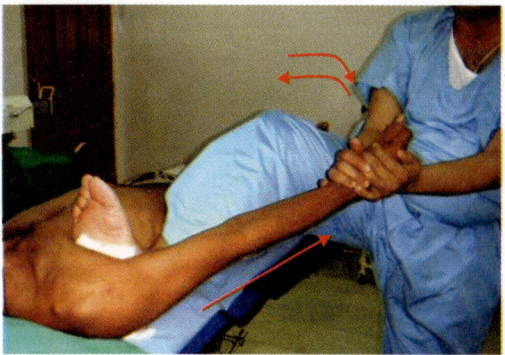

Fig. 8.6: Closed reduction technique

limb is allowed to hand down by the edge of the table by a weight.

- Traction and countertraction method is similar to Hippocratic method except for the surgeon using his foot, an assistant provides countertraction by a sheet of folded cloth across the armpit and chest wall.

After manipulation, the reduction is confirmed by X-rays.

Now the limb is immobilized in a position of adduction and internal rotation in anterior dislocations by strapping the arm to the front of the chest (Fig. 8.7).

In posterior dislocations, the position is of slight external or neutral rotation by a handshake cast.

The duration of immobilization lasts for three weeks after which physiotherapy is started to regain strength and range of motion.

Scapular Manipulation

The patient may be sitting up or lying prone. The health-care professional attempts to rotate the shoulder blade, dislodging the humeral head, and allowing spontaneous relocation. An assistant may be needed to help stabilize the arm.

External Rotation (Hennepin Manoeuvre)

With the patient lying flat or sitting up, the healthcare professional flexes the elbow to 90°

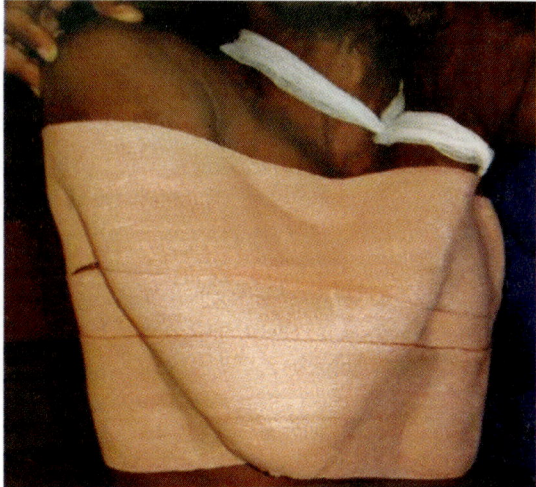

Fig. 8.7: Shoulder immobilizer

and gradually rotates the shoulder outward (external rotation). Muscle spasm may be able to overcome after 5 to 10 minutes of gentle pushing, allowing the shoulder to spontaneously relocate. The Milch technique adds gentle lifting of the arm above the head to achieve reduction.

Traction Countertraction

With the patient lying flat, a sheet is looped around the armpit. While the healthcare professional pulls down on the arm, an assistant, located at the head of the bed, pulls on the sheet to apply countertraction. As the muscles relax, the humeral head is able to return to its normal position.

A sling or shoulder immobilizer may be used as a reminder not to use the arm and allow the muscles that surround the joint to relax and not have to support the bones against gravity. The length of time a sling is worn depends upon the individual patient. A balance must be reached between immobilizing the shoulder to prevent recurrent dislocation and losing range of motion, if the shoulder has been kept still for too long.

In patients who suffer multiple dislocations or those who participate in contact sports, surgery is an option. The procedure involves repairing the labrum and capsule back to the glenoid so that the shoulder does not dislocate. The surgical procedure is usually able to be performed arthroscopically in an outpatient setting.

Complications

Recurrent instability.

Nonoperative treatment: Higher incidence of instability in younger patients with acute traumatic dislocations; 90% in athletic patients <20 years; 15% in patients >40 years; glenoid rim fractures.

- Axillary nerve palsy
- Brachial plexus palsy
- Axillary artery injury
- *Osteonecrosis:* Rare; generally associated with fracture dislocations.

Quick Facts
- >90% are anterior dislocations. <3% posterior dislocations.
- 85% associated with Bankart lesion.

- Anterior dislocations generally result from forced external rotation or extension in an abducted and externally rotated arm.
- *Posterior dislocations:* Associated with epileptic seizures, high-energy trauma, electrocution, or electroconvulsive therapy. Seizures may be associated with hypoglycaemia (diabetes) or drug withdrawal.
- Consider primary anteroinferior glenohumeral instability repair for highly athletic young (<25 years) patients with MRI confirmed Bankart lesion.
- Immobilization in 30° of external rotations has shown a decreased recurrence rate.

BIBLIOGRAPHY

- http://www.eorif.com/shoulder-dislocation-83101-s43016a
- https://www.shoulderdislocation.net
- http://www.radiologyassistant.nl/en/p4963d77684ef7/shoulder-mr-bankart-lesions.html
- www.radiologymasterclass.co.uk › Tutorial
- https://www.youtube.com/watch?v=xDePRKeB4kc

Recurrent Dislocation of the Shoulder

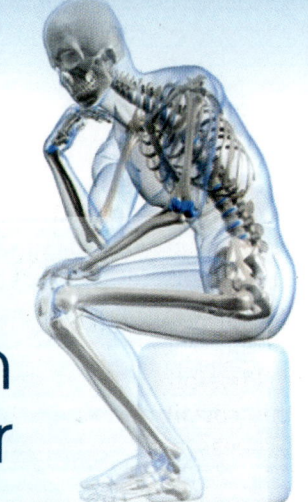

Young people are far more likely to have subsequent dislocations, and the risk of recurrence decreases as patients get older.

Athletes, who are at a higher risk for traumatic injury in general, also have a greater than usual chance of recurrent dislocation. Recurrence is also more likely in men than women.

Atraumatic instability is usually multidirectional and commonly occurs in individuals with generalized hyperlaxity due to connective tissue disorders, such as Ehlers-Danlos syndrome and Marfan syndrome.

A patient with recurrent dislocating tendency may have suffered a dislocation after an injury, following which repeated dislocations occur with relative ease (without any significant injury), present with a history of more than one episode of dislocation (usually a few) occurring following an episode of "first dislocation" occurring after a significant injury with subsequent dislocations occurring "with ease". Most of these patients are able to reduce (put back the dislocated shoulder) on their own or with some assistance.

There is also a small subset of patients who have what is described as voluntary instability, which may be either positional—as when a diver raises his arms and the shoulder pops out of place—or muscular, in which the patient can control the joint at will.

Physical examination will reveal an otherwise normal shoulder. The only positive finding is the 'apprehension test'. In this test, the arm is put in the vulnerable position of abduction and external position. This will cause pain or discomfort and the patient becomes apprehensive that the shoulder will re-dislocate (Fig. 9.1).

TREATMENT

The treatment options for repeated shoulder dislocations depend on the functional demands of the patient and the level of disability suffered by the patient due to these episodes of instability.

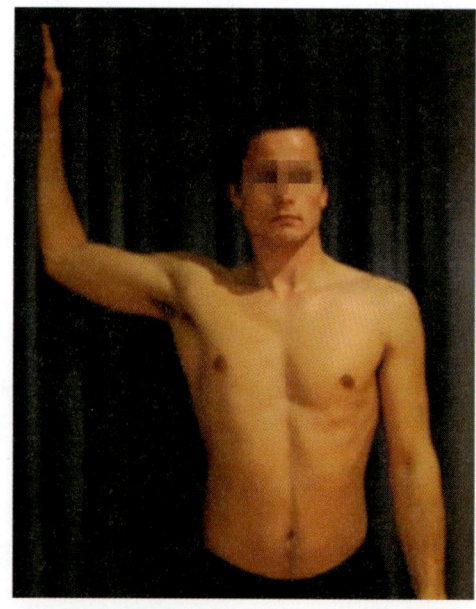

Fig. 9.1: Apprehension test—abduction and external rotation

Treatment for shoulder instability is based on a variety of factors including the severity of the condition, and the patient's age, activity level, occupation, and natural degree of looseness in the joint.

Physiotherapy treatment for patients with this condition is vital to hasten the healing process and ensure an optimal outcome (Fig. 9.2).

Surgical Treatment

- Putti-Platt procedure is performed by lateral advancement of subscapularis and medial advancement of the shoulder capsule.
- Magnuson-Stack procedure is performed with lateral advancement of subscapularis (lateral to bicipital groove and at times to greater tuberosity).
- Bristow-Latarjet procedure involves coracoid transfer to anterior inferior glenoid bone defect through a split in the proximal one-third of subscapularis (Fig. 9.3).

Surgery is very successful in preventing repeat dislocations and restoring motion. Arthroscopic surgery has the advantage of

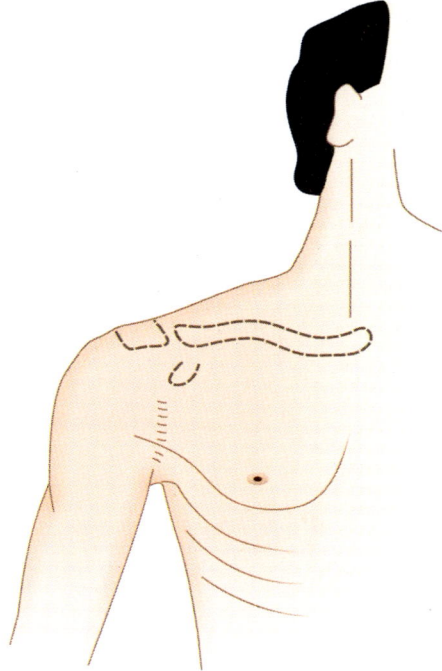

Fig. 9.3: Axillary incision

providing stability with minimizing loss of rotation often seen with an open procedure (Fig. 9.4). The success rate of surgery after a single dislocation is approximately 95% while that after numerous dislocations drops to at least 90–95%.

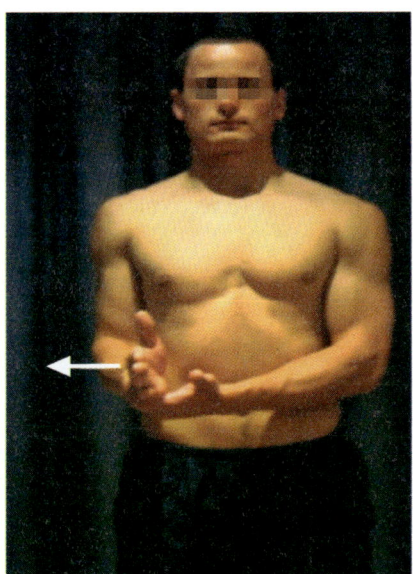

Fig. 9.2: Static rotator cuff strengthening exercises

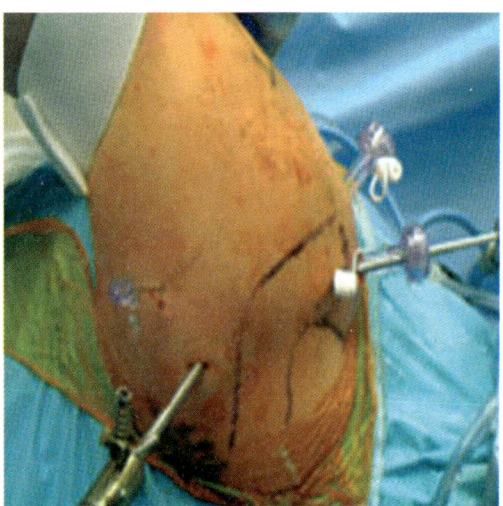

Fig. 9.4: Shoulder arthroscopy

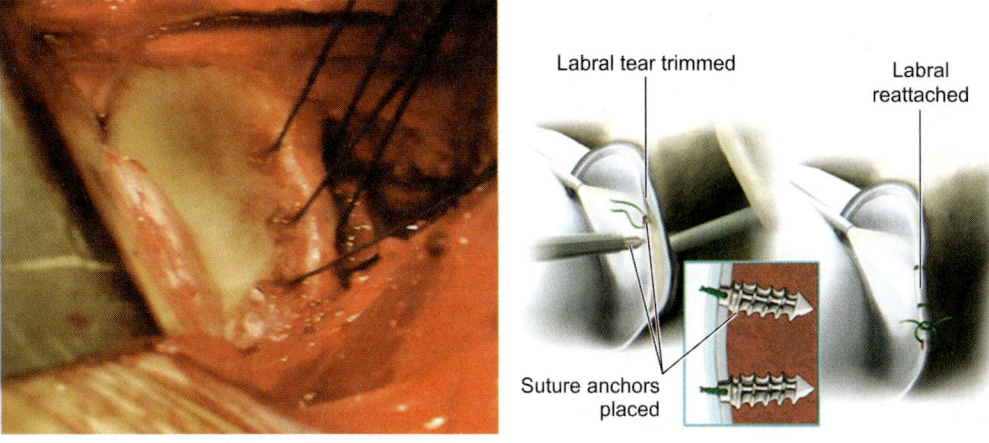

Fig. 9.5: Bankart repair

Operative treatment should aim at repairing or nullifying the effects of both types of lesions. For anterior detachment of the labrum, this involves either suturing the labrum back to the glenoid margin, or constructing some form of anterior buttress, fibrous or bony. For humeral head defects, it necessitates some procedure designed to limit external rotation, thus preventing the defect from coming into engagement with the glenoid cavity. Such limitation of external rotation does not constitute a significant disability.

Soft tissue surgery involves repair of Bankart's lesion, either arthroscopically or by open method.

Repair of Bankart Lesion (Fig. 9.5)

Once the glenoid rim has been prepared, three drill holes are made on the glenoid rim at the osteochondral junction, or just on the joint surface. If the anchors are placed too far medially, a residual Bankart lesion will be the result. The placement of the drill holes is critical. These will accommodate the three Mitek anchor sutures. The anchors should be distributed along the glenoid rim to allow all the detached capsule to be securely fixed to bone. The lower anchor should be introduced as low as possible, and the remaining two

about 1 to 1.5 cm apart. The recommended positions for three anchor sutures for a right shoulder are 5.30 to 6 o'clock, at 4.30 and at 2.30 to 3 o'clock.

Bony operations are indiacted with a large Hill-Sachs lesion. In such situations, a Bristow-Latarjet procedure (Fig. 9.6) (transfer of coracoid process to the glenoid defect) or a bone graft to the Hill-Sachs lesion needs to be performed.

For atraumatic instability, exercises are the first choice in treatment. When these are not successful the surgical approach needs to be

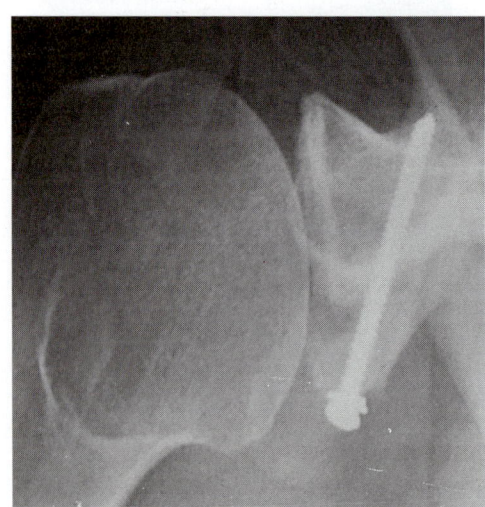

Fig. 9.6: Bristow-Latarjet procedure

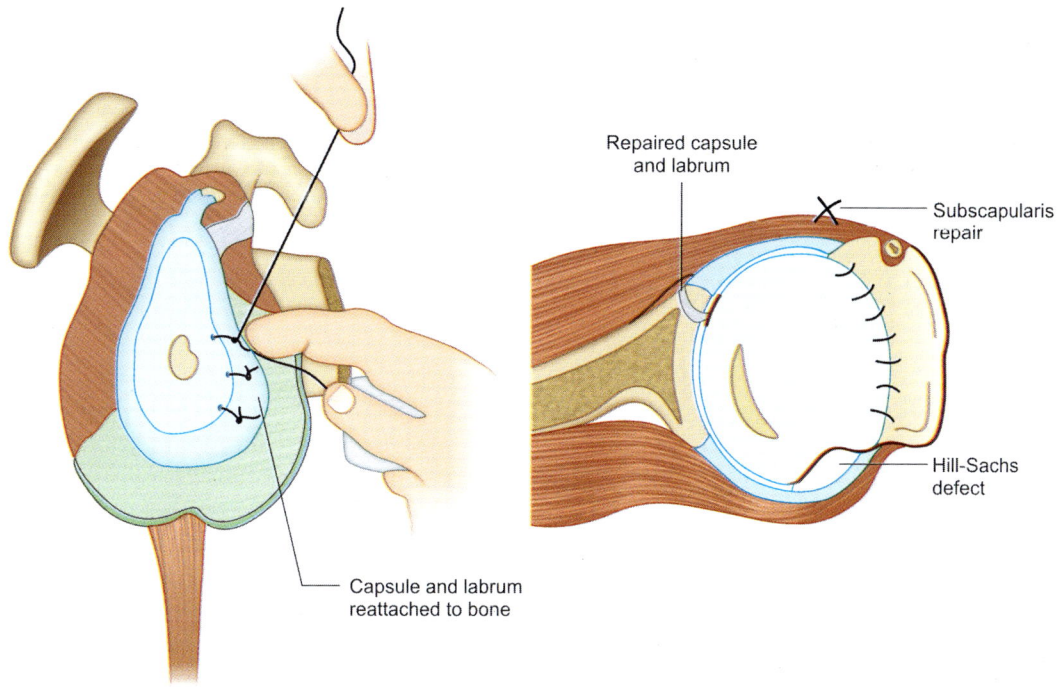

Repaired capsule
and labrum

Subscapularis
repair

Hill-Sachs
defect

Capsule and labrum
reattached to bone

Fig. 9.7: Capsular shift surgery

tailored to the specific circumstances. If the primary direction of atraumatic instability is posterior, a posterior glenoid osteoplasty provides a robust reconfiguration of the shape of the glenoid so that it provides additional stability. For multidirectional instability, a procedure to build up the glenoid labrum may increase the effective concavity of the glenoid socket. For patients with ligamentous hyperlaxity (excessive range of motion of the shoulder), a ligament and capsule tightening procedure is considered. This has been done with open surgery (known as a capsular shift—Fig. 9.7) and by arthroscopic surgery (e.g. by burning and scarring the capsule).

- 26–48% of those younger than 40 years will have a recurrence.
- 0–10% of those older than 40 years will have a recurrence.
- A single dislocation in a young man who plays contact sport may well merit referral to an orthopaedic surgeon to assess stability of the joint with a view to a stabilisation operation. Two dislocations in a young person certainly merit referral.
- There are several stabilisation procedures, dependent upon the nature of the lesion.

Summary
- Dislocation of the shoulder is often associated with damage to the joint capsule (as in Bankart's and Hill-Sachs lesions) and this can lead to instability and predispose to recurrent dislocation.
- 80–94% of patients who have a dislocation under the age of 20 years will have a recurrence of their dislocation.

BIBLIOGRAPHY
- http://www.orthop.washington.edu/?q=patient-care/articles/shoulder/bankart-repair-for-unstable-dislocating-shoulders.html
- http://www.radiologyassistant.nl/en/p4963d77684ef7/shoulder-mr-bankart-lesions.html
- https://www.youtube.com/watch?v=uObzRhWq7tk
- https://www.youtube.com/watch?v=a6BWiufgmsc
- https://www.youtube.com/watch?v=dzFyLuyiIAE

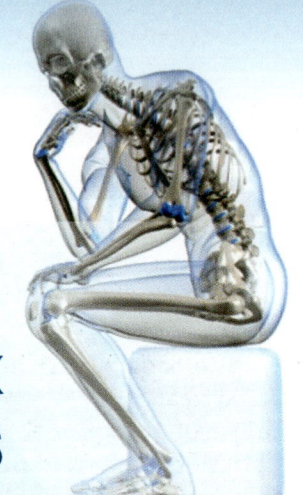

Fracture Surgical Neck of Humerus

- Third most common fracture pattern seen in elderly.
- 4–6% of all fractures.
- Incidence: 2:1 = M:F
- Approximately 75% of these fractures show only minor displacement and can be treated non-operatively.

CLASSIFICATION

- *Neer classification* (Fig. 10.1): Based on the four usual cleavage lines that occur due to the anatomy of the proximal head of the humerus (the articular segment or head, the lesser tuberosity, the greater tuberosity and the surgical neck/shaft), two-part, three-part and four-part fractures can occur. The fractures are then classified by their degree of displacement and angulation.
- Considered to be displaced, if there is more than 10 mm movement or angulation >45°.
- The AO classification for proximal humerus fractures was initially described by Muller in 1988 and divides the fracture patterns into the classic 27 subgroups based on the location, type, and severity of the fracture.

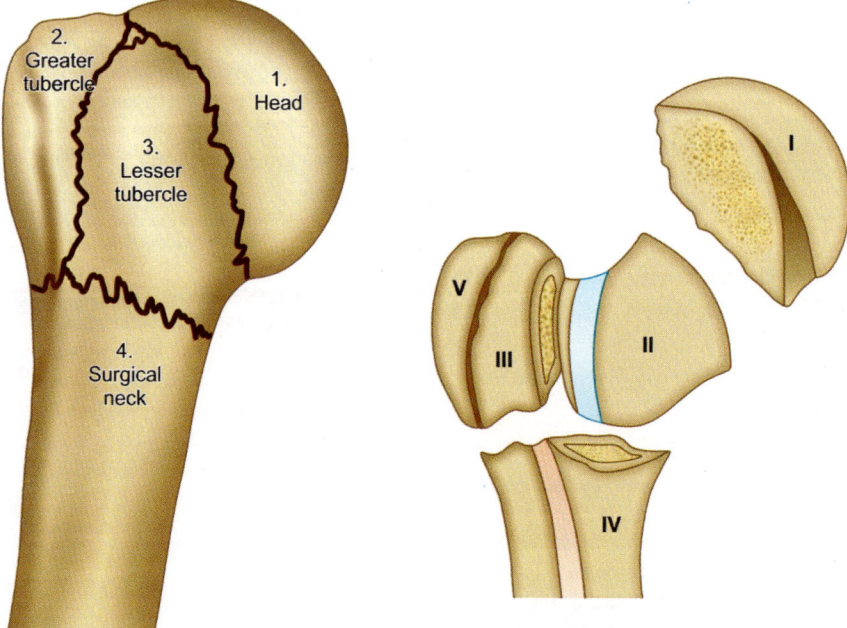

Fig. 10.1: Neer's classification

X-rays

The axillary view often is the most important view (since it tends to show the most displacement).

Up to 85% of proximal humeral fractures can be treated non-operatively. This involves the use of a sling or a shoulder immobiliser. A physiotherapy referral should be made.

Surgery involves either closed reduction with percutaneous fixation, open reduction and internal fixation, or proximal humeral head replacement. In general, unstable fractures are much more painful and often require surgical stabilization to achieve adequate pain relief.

Operative

The treatment approach to two-part fractures is multifactorial and must be individualized for each patient (Flowchart 10.1).

- *CRPP (closed reduction percutaneous pinning)*
  - Indications
    - 2-part surgical neck fractures
    - 3-part and valgus-impacted 4-part fractures in patients with good bone quality, minimal metaphyseal comminution, and intact medial calcar
- *ORIF*
  - Indications
    - Greater tuberosity displaced >5 mm
    - 2-, 3-, and 4-part fractures in younger patients
    - Head-splitting fractures in younger patients
- *Intramedullary nailing*
  - Indications
    - Surgical neck fractures or 3-part greater tuberosity fractures in younger patients
    - Combined proximal humerus and humeral shaft fractures
  - Outcomes
    - 85% success rate in younger patients

- *Hemiarthroplasty*
  - Indications
    - Anatomic neck fractures in elderly or those that are severely comminuted.
    - 4-part fractures and fracture-dislocations (3-part if stable internal fixation unachievable)
    - Rotator cuff compromise
    - Glenoid surface is intact and healthy
    - Chronic non-unions or malunions in the elderly
    - Head-splitting fractures with incongruity of humeral head
    - Humeral head impression defect of >40% of articular surface
    - Detachment of articular blood supply (most 3- and 4-part fractures)
- *Total shoulder arthroplasty*
  - Indications
    - Rotator cuff intact
    - Glenoid surface is compromised (arthritis, trauma)
- *Reverse shoulder arthroplasty*
  - Indications
    - Elderly individuals with non-reconstructible tuberosities

Complications

Neurovascular injury: Axillary nerve damage is most common. Suprascapular, radial and musculocutaneous nerves can also be affected. Axillary artery injury may (rarely) occur (look for expanding mass over the proximal shoulder girdle). The brachial artery is also rarely injured (Fig. 10.2).

Avascular necrosis of the humeral head: This is more common in complex fractures with multiple fragments.

Stiffness or frozen shoulder.

Malunion, mainly with fractures of greater tuberosity.
- Associated glenohumeral dislocation.
- Associated rotator cuff injury.

Flowchart 10.1: Algorithm of treatment

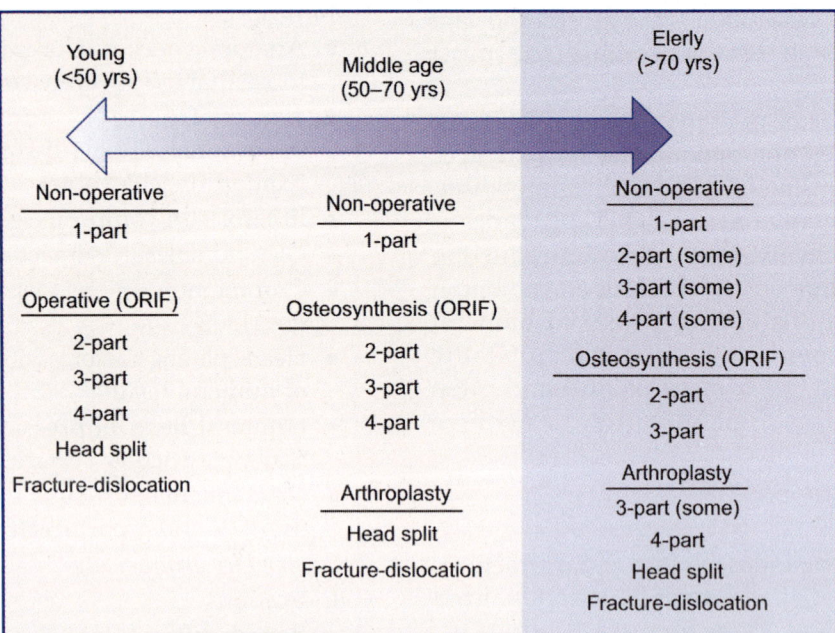

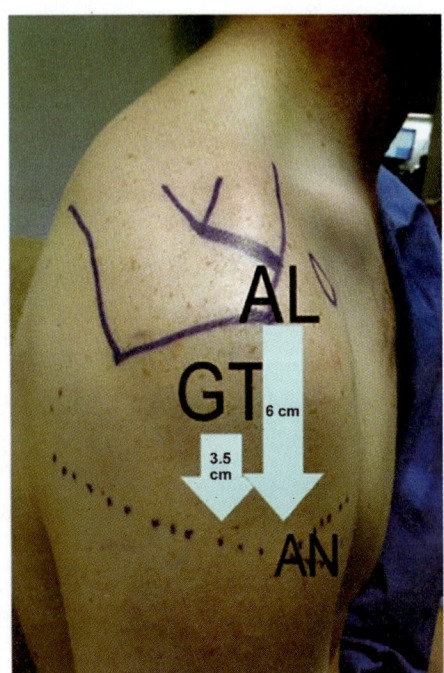

Fig. 10.2: Location of axillary nerve (AN) in relation to lateral border of acromion (AL) and greater tuberosity (GT)

The overall prognosis for proximal humerus fractures depends on numerous factors, including the following:

- Fracture pattern
- Patient's age
- Associated comorbidities
- Patient's expectations
- Willingness of the patient to undergo lengthy rehabilitation
- Ability to anatomically reduce the tuberosities in surgically managed fractures
- Presence or absence of inferomedial support

These fractures as a whole require at least 1 year for recovery.

- Compression fractures tend to be stable.
- Shear injuries tend to be unstable.

Summary
- The fracture is extracapsular, usually has an adequate blood supply and relatively low incidence of AVN.
- In contrast, anatomic neck fracture has much higher incidence of AVN.

- Associated undisplaced fractures into tuberosities are common, but they do alter natural history because the soft tissues are retained.
- Fractures with more than two fragments, those displaced more than 1 cm or associated with shoulder dislocation would most likely require an operation to assess the damage further.
- Successful internal fixation of fractures of the surgical neck of the humerus can be difficult to achieve because of osteopenia of the proximal aspect of the humerus.
- The development of intramedullary nails and minimally invasive locking plates provides greater ability to fix more complex fractures with less risk to the blood supply.
- Displaced and unstable humeral head fractures must be regarded as unsolved fractures, because existing surgical treatment modalities and implants have limitations.
- Modern implants such as intramedullary proximal humeral nails and anatomically designed proximal humeral angular stable plates offer high primary stability even in osteoporotic bone with preservation of periosteal blood supply to the humeral head.

BIBLIOGRAPHY

- https://www.youtube.com/watch?v=JHyYdlX1ibw
- https://www.youtube.com/watch?v=OybVbJfwxrU
- https://www.youtube.com/watch?v=IXCD_BcbgOw

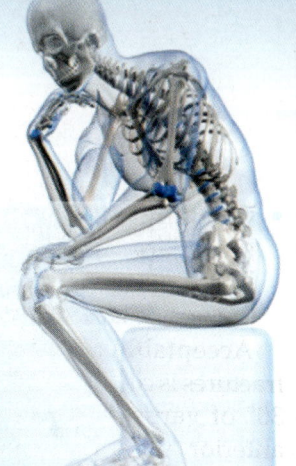

Fracture Shaft of Humerus

"A fracture of the shaft of the humerus is perhaps the easiest of major long bone fractures to treat by conservative means".

"If some shortening results, it is of no significance. If some angular deformity persists, it is usually concealed by muscle covering".

"These are facts which must be remembered when any elaborate or operative method for treating this bone is under consideration".

The Closed Treatment of Common Fractures

—John Charnley (1950)

Incidence

- 3–5% of all fractures.
- Bimodal age distribution
  - Young patients with high-energy trauma

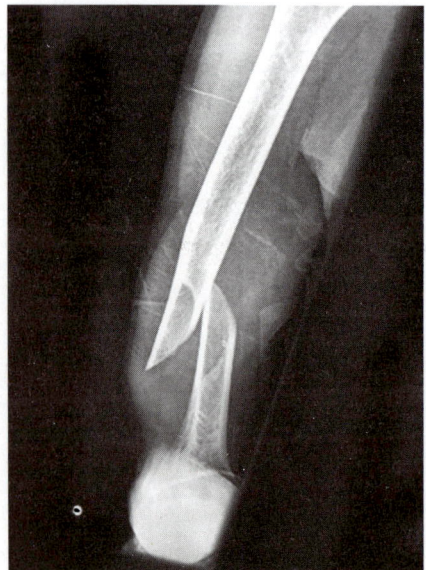

Fig. 11.1: Fracture of humeral shaft

- Elderly, osteopenic patients with low-energy injuries
- Holstein-Lewis fracture: A spiral fracture of the distal one-third of the humeral shaft (Fig. 11.1) commonly associated with neuropraxia of the radial nerve (22% incidence).

Report Checklist

In addition to reporting on the presence of a fracture, a number of features should be assessed and commented on:

- Fracture
  - Location and extension to metaphysis/epiphysis/articular surface
  - Type of fracture (transverse, spiral, oblique)
  - Comminution/segmental
  - Angulation, displacement and shortening
- Open vs. close; gas in soft tissues or foreign bodies
- Underlying bony lesions (i.e. pathological fractures)

- Carefully assess the elbow and shoulder for secondary injuries. (Be careful, as these will be suboptimally imaged unless dedicated views are obtained.)

Acceptable alignment of humeral shaft fractures is considered to be 3 cm of shortening, 30° of varus/valgus angulation, and 20° of anterior/posterior angulation. No set values for acceptable malrotation exist, but compensatory shoulder motion allows for considerable tolerance of rotational deformity.

Multiple closed techniques are available, including the following:

- Traction
- Hanging arm cast
- Coaptation splint
- Velpeau dressing
- Abduction humeral/shoulder spica cast
- Functional brace (Fig. 11.2)

Patients with large, pendulous breasts who are treated non-surgically are at increased risk of varus angulation.

Surgical options include external fixation, open reduction and internal fixation, minimally invasive percutaneous osteosynthesis, and antegrade or retrograde intramedullary nailing. Each of these techniques has advantages and disadvantages.

OPEN REDUCTION AND INTERNAL FIXATION
(Fig. 11.3)

- *Absolute indications*
  - Open fracture
  - Vascular injury requiring repair
  - Brachial plexus injury
  - Ipsilateral forearm fracture (floating elbow)
  - Compartment syndrome
- *Relative indications*
  - Bilateral humerus fracture
  - Polytrauma or associated lower extremity fracture
    - Allows early weight bearing through humerus
  - Pathologic fractures
  - Burns or soft tissue injury that precludes bracing
  - Fracture characteristics
    - Distraction at fracture site

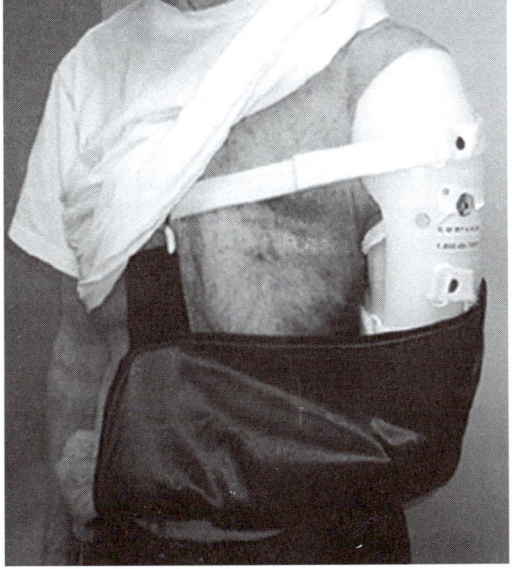

Fig. 11.2: Functional brace

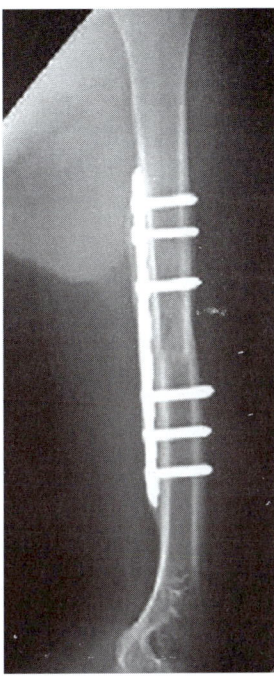

Fig. 11.3: Humeral plating

- Long oblique or spiral proximal fracture
- Intra-articular extension

Plating: "Effective and predictable", Rockwood and Green, 5th Ed.

The most common complications associated with plating procedures are iatrogenic nerve palsy (0–5%, with most cases being a transient problem that requires no further intervention) and infection (0–6%). The two approaches that are used for fracture exposure and plate application are the posterior approach and the anterolateral approach. Either is adequate for fractures in the midthird and distal third, but fractures in the proximal third often require the anterolateral approach.

Intramedullary nailing can be used to stabilize fractures that are 2 cm below the surgical neck to 3 cm proximal to the olecranon fossa. Standard locked intramedullary humeral nails can be inserted either antegrade or retrograde (Fig. 11.4). Antegrade intramedullary (IM) nailing of humeral shaft

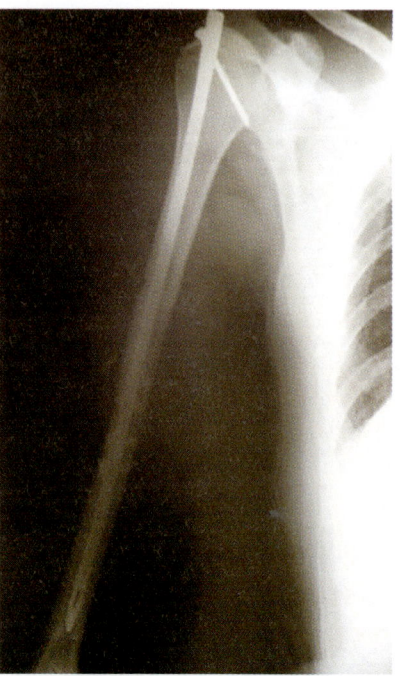

Fig. 11.4: Humeral nailing

fractures has been found to be associated with increased complication rates when compared with open reduction and internal fixation (ORIF).

Results comparing ORIF with locked intramedullary nailing have failed to demonstrate any difference in blood loss or operating room time.

Non-unions in humeral fractures after treatment with plate and screws typically respond well to replating with the addition of bone graft. A humeral non-union treated with an intramedullary nail is treated with open exchange nailing and bone grafting.

Traditionally, external fixation of humeral shaft fractures has been limited to open fractures.

Complications

Radial nerve injury occurs in as many as 18% of humeral shaft fractures. Although the oblique distal third humeral fracture (Holstein-Lewis) is better known for an association with radial nerve palsy than other humeral shaft fractures are, such palsy most commonly occurs with middle third humeral fractures. Most of these nerve injuries are neurapraxic or axonotmetic types, 90% of which resolve to at least grade IV strength in 3–4 months.

Observation

- Indicated as initial treatment in closed humerus fractures
- Obtain EMG at 3–4 months
- Wrist extension in radial deviation is expected to be regained first
- Brachioradialis first to recover, extensor indicis is the last.

Indications for early nerve exploration include a palsy associated with an open wound or penetrating injury.

Brachial artery injuries that are associated with humeral shaft fractures are uncommon. Surgical stabilization of fractures associated with arterial injury is mandatory at the time of vascular repair.

Non-union is defined as when a fracture shaft of humerus fails to heal in 4 months' time. The non-union rate reportedly ranges from 1 to 15%.

1. *Malunion:* Varus angulation is common but rarely has functional or cosmetic sequelae.
2. Adhesive capsulitis of shoulder leading to stiffness.
3. *Open fracture:* "Time to get the orthopod out of the gym and at the bedside".

Points to Note
- Each method of humeral shaft fracture treatment is associated with a union rate of higher than 90%. Each fracture must be considered separately and treated accordingly.
- The best operative treatment modality has still not been fully determined.

- Radial nerve injury has not been shown to be different between IM nailing and ORIF.
- No difference in union rates between the two modalities in prospective studies.
- *Radial nerve injury:* Occurs in 11.8% of fractures. It is most common in distal third fractures. It is more common in transverse or spiral fracture. Spontaneous recovery occurs in 70.7% treated conservatively. Initial expectant treatment may avoid unnecessary operations.

BIBLIOGRAPHY

- www.orthobullets.com/trauma/1016/humeral-shaft-fractures
- https://www2.aofoundation.org/wps/portal/surgery?...Humerus...Shaft
- https://www.youtube.com/watch?v=SRsCPFU94Mk
- https://www.youtube.com/watch?v=P_k-XTeIUc8

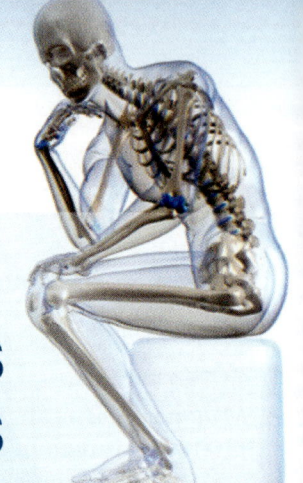

Intercondylar Fractures of Humerus

Fractures of the distal humerus account for 2% of all fractures and one-third of those at the elbow. Distal humeral fractures have a bimodal age distribution: High-energy injury generally occurs in younger patients, whereas low-energy fracture predominates in the elderly and are often associated with osteoporosis.

Riseborough and Radin Classification (Fig. 12.1)

- *Type I:* No displacement.
- *Type II:* The trochlear and capitellar fragments are separated but not appreciably rotated.
- *Type III:* As for type II but the fragments are also significantly rotated.
- *Type IV:* Severe comminution of the articular surface and wide separation of the humeral condyles.

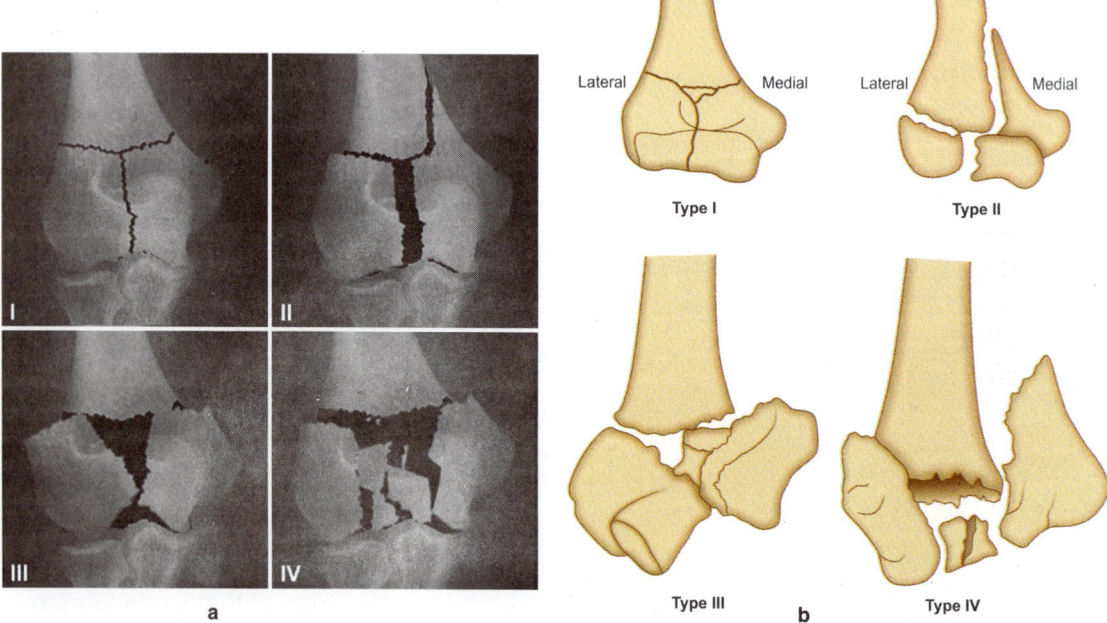

Fig. 12.1a and b: (a) Fracture patterns; (b) Riseborough and Radin classification of intercondylar fractures of the humers. (Reproduced with permission from Riseborough EJ and Radin EL. Intercondylar T fractures of the humerus in the adult. A comparison of operative and non-operative treatment in twenty-nine cases. J Bone Joint Surg Am 51, 130–141, 1969)

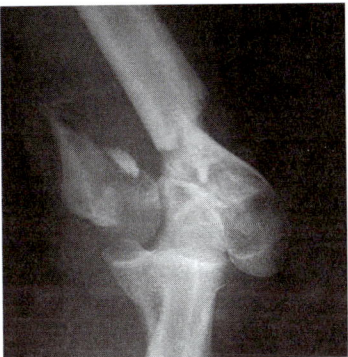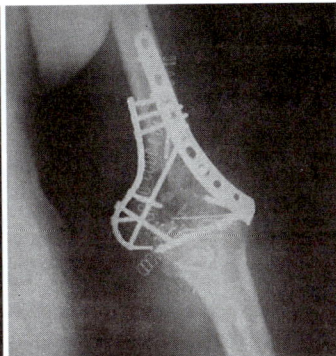

Fig. 12.2: Internal fixation

Intercondylar fractures of the distal humerus in adults are difficult fractures to treat because of their rarity and associated significant comminution.

Non-Operative Management

- Indicated for undisplaced fractures.
- In elderly patients with osteopenia and displaced fractures, careful decision making is required on non-operative and operative intervention—ORIF or arthroplasty.
- The trend in treatment of distal humeral fractures has shifted toward operative fixation.

Operative Management

- *The goals of treatment include:* Anatomic articular reduction, rigid internal fixation (Fig. 12.2) and early mobilization of the elbow.
- MUA and K-WIRE
- ORIF
- Arthroplasty

Principles of Internal Fixation

Two philosophies exist:

- AO 90/90 plating (Fig. 12.3)
- Restoring the arch concept

Fractures of the distal humerus are often complex and, therefore, challenging to treat. In elderly patients with decreased bone strength due to osteoporosis, strong fixation is crucial to allow resuming early motion that guarantees a good functional outcome as well as

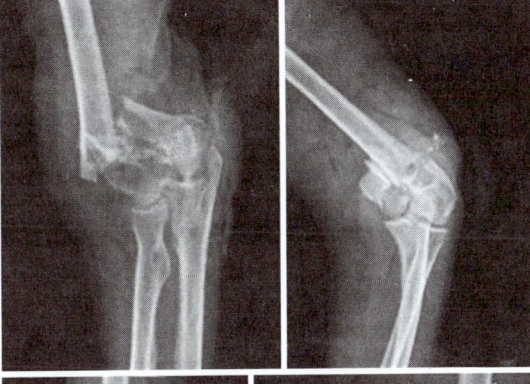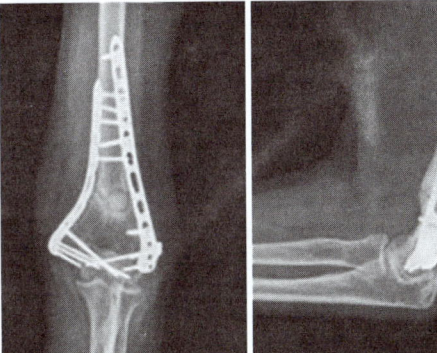

Fig. 12.3: Plating of intercondylar fracture of humerus

minimizing mechanical complications. Locked implants meet these requirements (Fig. 12.4).

Complications

- Superficial wound infection
- Contracture
- Non-union
- Hardware failure
- Malunion

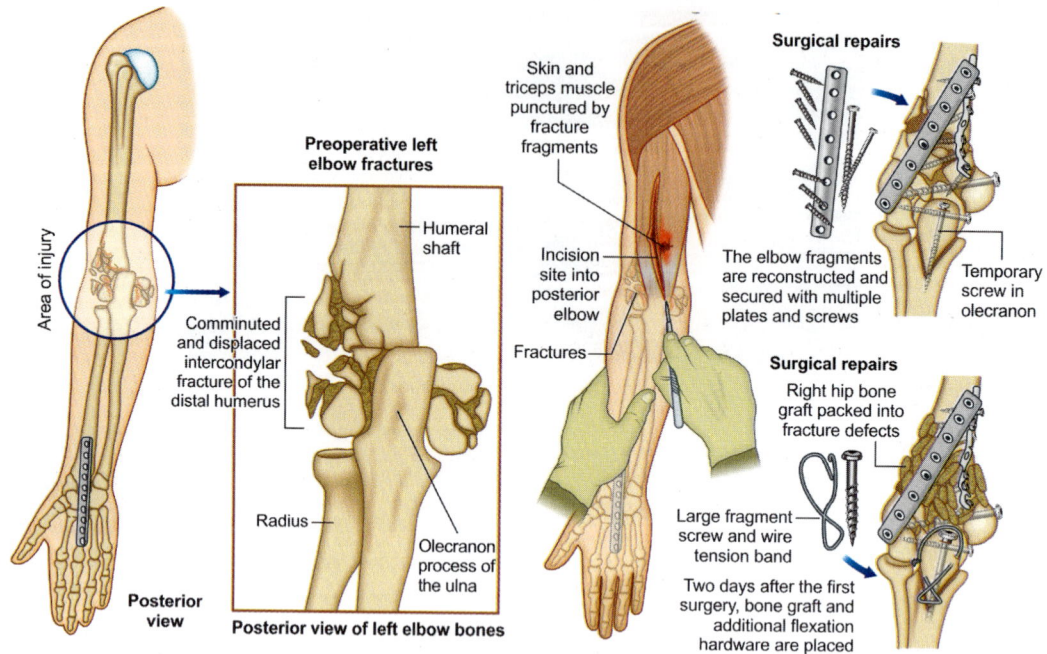

Preoperative left elbow fractures

Humeral shaft

Comminuted and displaced intercondylar fracture of the distal humerus

Radius

Olecranon process of the ulna

Posterior view

Area of injury

Posterior view of left elbow bones

Skin and triceps muscle punctured by fracture fragments

Incision site into posterior elbow

Fractures

Surgical repairs

The elbow fragments are reconstructed and secured with multiple plates and screws

Temporary screw in olecranon

Surgical repairs

Right hip bone graft packed into fracture defects

Large fragment screw and wire tension band

Two days after the first surgery, bone graft and additional flexation hardware are placed

Fig. 12.4: Comminuted left elbow fractures with surgical repairs

- Painful hardware
- Ulnar nerve palsy
- Radial nerve palsy
- Heterotopic ossification

Summary

Fractures of the distal humerus raise therapeutic challenges related to the complexity of the local anatomy. Internal fixation using two plates is the reference standard treatment. The specific anatomic characteristics of the distal humerus require fixation of both columns with transverse epiphyseal screws to rebuild the arch needed to restore sufficient regional stiffness and to reconstruct the articular surface.

The preferred treatment for displaced, intra-articular, intercondylar fractures of the distal part of the humerus is open reduction and internal fixation. Distal humerus fractures demand technically difficult operative treatment, often with relatively high morbidity.

Operative fixation of intra-articular fractures of the distal humerus requires adequate exposure. The transolecranon approach is a commonly used approach. The olecranon osteotomy has potential complications related to prominence/migration of hardware, displacement/non-union of osteotomy and triceps weakness.

An alternative exposure is the extensor mechanism—sparing paratricipital posterior approach to the distal humerus through a midline posterior incision, as suggested by O' Driscoll, et al. Triceps-reflecting anconeus pedicle (TRAP) approach avoids the olecranon osteotomy without compromising the operative exposure. TRAP approach incorporates modified Kocker's approach on lateral side and a triceps reflecting approach on the medial side. Both approaches converge distally at the tip of the anconeus.

BIBLIOGRAPHY

- www.powershow.com/.../Fractures_of_the_Distal_Humerus_powerpoint ww.rcsed.ac.uk/fellows/lvanrensburg/classification/.../distal_humerus
- www.orthopaedicclinic.com.sg/dictionary/intercondylar-elbow-fracture

Chapter 13

Dislocation of Elbow Joint

- Elbow dislocation (Fig. 13.1) is the most common dislocation in children; in adults, it is the second most common dislocation after that of the shoulder. Elbow dislocations constitute 10 to 25% of all injuries to the elbow.
- Posterior elbow dislocations comprise over 90% of elbow injuries. Posterolateral is the most common type of dislocation (80%). Anterior dislocations are seen much less commonly than posterior dislocations. Divergent dislocations, which result in the ulna and radius dislocating in opposite directions, are even rare (Fig. 13.2). In the paediatric population, radial head subluxation is the main cause of elbow dislocations.

- A fall on an outstretched hand is the usual mode of injury.
- Examination reveals a loss of the triangular orientation between the medial and lateral epicondyles of the humerus and the olecranon process of the ulna. X-rays of the elbow joint confirm a dislocation and may show a positive fat pad sign.

Report Checklist

In addition to reporting the presence of a dislocation, a number of features should be sought and commented upon.

- *Dislocation direction:* Posterior, posterolateral, posteromedial, lateral, medial or divergent
- *Associated fractures*
  - Most frequently the radial head and coronoid process

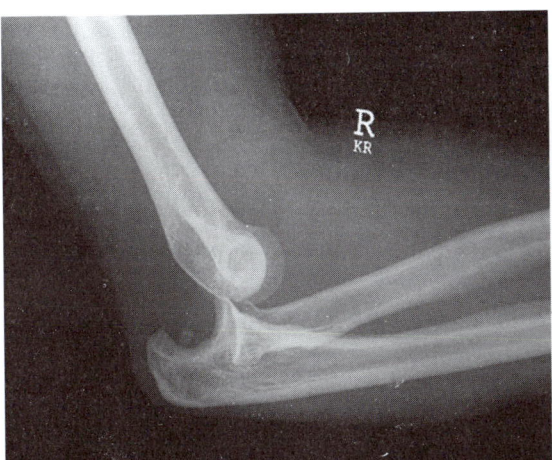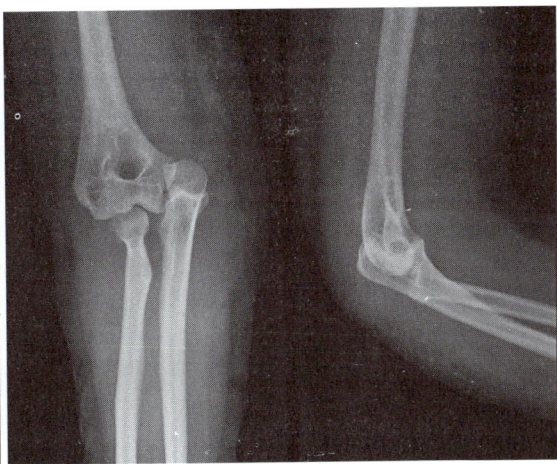

Fig. 13.1: Elbow dislocation

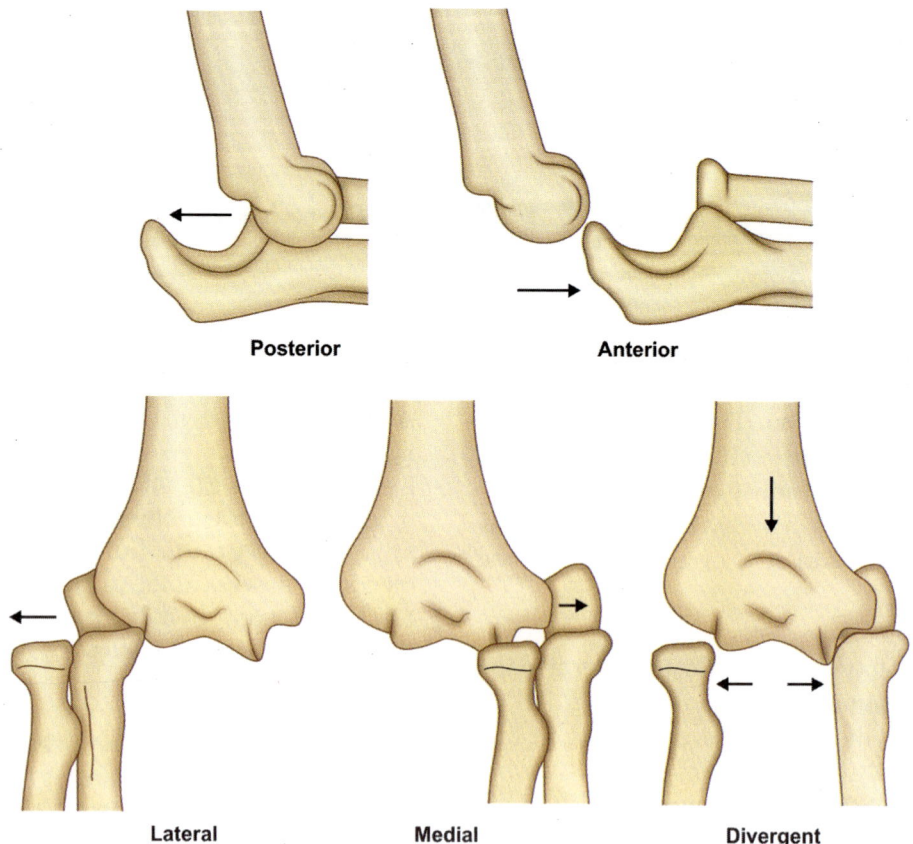

Posterior   **Anterior**

Lateral   **Medial**   **Divergent**

Fig. 13.2: Types of elbow dislocation

– Other fractures encountered include: Lateral condyle, capitellum, olecranon (Fig. 13.3).
• Wrist and shoulder may need to be imaged, if there is clinical concern.

MANAGEMENT

A dislocation with no fracture is simple which only requires close reduction (Figs 13.4 and 13.5), whereas an accompanying fracture makes the dislocation complex usually requiring surgical intervention. When elbow dislocation is simple (i.e. no associated fracture), then closed reduction and a brief period (e.g. <2 weeks) of immobilization at 90° of flexion usually suffices. If the reduction is concentric and the joint is stable, the elbow should be splinted in 90° of flexion. Patients should be followed up in 3–5 days with repeat X-rays to check reduction.

Complex fracture dislocations of the elbow require operative management, consisting reduction of the dislocation, management of the fracture and repair of surrounding damaged soft tissues (ORIF) (Fig. 13.6). They are far more likely to have a poor outcome, including secondary osteoarthritis, limited range of motion, instability and recurrent dislocation as well as pain.

The terrible triad consists of dislocation with associated radial head and coronoid process fracture.

COMPLICATIONS

• *Varus posteromedial instability*
  – Injury to the LCL and fracture of the anteromedial facet of the coronoid.

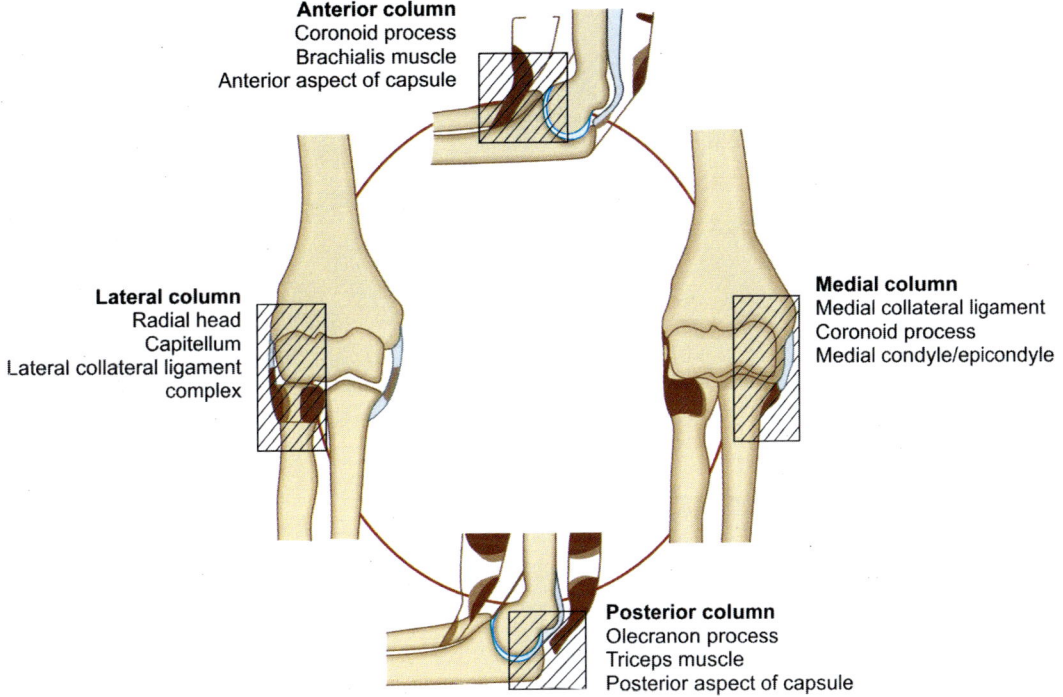

Anterior column
Coronoid process
Brachialis muscle
Anterior aspect of capsule

Lateral column
Radial head
Capitellum
Lateral collateral ligament
complex

Medial column
Medial collateral ligament
Coronoid process
Medial condyle/epicondyle

Posterior column
Olecranon process
Triceps muscle
Posterior aspect of capsule

Fig. 13.3: Columns of the elbow joint

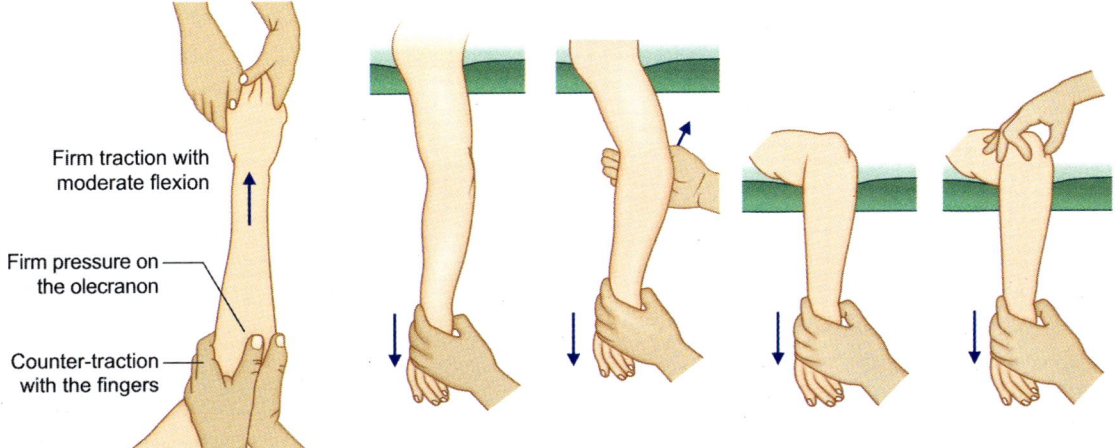

Firm traction with
moderate flexion

Firm pressure on
the olecranon

Counter-traction
with the fingers

Fig. 13.4: Closed reduction

- Solid fixation of the anteromedial facet is critical for functional outcome and prevention of arthrosis.
- *Loss of motion*
  - Loss of terminal extension is the most common sequelae after closed treatment of a simple elbow dislocation.
  - Early active ROM can help prevent this from occurring.
  - Static, progressive splinting can be utilized after inflammation has diminished.

Neurovascular injuries (ulnar/median nerves): Arterial injuries occur in 5 to 13% of

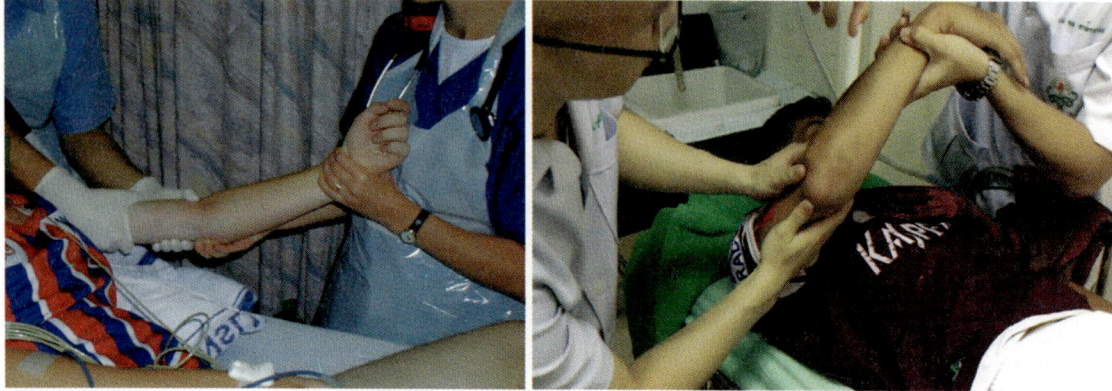

Fig. 13.5: Technique of closed reduction

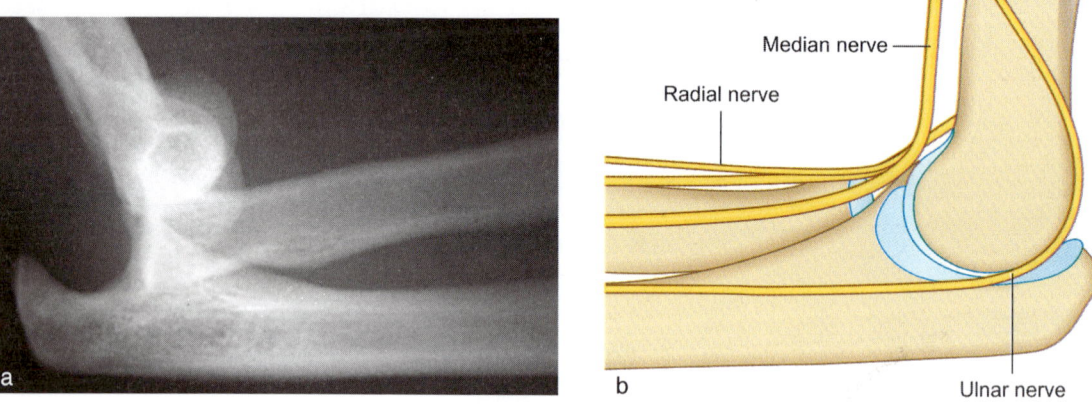

Fig. 13.6a and b: (a) Dislocation of elbow; (b) Nerves around elbow joint

elbow dislocations, mostly in cases of open dislocations or penetrating injuries (Fig. 13.7).

- Compartment syndrome
- Damage to articular surface
- Chronic instability
- Heterotopic ossification
- Contracture/stiffness
  - Correlated with immobilization beyond 3 weeks

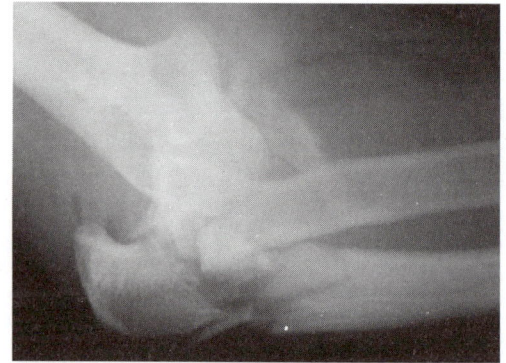

Fig. 13.7: Fracture dislocation of elbow

BIBLIOGRAPHY

- https://www.orthobullets.com
- https://www.youtube.com/watch?v=WZagUe4GvOQ
- https://www.youtube.com/watch?v=uWAAnvTPpO0
- https://www.youtube.com/watch?v=mlAOGgocRnk
- https://www.youtube.com/watch?v=g4Fw1IsmVRU

Fractures of Radial Head

Radial head fractures are common injuries, occurring in about 20% of all acute elbow injuries. Many elbow dislocations also involve fractures of the radial head. Fractures of the radial head occur primarily in adults, whereas fractures of the radial neck are more common in children.

Radial head fractures are more frequent in women than in men, and are more likely to happen in people who are between 30 and 40 years of age (Fig. 14.1).

Injuries associated with radial head fractures include the Essex-Lopresti lesion (tear of the interosseous membrane, distal radioulnar joint disruption) and the so-called terrible triad of the elbow (elbow dislocation, coronoid fracture, and radial head fracture).

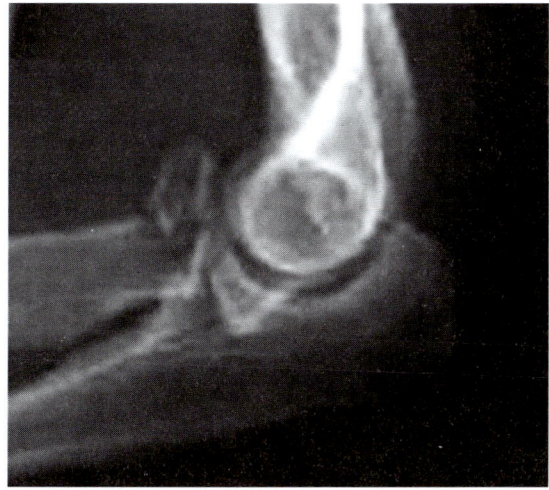

Fig. 14.1: Fracture of radial head

While the majority radial head fractures are isolated, a number of other injuries may also be seen:
• Fracture of the coronoid process of the ulna
• Medial collateral ligament tear
• Interosseous membrane injury
• Triangular fibrocartilage complex injury at the wrist (Essex-Lopresti fracture dislocation)

Even the simplest of fractures may result in some loss of movement in the elbow.

Radial head fractures can be subtle and easily missed on plain films. It is important to assess the film for a joint effusion and where one exists, to take extra care in assessment of the radial head. Even when a fracture cannot be identified, the presence of a joint effusion in adults should be treated as a non-displaced radial head fracture.

In addition to reporting the presence of a radial fracture, a number of specific features should be sought +/- commented upon.
• *Fracture*
  – Location
  – Involvement of the articular surface
  – Articular step-off/gap
  – Comminution
  – Impaction, displacement and impaction
• *Associated injuries*
  – Evaluate rest of elbow for
    ▪ Coronoid process fractures
    ▪ Capitellum osteochondral injuries
    ▪ Elbow dislocations

- Olecranon fracture
- Ligamentous injury (widening of joint space due to medial collateral tear) (Fig. 14.2)
- Evaluate wrist
– Wrist X-rays should be obtained, if any clinical suspicion exists or where assessment is difficult to assess for presence of Essex-Lopresti fracture dislocation.

The physical examination of elbow injuries always must include the wrist, because injury to the radial head may also involve the distal radioulnar joint.

Treatment options for radial head fractures or dislocations include closed reduction with casting or early motion or open reduction with internal fixation, replacement, or resection.

Non-displaced and minimally displaced radial head fractures can be treated with a sling or splint for a few days followed by early ROM.

Long-term disability following a fracture is almost never the result of damage to the bone. It is the result of damage to the soft tissues and stiffness of neighbouring joints.

In the Mason classification, the fracture is type I, if it is undisplaced; type II, if a single fragment is displaced; and type III, if it is comminuted (Fig. 14.3). Type I (non-displaced) is generally treated non-operatively. Type II

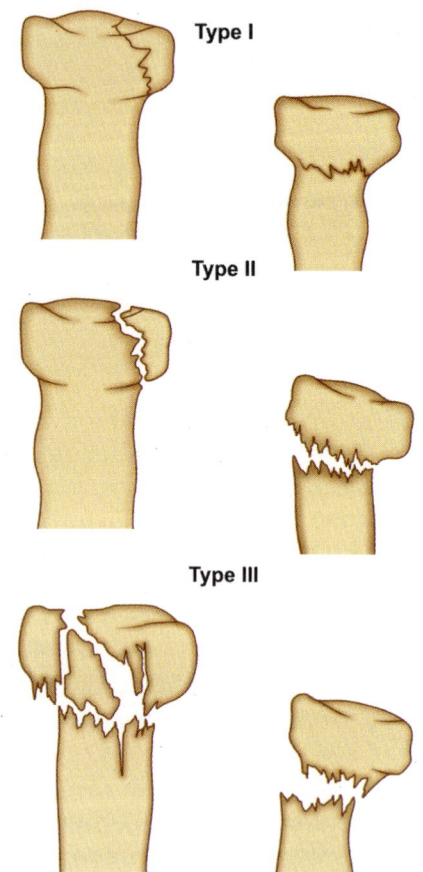

Fig. 14.3: Mason's classification

may be treated non-operatively, if the displacement is minimal. The rule of thirds is used: Non-surgical treatment can be considered, if the fracture involves less than one-third of the articular surface, if there is less than 30° of angulation, and if displacement is less than 3 mm. Type III fractures usually require operative intervention but may occasionally be treated closed with early motion, if the radial head is not reconstructible.

MASON CLASSIFICATION OF RADIAL HEAD FRACTURES

- *Type I:* Non-displaced radial head fractures (or small marginal fractures), also known as a "chisel" fracture—conservative management.

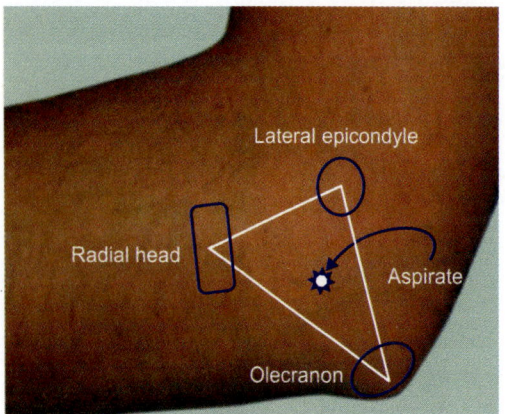

Fig. 14.2: Bony landmarks around elbow

- **Type II:** Partial articular fractures with displacement (>2 mm)—require open reduction and internal fixation (ORIF).
- **Type III:** Comminuted fractures involving the entire radial head—often require early complete excision of the radial head.

Mason Classification (Modified by Hotchkiss and Broberg-Morrey)

Type I: Non-displaced or minimally displaced (<2 mm), no mechanical block to rotation.

Type II: Displaced >2 mm or angulated, possible mechanical block to forearm rotation.

Type III: Comminuted and displaced, mechanical block to motion.

Type IV: Radial head fracture with associated elbow dislocation.

Once the fracture is opened, the final decision is made regarding fixation, replacement, or excision. When possible, best results are obtained with anatomic reduction and fixation. Fixation options include minifragment plates and screws and Herbert screws.

When radial head excision is chosen, the surgeon must not excise distal to the annular ligament because this results in an unstable proximal radioulnar joint. If comminution extends distal to the annular ligament, then replacement with a spacer should be strongly considered (Fig. 14.5).

If radial head replacement is chosen, metallic implants offer better biomechanical properties and biologic compatibility than alternatives such as silicone (Fig. 14.6).

Radial head replacement designs such as bipolar designs and radial head and capitellar replacements are currently available, but there have been limited studies concerning results with these designs.

COMPLICATIONS

Early complications include: Compartment syndrome, neurovascular injury, and infection. Late complications include: Non-union, hardware failure, malunion, infection, synostosis, and persistent pain.

Persistent pain after radial head fracture may be due to the hardware, intra-articular cartilage injury and post-traumatic arthritis, adhesions, malalignment, or associated nerve or muscle injuries.

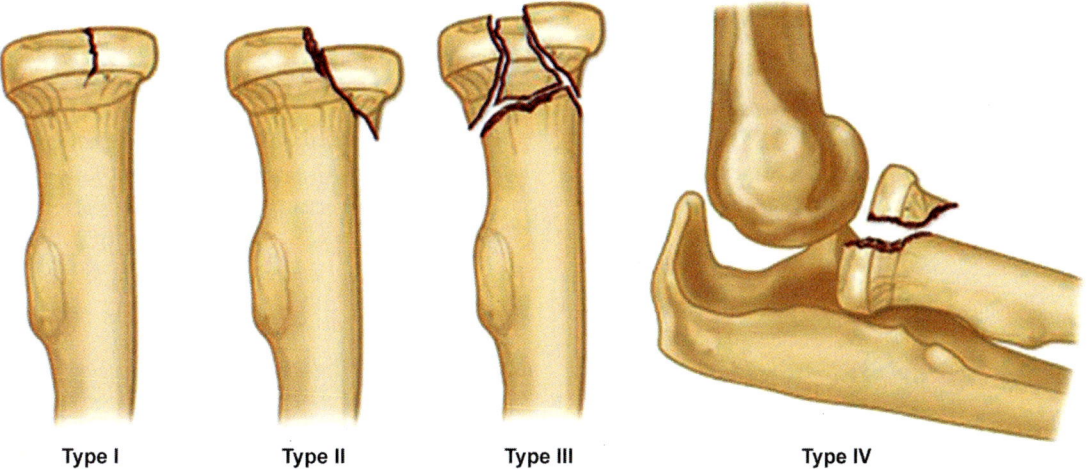

| Type I | Type II | Type III | Type IV |

Fig. 14.4: Modified Mason's classification

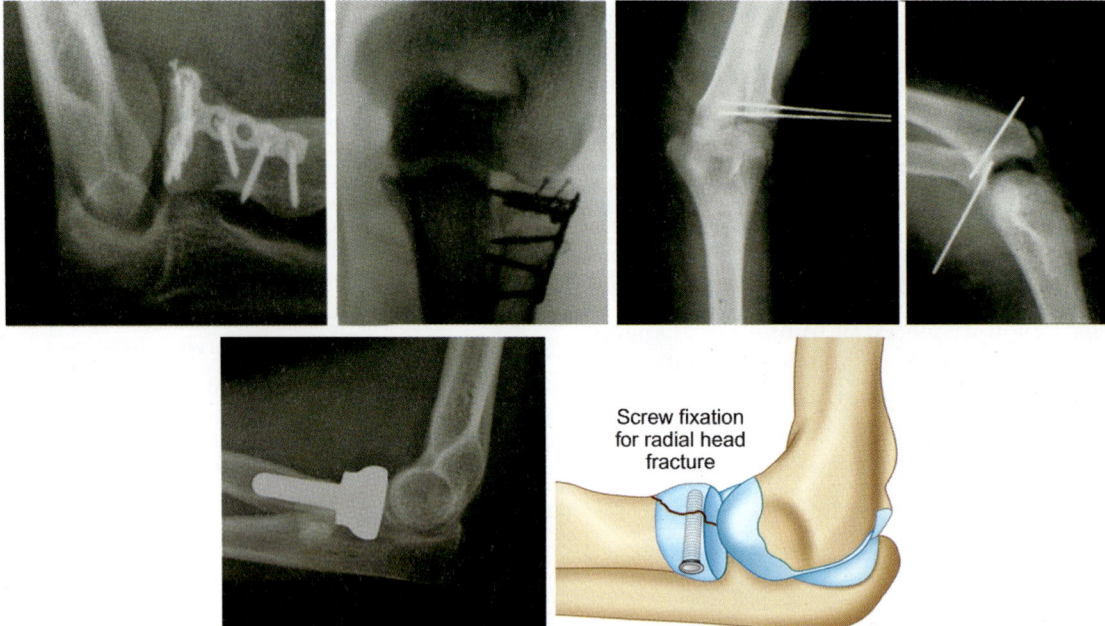

Fig. 14.5: Surgical treatment options

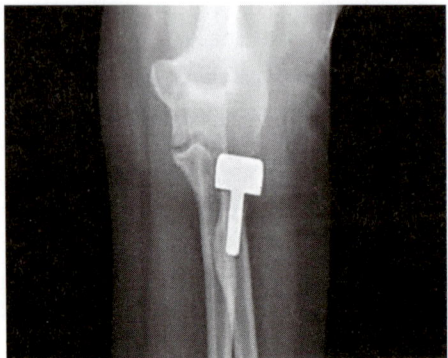

Fig. 14.6: Replacement of radial head

BIBLIOGRAPHY

- http://emedicine.medscape.com/article/1240337-treatment#a28
- www.ncbi.nlm.nih.gov › NCBI › Literature › PubMed Central (PMC)
- https://www.youtube.com/watch?v=M2pvYTLNq14
- https://www.youtube.com/watch?v=xJL9l7hFIZ0
- https://www.youtube.com/watch?v=jEA
- http://torontofirstaidcpr.ca/management-of-adult-forearm-fractures/

Fractures of Radial Neck

Radial neck fractures are more common in children, whereas fractures of radial head occur primarily in adults. In adults, isolated radial neck fractures are very rare with incidence of 1% of all fractures.

Radial neck fractures (Fig. 15.1) are uncommon and account for 8% of all elbow fractures in children. Median age of incidence is 9–10 years. The incidence of radial neck fracture is around 1% of all paediatric fractures and between 5 and 10% of all paediatric elbow fractures. 90% of cases are Salter and Harris type II epiphyseal injuries.

The most common mechanism is a fall onto the outstretched arm with a valgus stress at the elbow. Force applied along the radius results in impaction of the radial head against the capitellum. They can also occur as a result of a posterior dislocation or reduction of the elbow joint.

Associated elbow injuries occur in 50% of radial neck fractures, which include: Avulsion fracture of medial humeral epicondyle, olecranon fracture, fracture of proximal ulna or elbow dislocation.

CLASSIFICATION (Figs 15.2 and 15.3)

O'Brien classification	
Type I	<30°
Type II	30–60°
Type III	>60°

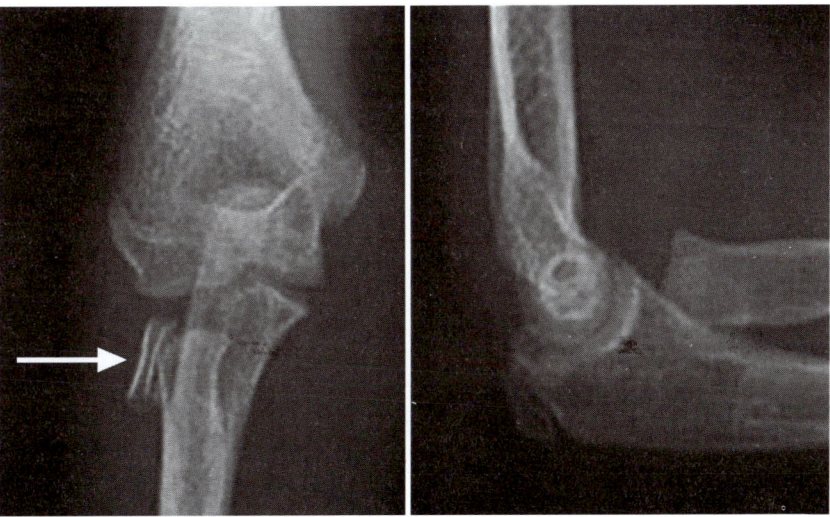

Fig. 15.1: Fracture of radial neck

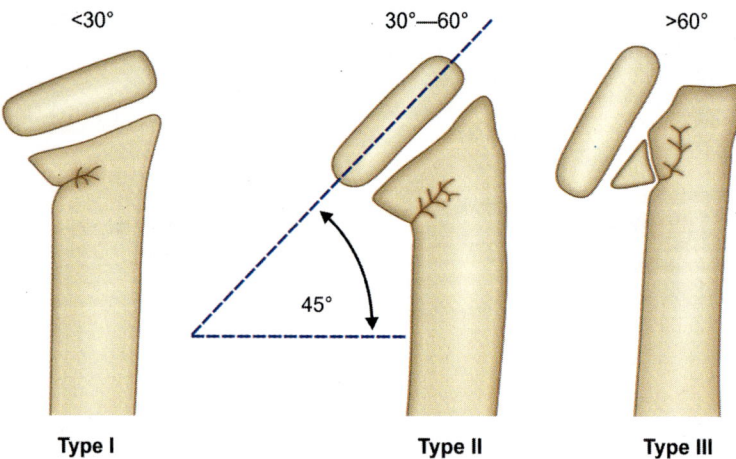

Fig. 15.2: O'Brien classification

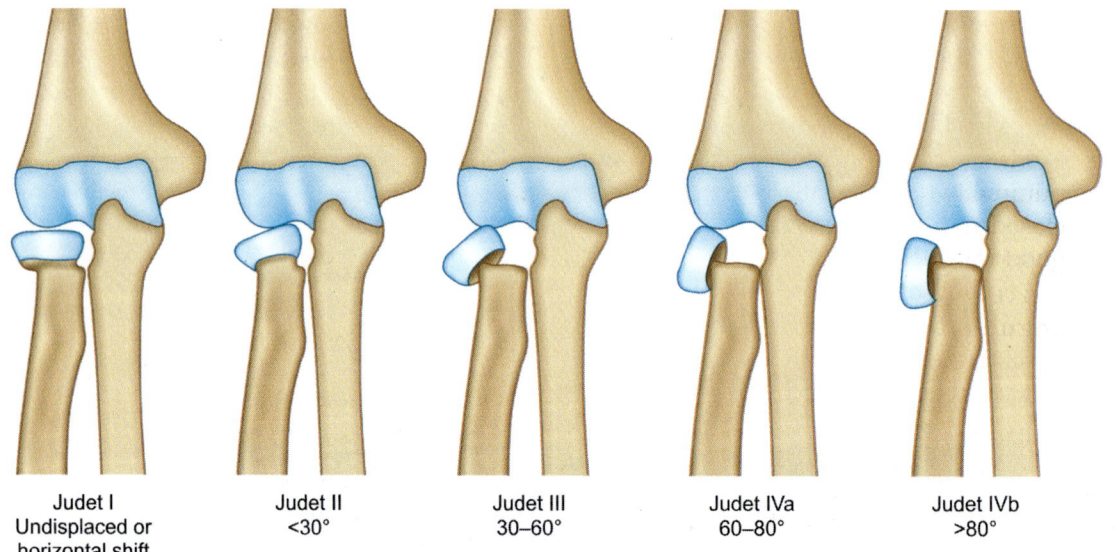

Fig. 15.3: Judet classification

Judet classification	
Type I	Undisplaced
Type II	<30°
Type III	30–60°
Type IVa	60–80°
Type IVb	More than 80°

The radial head should point to the capitellum in all views (Fig. 15.4).

It is recommended that displacement be measured as the angle between a line perpendicular to the articular surface with another down the shaft of the proximal radius (Fig. 15.5).

TREATMENT

The treatment of radial neck fractures in children varies according to the displacement, angulation, and skeletal maturity. Restoration of radial neck angulation and displacement is essential to restore the normal biomechanics and stability of the elbow.

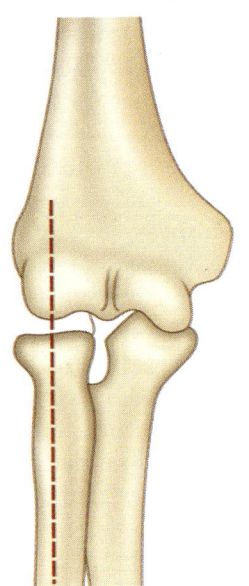

Fig. 15.4: Normal position of radial head

Most fractures are undisplaced or minimally displaced and can be treated with closed reduction (Fig. 15.6) and casting with good outcome.

Treatment depends on the degree of angulation and is surgical, if angulation remains greater than 30° after closed reduction is attempted.

Fractures with angulation >30° and translation >3 mm (>50%) should initially be treated with attempted closed reduction under sedation or anaesthesia. If closed reduction is unsuccessful, then percutaneous-assisted reduction should be attempted. This can be performed with direct manipulation of the fragment with a Kirschner wire (Fig. 15.7).

Another option is the Metaizeau technique which utilizes an elastic nail in a retrograde fashion, engaging the proximal fragment for manipulation and fixation (Fig. 15.8).

Studies reveal that paediatrics Judet type II–type IV fractures have been successfully treated with intramedullary TEN (Metaizeau) techniques and results are promising.

Irreducible or unstable fractures should be treated with open reduction and internal fixation or open reduction with percutaneous fixation (Fig. 15.9).

There are several treatment possibilities for grossly displaced fractures including percutaneous pin reduction, elastic stable intramedullary nailing (ESIN), and open

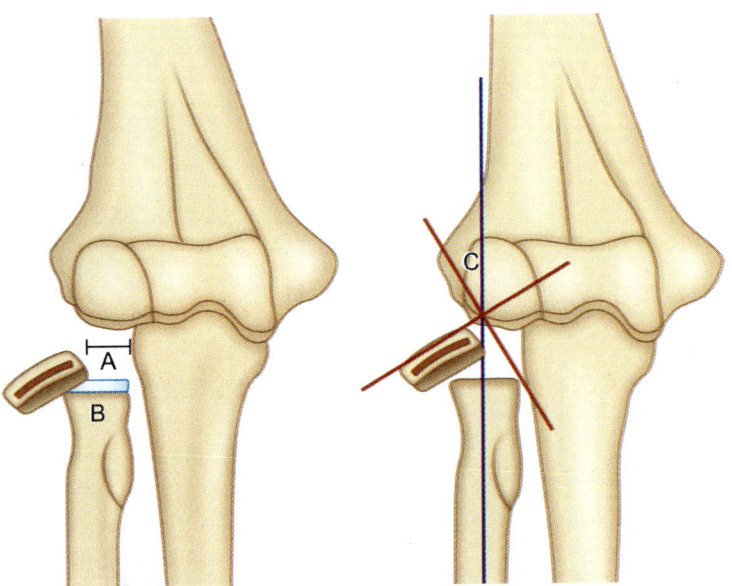

Fig. 15.5: Measurement of displacement of radial head and neck

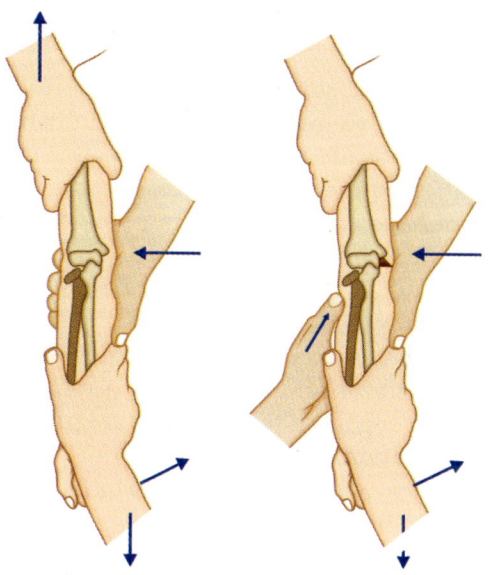

Fig. 15.6: Closed reduction

reduction with or without internal fixation. The standard procedure accepted for isolated radial neck in paediatric age group is centro-medullary pinning (Metaizeau technique).

The optimal treatment method of displaced radial neck fracture in adults remains a matter of controversy. The treatment options include open reduction and internal fixation using antegrade crossed countersunk headless screws, or low-profile plate and screws and radial head excision with or without prosthetic replacement (Fig. 15.10).

Although osteosynthesis yields result superior to radial head excision, it carries the risk of joint stiffness, loss of reduction, and implant failure especially when plate fixation is performed. Hardware removal is sometimes indicated in an attempt to improve range of motion. Radial head resection has been observed to be complicated by instability, symptomatic proximal migration of the radius, and late post-traumatic arthritis when performed in the setting of associated disruption of the medial collateral ligament or interosseous membrane.

Open reduction and internal fixation (ORIF) is associated with non-union, implant-related complications, reduced range of motion, heterotopic bone formation and avascular necrosis of the radial head.

COMPLICATIONS

Overall 20–60% complication rate. Complications are thought to be a result of aggressive treatment and a result of the initial severity of

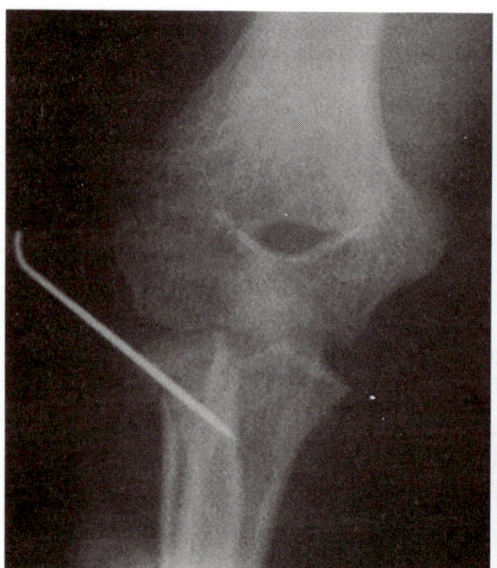
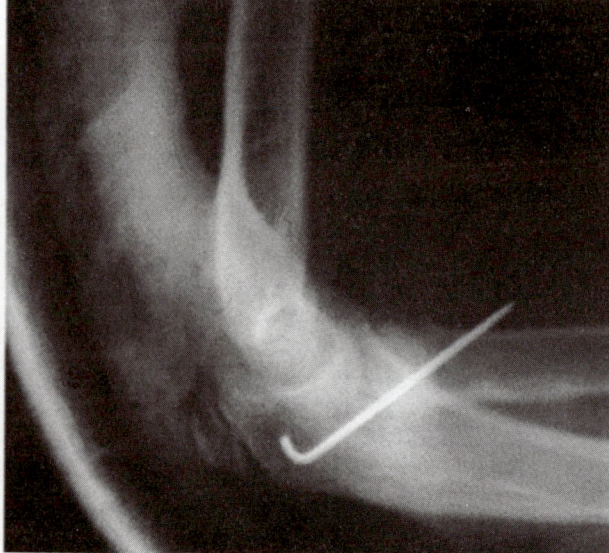

Fig. 15.7: Percutaneous 'K' wiring

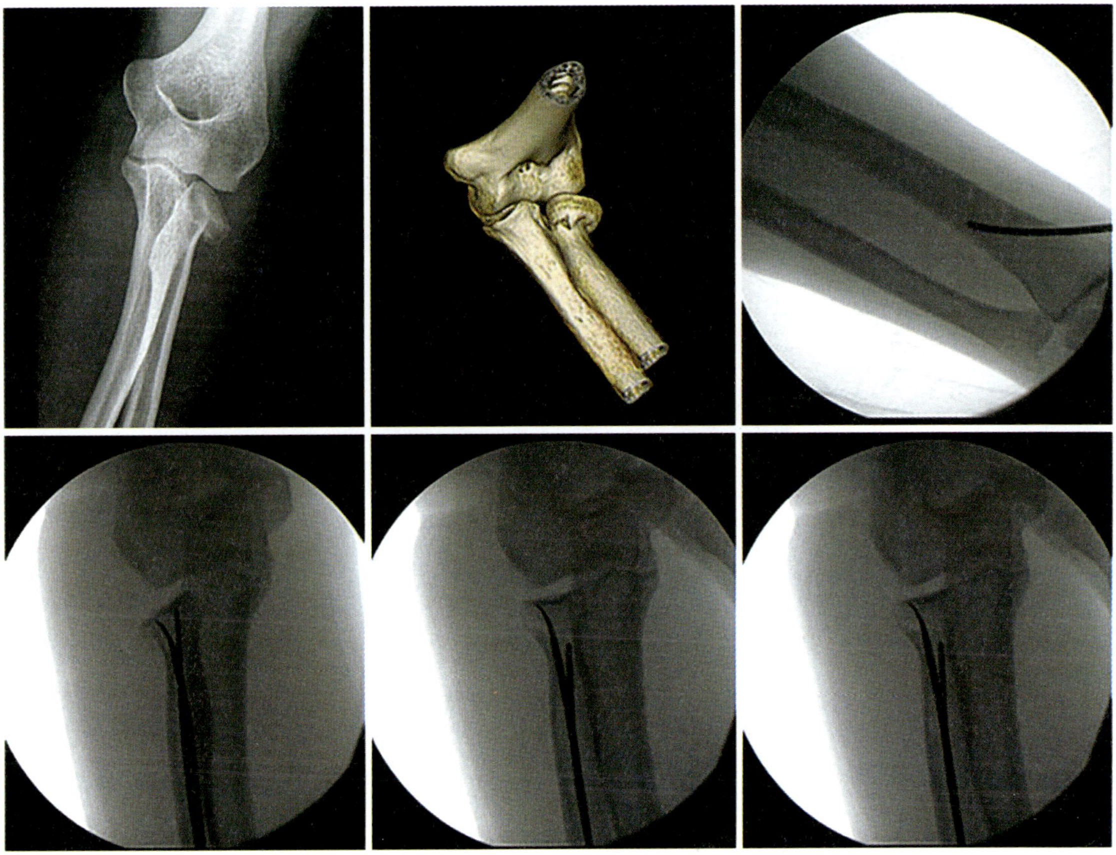

Fig. 15.8: Elastic nailing

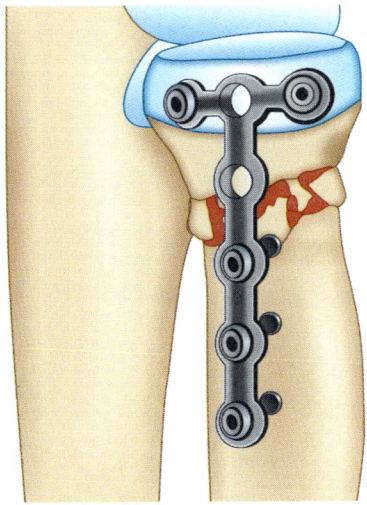

Fig. 15.9: Plating

the fracture, particularly vascular and physeal injury.

Common Complications

- Loss of motion (0–79%)
- Pain (9–66%)
- Avascular necrosis (7–44%)
- Premature physeal closure (0–31%)
- Periarticular ossification (2–13%)
- Non-union
- Malunion
- Radioulnar synostosis
- Residual angulation
- Cubitus valgus

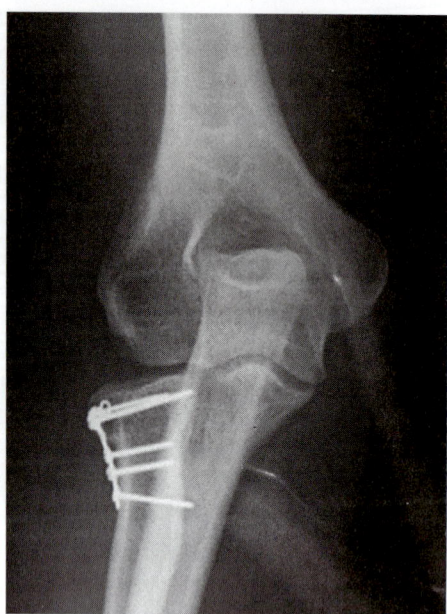

Fig. 15.10: Plate and screws

- Nerve palsy
- Pin tract infection
- Hardware breakage (after transarticular fixation)
- Compartment syndrome

BIBLIOGRAPHY

- https://www.rch.org.au/clinicalguide
- https://www.orthobullets.com
- https://www.youtube.com/watch?v=Pgsk2K_MQ6E

Olecranon Fractures

Olecranon fractures (Fig. 16.1) are rare in children, constituting only 5 to 7% of all elbow fractures. But in adults, they are one of the most common elbow fractures.

CLASSIFICATION

There are several classifications.

Mayo Classification

Based on the stability, the displacement and the comminution of the fracture. It is composed of three types. And each type is divided in two subtypes: Subtype A (non-comminuted) and subtype B (comminuted).

- **Type I:** Non-displaced fractures: It can be either non-comminuted ones (type IA) or comminuted (type IB).
- **Type II**: Displaced, stable fractures: In this pattern, the proximal fracture fragment is displaced more than 3 mm, but the collateral ligaments are intact. That is why there is no elbow instability. It can be either non-comminuted ones (type IIA) or comminuted (type IIB).
- **Type III**: Displaced instable fracture: In this case, the fracture fragments are displaced and the forearm is instable in relation to the humerus. It is a fracture dislocation. It also may be either non-comminuted (type IIIA) or comminuted (type IIIB).

AO Classification

This classification incorporates all fractures of the proximal ulna and radius into one group. And this one is subdivided into three patterns:
- **Type A:** Extra-articular fractures of the metadiaphysis of either the radius or the ulna.
- **Type B:** Intra-articular fractures of either the radius or ulna.
- **Type C:** Complex fractures of both the proximal radius and ulna.

TREATMENT

The goals of olecranon fracture treatment must be individualized to the needs of the patient. In young active individuals, restoration of the articular surface, preservation of motor power, restoration of stability, and prevention of joint stiffness are important. In older patients,

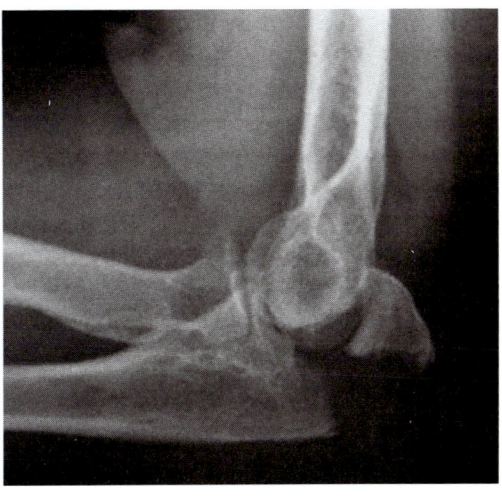

Fig. 16.1: Olecranon fracture

minimization of morbidity is the most important goal.

Non-displaced fractures (with <1–2 mm displacement) with intact extensor mechanisms may be treated non-operatively.

In fractures with a little or no displacement, the immobilization for 4 to 6 weeks can be sufficient. But for the rest of the cases it needs surgery, using pins, wires, screws only or plates and screws. Open reduction and internal fixation (Fig. 16.2) is preferred for displaced intra-articular fractures. Tension band wiring is especially useful for transverse fractures. Plate fixation with a lag screw provides excellent stability for oblique fractures. Plate fixation is especially recommended for extensive comminuted or unstable oblique fractures not amenable to other types of treatment. Plate fixation may also be preferable in the face of an associated coronoid fracture.

When determining the appropriate surgical approach, consider patient age, health, bone quality, fracture pattern, and ligamentous stability. Careful evaluation of the dorsal cortex on preoperative X-rays assists in pre- operative planning to choose the surgical technique. The tension band techniques convert dorsal distraction forces to compressive forces at the articular surface and fracture site. If the dorsal cortex is comminuted, mechanical stability is lost. Therefore, if there is an intact dorsal cortex, tension band wiring is an excellent choice for fixation, but if the dorsal cortex is comminuted, the surgeon should consider a plate or intramedullary device instead.

Approximately 70% of the extensor power is estimated to be lost when the fracture is displaced more than 1.5 cm.

COMPLICATIONS

Symptomatic hardware requiring removal is the most frequent complication following internal fixation occurring in 22–80% of patients. Hardware problems have occurred in up to 80% of patients with Kirschner tension band wires. Wire migration occurs with soft tissue irritation, wire breakage, or fracture displacement.

Loss of motion is a common problem following fractures of the elbow but is usually

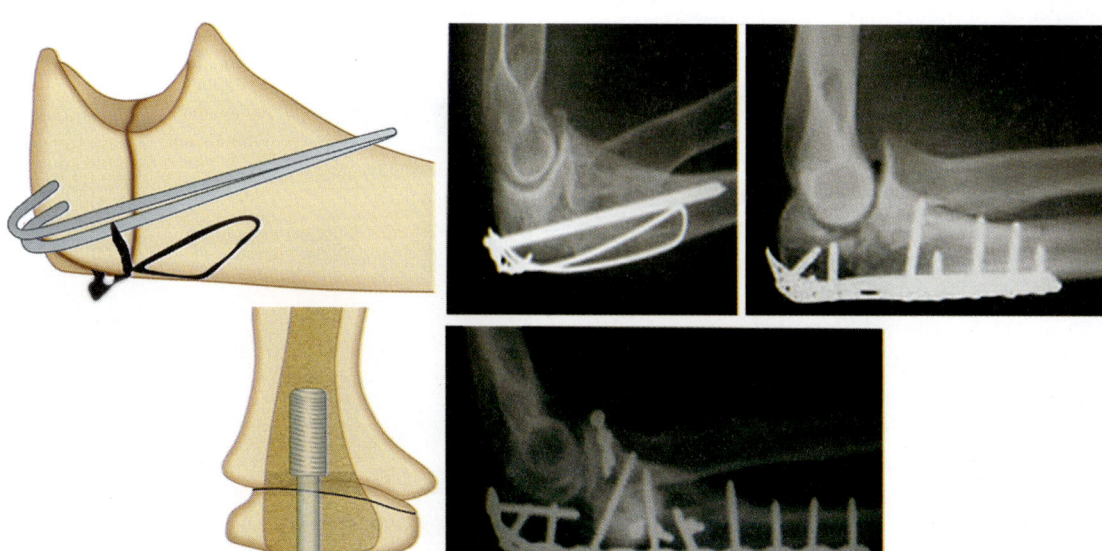

Fig. 16.2: Internal fixation technique

not a significant issue for olecranon fractures. Generally, patients lose 15° of extension and, occasionally, a small amount of supination. Motion tends to improve progressively with time for up to 2 years.

Heterotopic ossification occurs in 13–14% of patients. The range of reported rates of infection following operative treatment is 0–6%. Reflex sympathetic dystrophy occurs on rare occasions. Ulnar neuritis occurs in 2–12%.

Generally, non-union occurs in fewer than 5% of patients. When non-unions are treated by internal fixation +/– bone grafting, good to excellent results occur in approximately two-thirds of cases. Non-union can occur even in patients treated non-operatively.

95% of patients with olecranon fractures are expected to have near-normal function. 20–25% of patients will develop radiographic evidence of arthrosis at 15–20 years follow-up but these patients are usually asymptomatic.

Occasionally ulnar nerve injury can result in long-term sensory and motor impairment, most marked in the hand.

BIBLIOGRAPHY

- en.wikipedia.org/wiki/Olecranon_fracture
- http://emedicine.medscape.com/article/1231557-treatment#a1133
- https://www.youtube.com/watch?v=GauDxDVWnP4

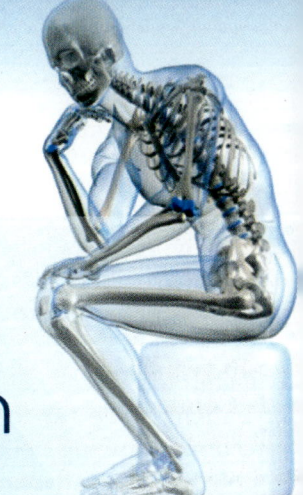

Chapter 17

Elbow Injuries in Children

INJURIES AROUND THE ELBOW IN CHILDREN

Elbow fractures are common childhood injuries, accounting for about 10% of all childhood fractures (Table 17.1). Upper extremity injuries account for 65% of injuries in children, of which fractures and dislocations of the elbow are the second most common. Children regularly engage in many activities that put them at risk for injuries to the elbow. Many stable fractures heal successfully with cast or splint immobilization. If the bone fragments are displaced, surgery may be required to ensure that the fracture heals fully through closed reduction and percutaneous pinning or by open reduction and internal fixation. In most cases, the elbow's range of motion returns to normal, or has just a mild limitation.

The assessment of the elbow can be difficult because of the changing anatomy of the growing skeleton and the subtility of some of these fractures.

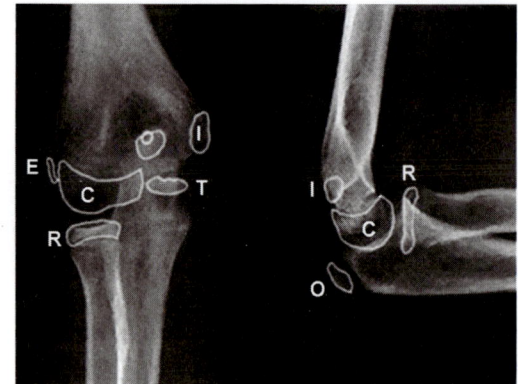

Fig. 17.1: X-rays showing ossification centres around elbow

The mnemonic "CRITOE" allows for remembering the progression of ossification of the elbow's secondary ossification centres (Fig. 17.1):

- C: Capitellum (1 to 2 years)
- R: Radial epiphysis (3 to 4 years)

Table 17.1: Paediatric elbow injury frequency

Fracture type	% Elbow injuries	Peak age	Requires OR
Supracondylar fractures	41%	7	Majority
Radial head subluxation	28%	3	Rare
Lateral condylar physeal fractures	11%	6	Majority
Medial epicondylar apophyseal fracture	8%	11	Minority
Radial head and neck fractures	5%	10	Minority
Elbow dislocations	5%	13	Rare
Medial condylar physeal fractures	1%	10	Rare

- I: Inner epicondyle (medial epicondyle, 5 to 6 years)
- T: Trochlea (9 to 10 years)
- O: Outer epicondyle (lateral epicondyle, >10 years)
- E: Common epiphysis (14 to 16 years)

It is not important to know these ages, but as a general guide you could remember 1-3-5-7-9-11 years.

Four important questions
- Joint effusion?
- Normal alignment?
- Ossification centres normal?
- Subtle fracture?

Positive Fat Pad Sign

Distention of the joint will cause the anterior fat pad to become elevated and the posterior fat pad to become visible.

An elevated anterior lucency or a visible posterior lucency on a true lateral radiograph of an elbow flexed at 90° is described as a positive fat pad sign.

Displacement of the elbow fat pads is an important indicator of an elbow joint effusion (Fig. 17.2).

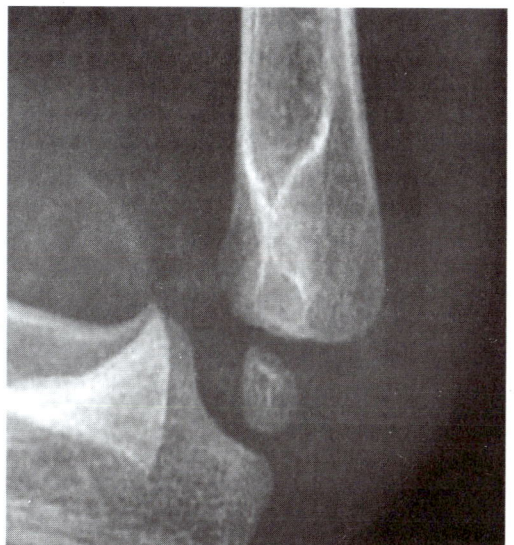

Fig. 17.2: Fat pads at the elbow joint

A visible fat pad sign without the demonstration of a fracture should be regarded as an occult fracture. Approximately 70–90% of children with an elbow joint effusion following trauma have a fracture as demonstrated on the initial or follow-up radiographs.

ALIGNMENT

There are two important lines which help in the diagnosis of dislocation and fracture.

These are the radiocapitellar line and the anterior humeral line.

Radiocapitellar Line (Fig. 17.3)

A line drawn through the centre of the radial neck should pass through the centre of the capitellum, whatever the positioning of the patient, since the radius articulates with the capitellum.

In dislocation of the radius, this line will not pass through the centre of the capitellum.

Anterior Humeral Line (Fig. 17.4)

A line drawn on a lateral view along the anterior surface of the humerus should pass through the middle third of the capitellum.

This line is called the anterior humeral line. In cases of a supracondylar fracture, the anterior humeral line usually passes through the anterior third of the capitellum or in front of the capitellum due to posterior bending of the distal humeral fragment.

Whenever the radius is fractured or dislocated, always study the ulna carefully.

Ultrasonography is highly sensitive for elbow fractures, and a negative ultrasound may reduce the need for radiographs in children with elbow injuries.

Common elbow fractures
- Supracondylar — >60%
- Lateral condyle — 10–20%
- Medial epicondyle — 10%
- Radial neck
- Olecranoan

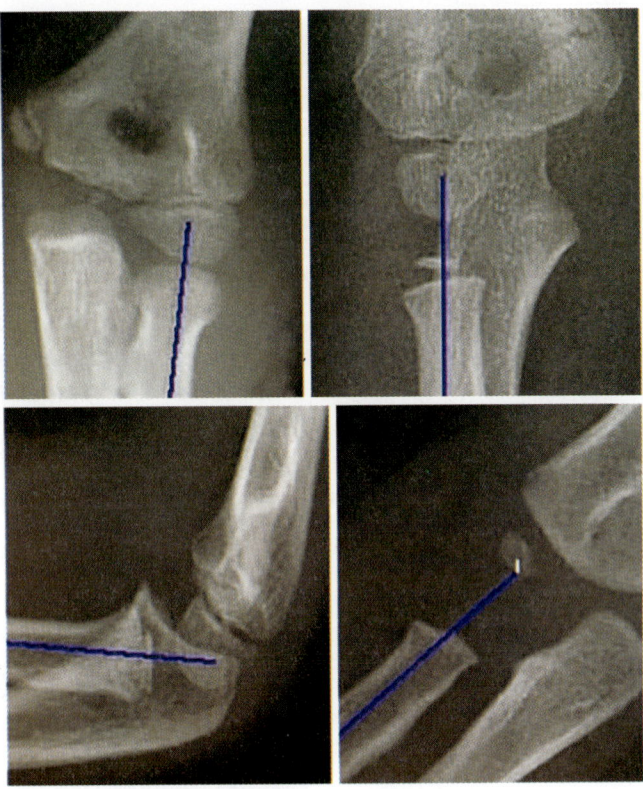

Fig. 17.3: Radiocapitellar line

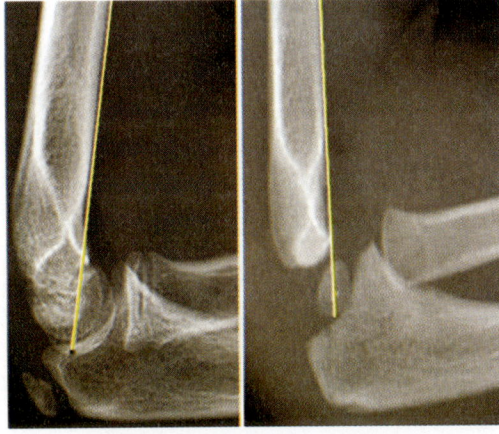

Fig .17.4: Anterior humeral line

Points to Remember
The evaluation of paediatric elbow radiographs in the setting of acute trauma may be challenging for many emergency department physicians, orthopaedic surgeons, and radiologists. Diagnostic difficulties stem both from the complex developmental anatomy of the elbow and from significant differences between children and adults in the patterns of injury after elbow trauma.

Whenever you study a radiograph of the elbow of a child, always look for:
• Supracondylar fracture with minimal displacement
• Lateral condyle fracture
• Slipped radial epiphysis
• Radial dislocation
• Position of the medial epicondyle.

BIBLIOGRAPHY

• https://www.youtube.com/watch?v=VEg2rReyM6k
• http://www.radiologyassistant.nl/en/p4214416a75d87/elbow-fractures-in-children.html
• https://www.youtube.com/watch?v=XRgjhQYUJlA

SUPRACONDYLAR FRACTURES OF HUMERUS

"Nightmare of a young Orthopaedic Surgeon!"

Of the upper limbs in children, the elbow is the second most common site of occurrence of fractures, surpassed only by forearm fractures.

Supracondylar fractures of the humerus are a common paediatric elbow injury that are historically associated with morbidity due to malunion, neurovascular complications, and compartment syndrome.

This is the most common elbow fracture in children, about 60% of fractures in children. Supracondylar fractures are a common elbow injury in children accounting for 16% of all paediatric fractures and two-thirds of all hospitalizations for paediatric elbow injuries. It is most common in children <10 years, peak incidence is between the ages of 5 and 8 years. Primarily in children who are around age 7 years, which is often a period of maximum

ligamentous laxity; therefore, the elbow hyperextends when the child tries to catch himself or herself during a fall. During the hyperextension process, the olecranon (elbow bone) process is forced against the weaker, immature metaphyseal bone of the distal humerus, producing the typical extension-type supracondylar fracture.

It may be of a flexion type or an extension type, depending upon the displacement of the distal fragment of bone (Kocher).

Extension type: The most common type, accounting for 95% of all supracondylar fractures. The distal fragment is displaced posteriorly (Fig. 17.5).

Flexion type: The least common variety (5%), where the distal fragment is displaced anteriorly relative to the proximal segment (Fig. 17.6).

CLINICAL EXAMINATION

A pucker, dimpling, or ecchymosis of the skin just anterior to the distal humerus may

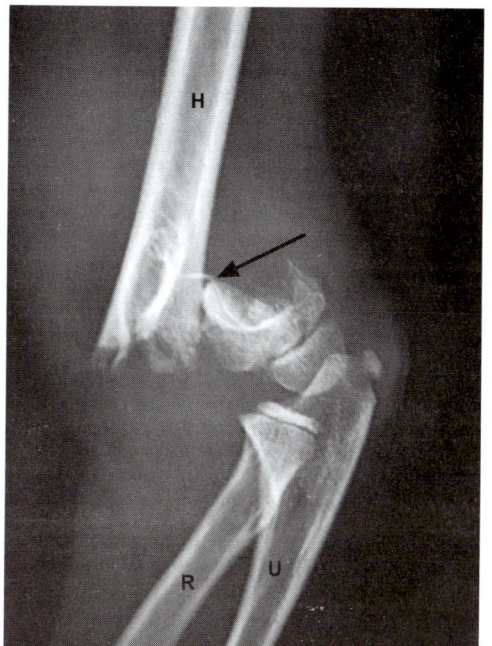

Fig. 17.5: Supracondylar fracture of humerus (extension type)

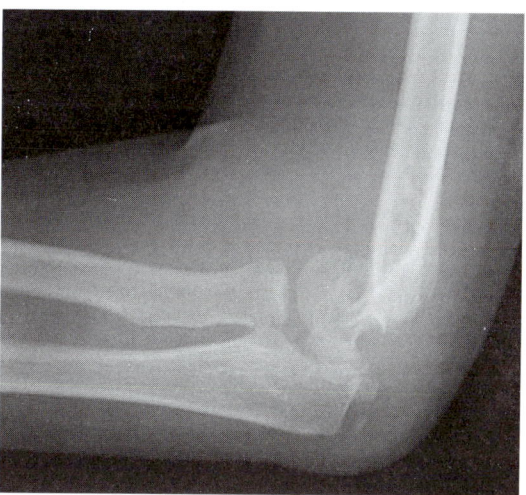

Fig. 17.6: Supracondylar fracture of humerus (flexion type)

indicate that the proximal, anteriorly directed fragment has penetrated the brachialis muscle and possibly the subcutaneous layer as well (Pucker sign) (Fig. 17.7a). Up to 20% of patients with a supracondylar humerus fracture may not have a radial pulse at wrist.

Clinically deformed elbow should be immobilized in about 30° short of full extension, prior to X-ray evaluation. This is important for pain management.

- Vascular status classification:
  - Class I—well perfused (warm and red) with radial pulse
  - Class II—well perfused but radial pulse absent
  - Class III—poorly perfused (cool and blue or blanched) and radial pulse absent.
- Neurologic status—especially ulnar nerve
- Compartment syndrome—swelling and/or ecchymosis, anterior skin puckering, and absent pulse.
- Injury to the brachial artery (Fig. 17.7b) can have potentially serious consequences, such as Volkmann ischaemia, loss of limb, and retarded development of the limb.
- The common practice of watchful waiting for pulseless and perfused supracondylar fractures may be open to question in favour of a more aggressive approach.

- Doppler ultrasound may be useful in differentiating patients at risk and can be part of an effective vascular evaluation.
- Prospective studies are needed to provide more definitive information on management of supracondylar humerus fractures.

Pale, Pulseless Hand

Approximately 10–20% of Gartland III fractures present with an absent pulse. As the hand is also pale, the circulation is not maintained by the collateral supply and emergent (immediate) reduction of the fracture is required with percutaneous pinning. An arm that is pulseless with poor perfusion is an emergency.

From the literature, reduction and fixation restores the pulse in the majority of cases (75%) with the artery in spasm or trapped in the fracture site. If the pulse is not restored following reduction and percutaneous pinning open exploration of the artery is required with the vascular team.

Pink, Pulseless Hand with Nerve Injury

In this case, the rich collateral blood supply maintains circulation to the hand despite vascular injury. An absent radial pulse is not in itself an emergency as the collateral circulation keeps the arm perfused.

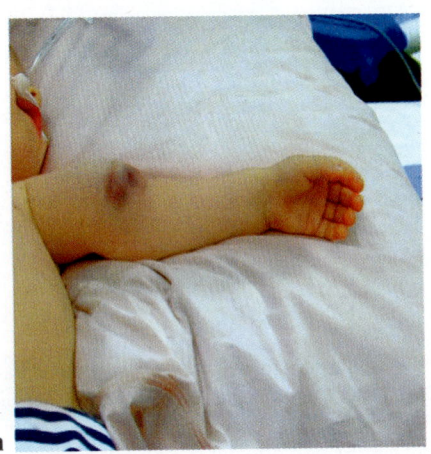
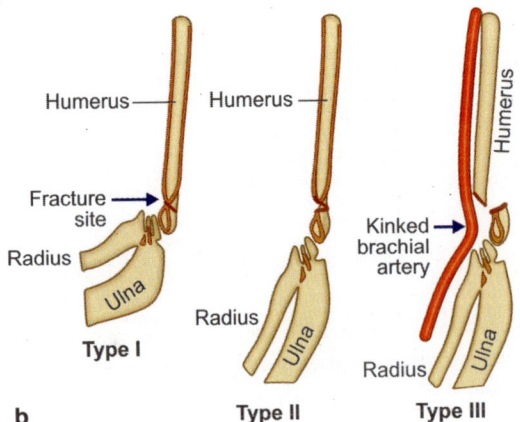

Fig. 17.7: (a) Injury to brachial artery; (b) Pucker sign

There is some controversy in the literature as to the most appropriate course of action. Presently urgent but non-emergent reduction and pinning is advised though more recent studies suggest a concurrent nerve injury may indicate a co-existing vascular tethering at the fracture site due to the proximity of vessels advising immediate reduction and early exploration to untether vessels, if the pulse does not return.

Pink, Pulseless Hand without Nerve Injury

This remains the most controversial area in the literature. Urgent but non-emergent reduction and fixation is required.

If the pulse does not return after surgery but the hand remains perfused most centres advocate monitoring the patient for 48 hours. If the hand becomes pale, exploration is then required with the vascular team.

In practical terms, most supracondylar injuries present towards the end of the day and provided the patient is starved fixing them in twilight hours is sensible.

CLASSIFICATION

The Gartland type classification (Fig. 17.8 and Table 17.2) is based on the lateral X-ray,

identifying where the capitellum sits in relation to a line drawn down the anterior aspect of the humerus—the anterior humeral line.

Wilkin's Modification of Gartland's Classification (1984)

Type 1: Undisplaced fracture.

Type 2: 2A: Intact posterior cortex + angulation only.

2B: Intact posterior cortex + angulation + rotation

Type 3: 3A: Completely displaced (postero-medially)

3B: Completely displaced (postero-laterally).

Displacements: The displacements may present in one of a number of ways: Posterior shift, posterior tilt, lateral or medial shift, proximal shift or internal rotation.

Supracondylar fractures can also be categorized by the Gartland classification system, based upon the degree of displacement of the distal fragment.

MANAGEMENT

It depends on the type and degree of angulation.

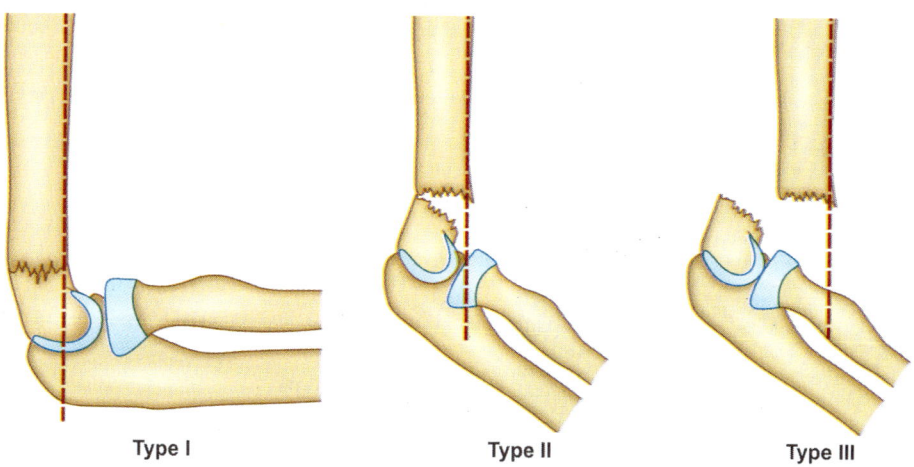

Type I   Type II   Type III

Fig. 17.8: Gartland's classification

Table 17.2: Gartland classification (1959)
(may be extension or flexion type)

Type I	Non-displaced, beware of subtle medial comminution leading to cubitus varus
Type II	Displaced, posterior cortex intact
Type III	Completely displaced
*Type IV	Complete periosteal disruption with instability in flexion and extension

*Not a part of original Gartland classification

Type I

Type I (undisplaced) fractures are stable and can be treated with cast immobilization for approximately 3 weeks.

Type II

Type II usually require reduction (especially when angulation is more than 20°). Although traditionally these fractures were treated non-operatively with cast immobilization of the flexed arm to 120°, this, however, dramatically increases risk of ischaemic contracture (Volkmann contracture), as such most authors recommend percutaneous pinning and cast immobilization with less than 90° flexion.

Type III

Type III fractures can sometimes be treated similarly to type II (closed reduction and

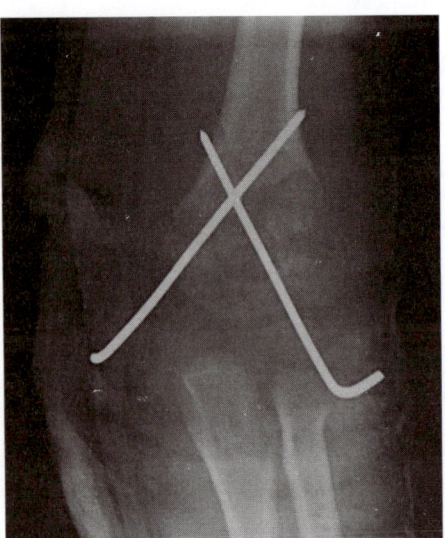

Fig. 17.9: Percutaneous 'K' wiring

percutaneous pinning) although frequently the fracture is held open by interposed soft tissues requiring open reduction.

Risk of iatrogenic ulna nerve injury is increased, if the medial wire is inserted when the elbow is hyperflexed rather than extended (Fig. 17.9).

Acceptable Reduction

On lateral X-ray post-reduction, it is acceptable for the fracture to remain in a degree of extension to the extent that it would still be classified as a type II fracture.

Alignment in the AP X-ray is more important. No degree of tilt can be accepted on the post-reduction films. Such displacement would imply a more unstable fracture requiring surgical reduction.

True vascular insufficiency after reduction calls for surgical exploration.

Clinical signs that indicate urgent orthopaedic review in the emergency department include:
- Absence of radial pulse
- Ischaemia of hand: Pale, cool
- Severe swelling in forearm and/or elbow
- Skin puckering or anterior bruising
- Open injury
- Neurological injury

Reduction Technique

The below steps summarise the reduction manoeuvre:
1. *Traction:* Disengages the proximal fragment from the brachialis muscle.
2. *Coronal plane correction:* Medial or lateral translation.

3. *Axial plane correction:* Correction of internal rotation deformity.
4. *Distal fragment reduced:* Push with thumb on olecranon.
5. *Elbow flexion:* >100°
6. *Pronation:* Tightens medial periosteal sleeve

MANAGEMENT OF PULSELESS SUPRACONDYLAR FRACTURE

1. **On presentation**
   - Urgent closed reduction + K wire
   - Position at 90°
   - Ensure pulse returns and hand pink
   - Observe if not pulse but hand pink
   - Close monitoring/ensure cast not too tight/minimal flexion

2. **No pulse and white after reduction**
   Scenarios:
   A. *Pulse present premanipulation/pulse lost and hand white post-reduction*
      - Likely brachial artery entrapped in fracture
      - Anterior lazy S approach
      - Expose artery
      - Open reduction and 'K' wire
   B. *No pulse before or after closed reduction:*
      - Artery either in spasm or has intimal tear
      - Open artery exploration
      - Antispasmodics trialled
      - If this fails, it requires vascular surgeon's help
      - Intraoperative angiogram may be required to diagnose thrombus/intimal tear
      - Thrombectomy/microvascular repair
      - Lazy S anterior approach
      - Transverse component just proximal to transverse crease
      - Proximal limb medial over brachial artery
      - Distal extension Henry approach

3. **No pulse and pink after reduction**
   Controversial
   - Observe for 24 hours
   - Arm kept warm
   After 24 hours
   - Colour duplex ±MRI angiogram
   - Vascular consult
   - Up to 70% will have a vascular injury
   - Risk is late Volkmann's contracture

4. **Too swollen/skin abraded**
   1. *Skin traction:*
      - Arm straight
      - Weight over pulley
      - Body weight countertraction
   2. *Dunlop traction:*
      - Screw in olecranon
      - Bent arm traction
      - Difficult to control rotation

   Postoperative results are shown in Fig. 17.10.

Complications

- Malunion—resulting in cubitus varus (varus deformity of the elbow, also known as gunstock deformity) (Fig. 17.11). Incidence is 10–60%. Remodelling of the angulation in the sagittal plane can occur, but angular deformities in the coronal plane are less likely to remodel—resulting in a cubitus varus or valgus deformity. Horizontal rotation in a medial direction or internal rotation of the distal fragment is believed to predispose to distal fragment varus angulation. Eccentric position of the biceps has been suggested as a cause of varus tilting by the distal fragment. Avascular necrosis of the trochlea or medial portion of the distal humeral fragment can result in progressive varus (gunstock) deformity.
- Ischaemic contracture (Volkmann contracture) due to damage/occlusion to the brachial artery and resulting in volar compartment syndrome. Vascular insufficiency resulting from supracondylar fractures has been reported to range from 5 to 12%. "The radial

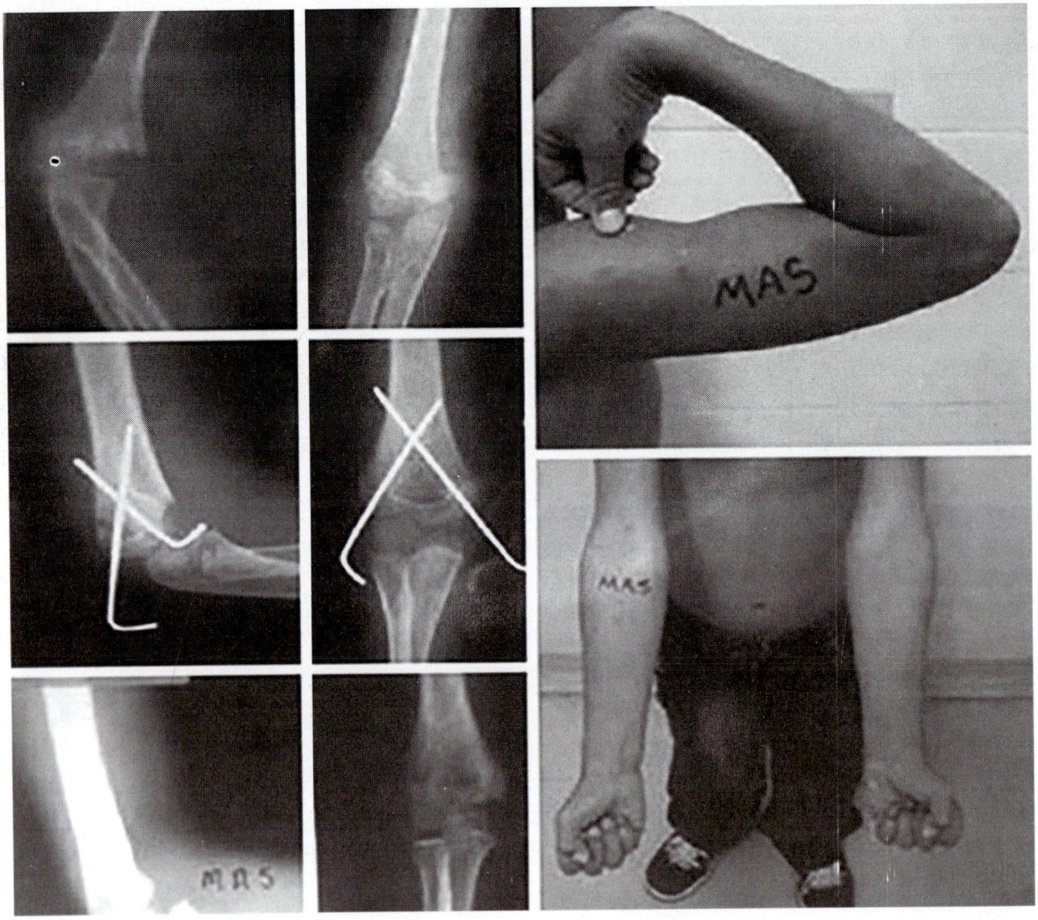

Fig. 17.10: Postoperative results

pulse is unreliable as a danger signal. Its absence is not an indication for surgery, nor its presence a guarantee that ischaemia will not develop" (BLOUNT).

- The signs of acute Volkmann's ischaemia include: **P**ain (stretch pain in fingers), **P**uffiness (swollen and tense forearm), **P**araesthesia, **P**allor, **P**ulselessness and **P**aralysis.
- Damage to the ulnar nerve (most common), median nerve or radial nerve. The incidence of traumatic and iatrogenic nerve injures with this type of fracture have been recorded as 12–20% and 2–6%, respectively. The median nerve, specifically the anterior interosseous nerve (52%), and radial nerve

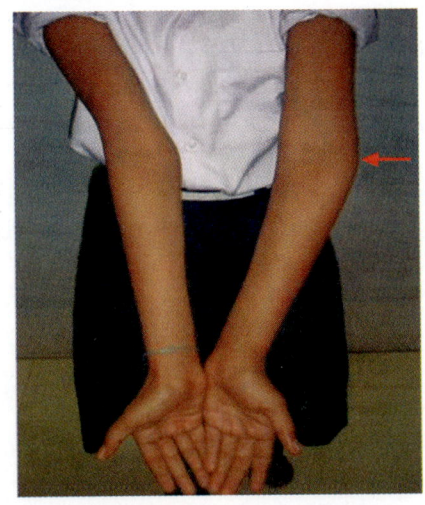

Fig. 17.11: Cubitus varus

(32%) are most frequently injured in the course of the injury.

- *Myositis ossificans:* The condition tends to present with pain, tenderness, focal swelling, and joint/muscle contractures. Avoid excessive physiotherapy, rest the joint until pain subsides, NSAIDs may be helpful and consider excision after the lesion has stabilised (usually 6–24 months).
- Elbow stiffness
- Non-union—very rare.

Summary

This is a fracture that occurs more frequently in skeletally immature children than adults.

Splinting in full elbow extension is contraindicated because it stretches the neurovascular bundle over the fracture site in displaced or unstable fractures.

Management
- Type I: POP slab/cast for 3 weeks (elbow at 90–100° flexion)
- Type II: MUA; Percutaneous. 'K' wiring
- Type III: Closed/open reduction + 'K' wiring

Other methods: Dunlop traction

Iatrogenic nerve deficits often affect the ulnar nerve and result from a pin impinging on the nerve.

BIBLIOGRAPHY

- https://www.youtube.com/watch?v=xG-ZmNUs6ZY
- https://www.youtube.com/watch?v=oTYjm2HO5Zo
- http://radiologymasterclass.co.uk/gallery/trauma/x-ray_arm_1/fractures_8.html#top_first_img
- http://www.orthointerview.com/News/files/Core-Knowledge-Supracondylar-Fractures.html

FRACTURE LATERAL CONDYLE OF HUMERUS

Accounts for 17% of all distal humerus fractures and 54% of distal humeral physeal fractures. The frequency of lateral condyle fractures peaks in children aged 6 years. Most fractures occur in children aged 5–10 years. The lateral condyle fracture is a Salter-Harris IV fracture pattern and follows physeal injury principles. In lateral condyle fractures, the displacement is greater than appreciated, and incongruity of the articular surface is present. Fractures with minimal displacement must be carefully monitored, as they have a high tendency to displace. Surgical reduction should be performed and is recommended within the first 48 hours post fracture, because a malunited fracture is difficult to treat and is associated with many complications.

MILCH (1968) CLASSIFICATION

Milch I: Fracture extends through the ossification center of the lateral condyle and exits at the radiocapitellar groove. The lateral crista of the trochlea remains intact and therefore has less tendency to dislocate laterally. This pattern is less common (Fig. 17.12).

Milch II: Fracture extends across the physis and exits through the apex of the trochlea. The lateral crista is in the fracture fragment, and the trochlea is no longer intact, rendering the elbow unstable. This is the more common fracture pattern (Fig. 17.13).

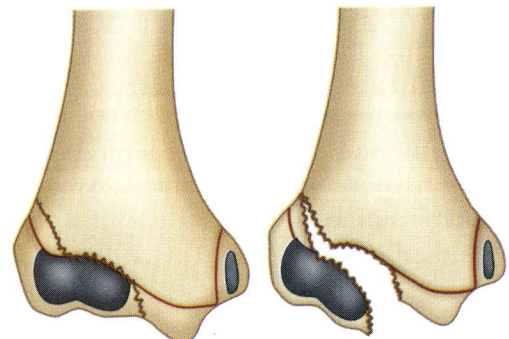

Fig. 17.13: Milch type II fracture

Milch Classification

Type I   Fracture line is lateral to trochlear groove (considered an SH IV fracture)

Type II   Fracture line into trochlear groove (considered an SH II fracture)

Fracture Displacement Classification (Lagrange and Rigault) (Fig. 17.14)

Type I   <2 mm, indicating intact cartilaginous hinge

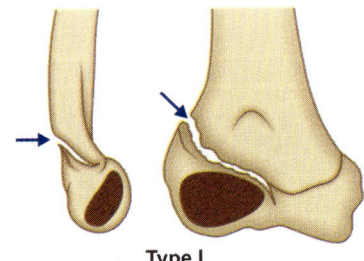

Type I

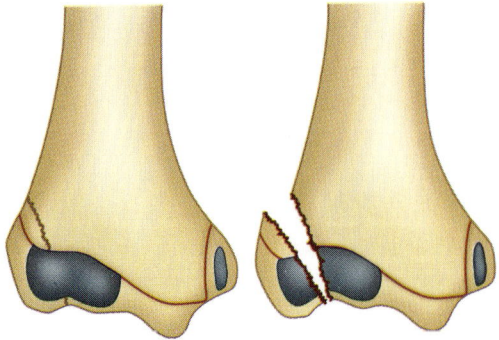

Fig. 17.12: Milch type I fracture

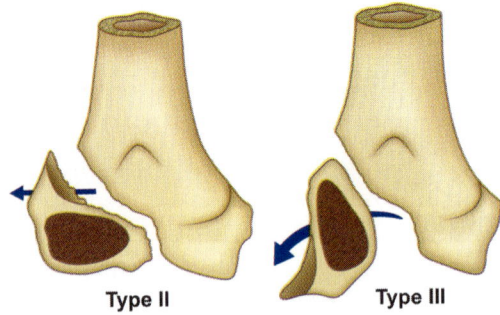

Type II   **Type III**

Fig. 17.14: Lagrange and Rigault classification (1962)

Type II   2–4 mm, displaced joint surface
Type III   >4 mm, joint displaced and rotated

JACOB (1975) TYPES

Stage I: Fracture is nondisplaced with an intact articular surface.

Stage II: The fracture extends through the articular surface, and there is moderate rotational displacement.

Stage III: Complete displacement and capitellar rotation with elbow instability.

Stage I or type I lateral condyle fractures with less than 2 mm of displacement may be treated with immobilization. Maintain cast immobilization for 3–4 weeks at 90° of flexion and forearm supination. Close follow-up is necessary because of the high incidence of late displacement and subsequent malunion. If fracture identification is delayed by 6 weeks or longer, continue closed treatment regardless of displacement. A high incidence of avascular necrosis occurs with delayed open reduction and fixation.

Open reduction is indicated for all displaced type II and type III fractures. Fragment stabilization is most frequently performed using two percutaneously placed smooth Kirschner wires (Fig. 17.15). Fixation consists of two laterally placed pins.

COMPLICATIONS

Lateral condylar overgrowth or spur formation (30%), cubitus varus, non-union, malunion, valgus angulation, ulnar nerve palsy, myositis ossificans and avascular necrosis.

A non-union is considered present, if no healing is evident at 12 weeks following injury. If the non-union is well established, exploration and removal of the interposed fibrous tissue is recommended, followed by insertion of 1 or 2 compression screws. Perform bone grafting, if significant fragment separation exists. Definitive treatment can safely be delayed until the patient becomes symptomatic or reaches skeletal maturity.

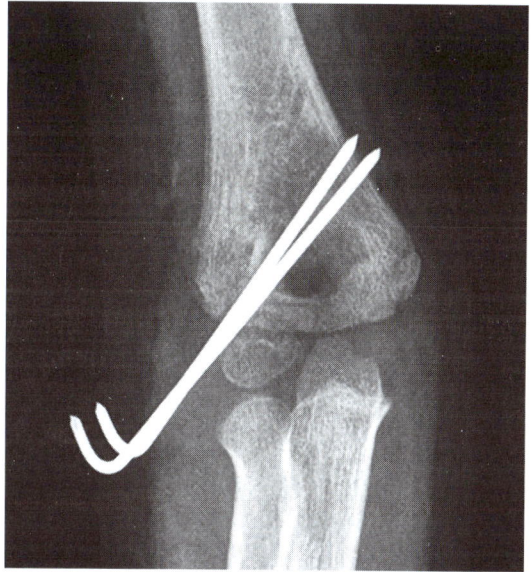

Fig. 17.15: 'K' wiring

A cubitus valgus deformity may occur, if there is non-union or malunion of a lateral condyle fracture. In simple valgus malunion cases, a medial closing wedge osteotomy is performed. In cases of angular deformity and non-union, treatment is complex and difficult. Tardy ulnar nerve palsy occurs late in the treatment and follow-up of lateral condyle fractures and usually is due to cubitus valgus. This ulnar neuropathy can be treated with ulnar nerve transposition, cubital tunnel release, or medial epicondylectomy.

Occasionally, a fishtail deformity of the distal humerus is seen because of the loss of ossific contact between the capitellum and trochlea. This results in a gap or a deficiency of the lateral trochlear buttress. This deformity usually does not result in any significant dysfunction and is treated non-operatively.

BIBLIOGRAPHY

• emedicine.medscape.com/article/1231199-overview
• www.orthobullets.com/pediatrics/4009/lateral-condyle-fracture--pediatric
• radiopaedia.org/articles/lateral-epicondyle-fracture

FRACTURES OF MEDIAL EPICONDYLE OF HUMERUS

In 1818, Granger reported the first unequivocal description of a medial epicondyle fracture (Fig. 17.16).

Medial epicondyle fractures must not be confused with medial condyle fractures that involve the medial column but are extra-articular. These two fracture patterns are separate entities and are treated differently. Both fracture patterns may be difficult to diagnose in young children, especially before the secondary ossification centres have formed. Medial epicondyle fractures are much more common than medial condyle fractures. Medial epicondyle fractures are four times as likely to occur in males, and most cases occur in children aged 9–14 years. The reported incidence of association with elbow dislocation reaches 55% in some series, and the fragment may be incarcerated in the joint in approximately 15–18% of cases.

For non-displaced or minimally displaced fractures, non-operative management is the procedure of choice. More controversy exists with displacement of 5–15 mm. The only absolute indications for operative management of closed medial epicondyle fractures are the incarceration of the medial epicondyle fragment within the joint and an open fracture (Fig. 17.17).

Several closed means of reduction can be used, and the success rate with these methods approaches 40%. One such manoeuvre (Roberts' manipulative technique) is performed under sedation and involves placing a valgus stress on the elbow while supinating the forearm and simultaneously dorsiflexing the wrist and fingers to place the forearm flexor muscles on stretch. Initially, the arm should be splinted in 90° of elbow flexion. Gentle active range-of-motion exercises may begin within 1 week after injury. Protective splinting may be continued for 3 weeks, if necessary.

COMPLICATIONS

Failure to recognize incarceration into the joint with functional loss and ulnar or median nerve dysfunction. Most of the other complications associated with medial epicondyle fractures,

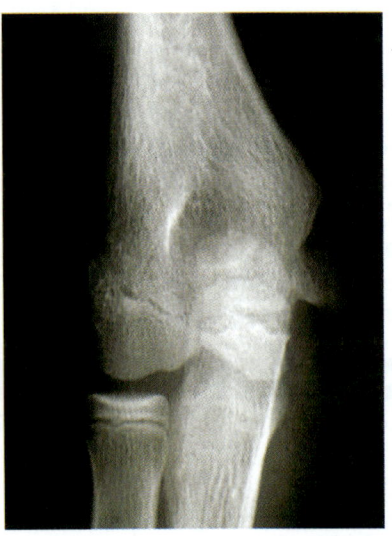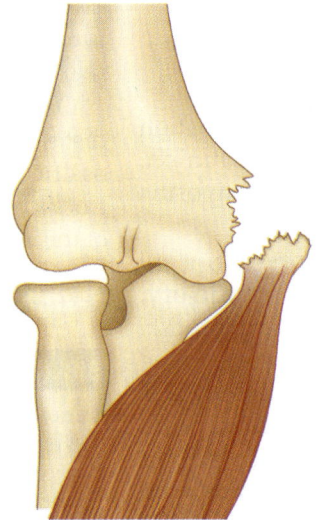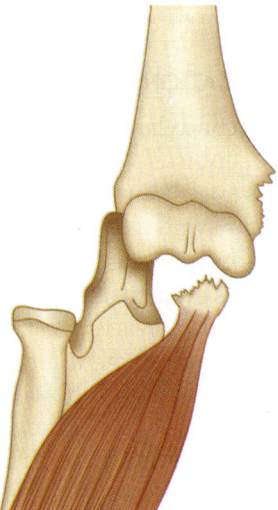

Fig. 17.16: Fractures of medial humeral epicondyle

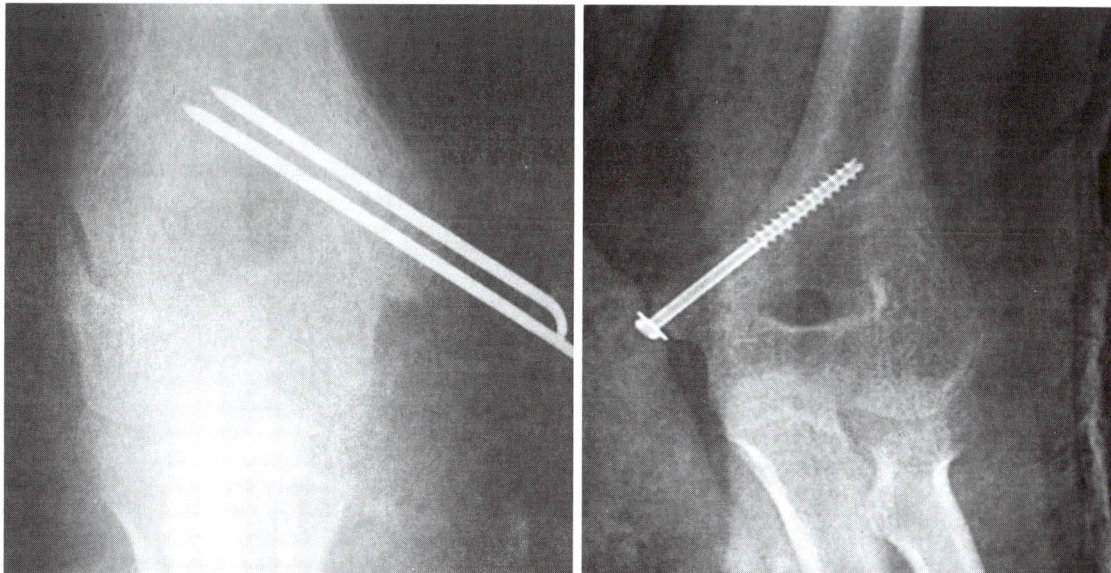

Fig. 17.17: Internal fixation

including non-union, are considered minor and do not result in a loss of function.

Points to Remember
- Most children with medial epicondyle fractures treated either non-surgically or surgically end up with good long-term functional results.
- ORIF is required in children with medial epicondyle fractures and incarcerated fragments (Fig. 17.18) that block motion. Comminuted medial epicondyle fractures appear to do worse, if the epicondyle is excised as opposed to non-surgical fracture treatment.

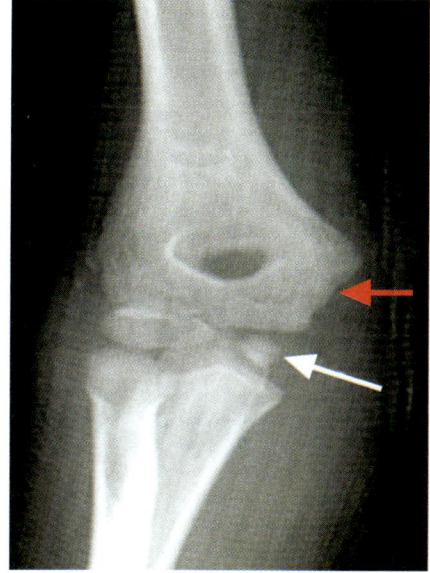

Fig. 17.18: Incarcerated fracture fragment

BIBLIOGRAPHY

- https://www.youtube.com/watch?v=T-Qvmh6jHiE
- http://www.rch.org.au/clinicalguide/guideline_index/fractures/Medial_epicondyle_emerg/

FRACTURES OF NECK OF RADIUS

In children, proximal radial epiphysis is cartilaginous and is more prone to fracture than hard articular surface of radial head. It is a comparatively rare injury and constitutes 5–10% of all elbow fractures. Radial neck fractures are more common in children, whereas fractures of radial head occur primarily in adults. 90% of cases are Salter-Harris type II fractures.

This fracture occurs on average at age of 10 years, after ossification centre of the proximal radial epiphysis appears. Physical examination should include careful assessment of function of posterior interosseous nerve.

X-rays: The radial head should point to the capitellum in all views (Figs 17.19 to 17.21).

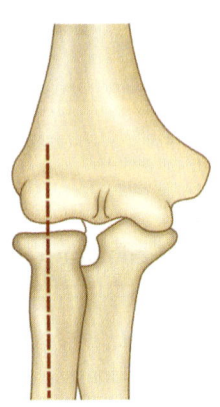

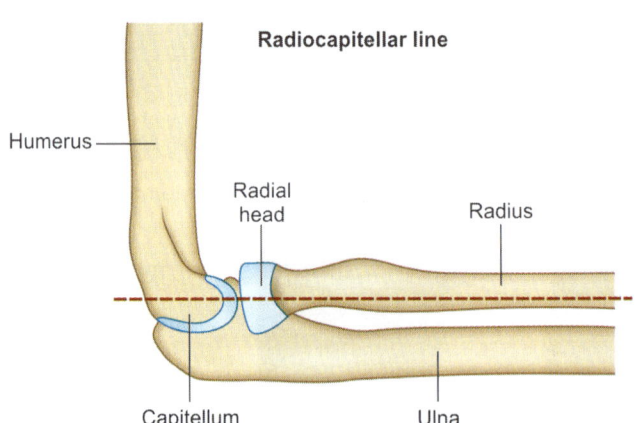

Fig. 17.19: Radiocapitellar line

CLASSIFICATION

- Classification of most authors is based on the amount of initial angulation.
- Mild (0°–30°), moderate (30°–60°) and severe (>60°).
- Some authors include the combination of angulation and/or translation in their classification system.

Steinberg et al and Rodríguez-Merchán Classification

Mild (10°–29°, <30% translation), moderate (30°–59°, <50% translation) and severe (60°–90°, >50% translation).

Steele and Graham Classification

- Grade 1 (0°–30°, 0–10% translation)

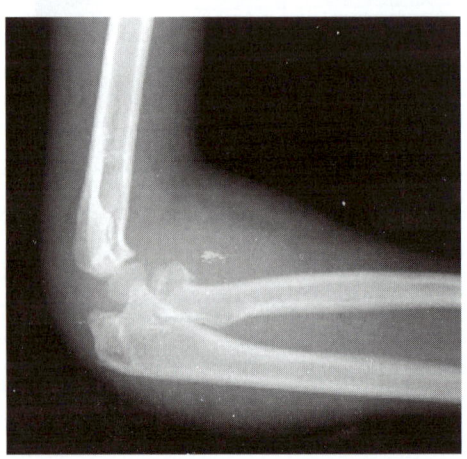

Fig. 17.20: Type II epiphyseal injury

- Grade 2 (31°–60°, 11–50% translation)
- Grade 3 (61°–90°, 51–90% translation)
- Grade 4 (>90°, >90% translation)

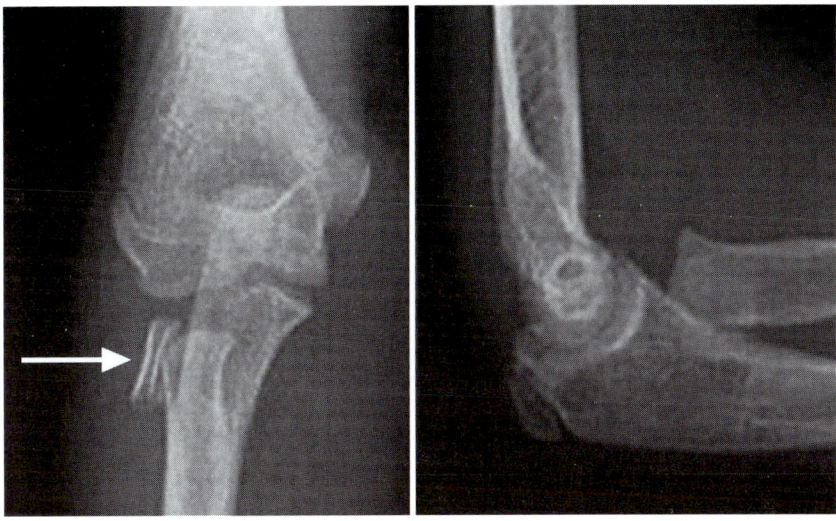

Fig. 17.21: A completely displaced fracture

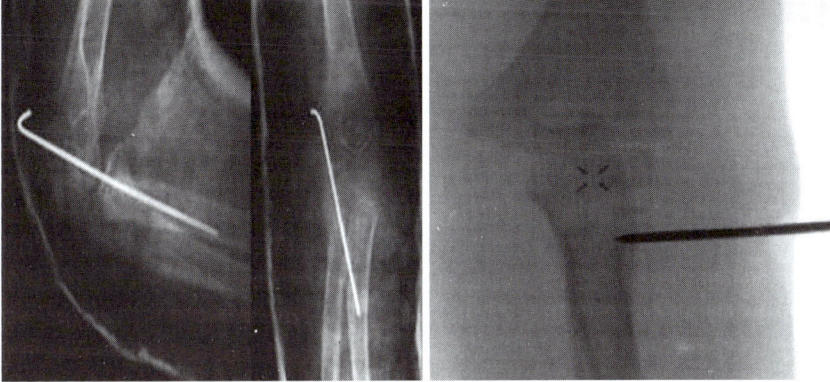

Fig. 17.22: 'K' wiring

Metaizeau et al and Judet et al Classification

- Grade 1 (0°, with translation)
- Grade 2 (<30°)
- Grade 3 (30°–60°)
- Grade 4a (60°–80°)
- Grade 4b (80°–90°).

MANAGEMENT

Management of pediatric radial neck fractures is controversial regarding acceptable alignment, variable reduction techniques, and suboptimal outcomes.

Minimally displaced fractures may be treated in an above-elbow plaster cast for about 2–3 weeks. Displaced fractures (including cases with more than 30° of angulation and displacements more than 3 mm) need closed/open reduction. Fracture is best fixed with 'K' wires (Fig. 17.22).

A 'K' wire may also be used as a joystick to aid in reduction of the fracture.

In January 1980, Metaizeau proposed intramedullary nailing as a surgical option for the treatment of radial neck fractures. The main advantage of intramedullary nailing is

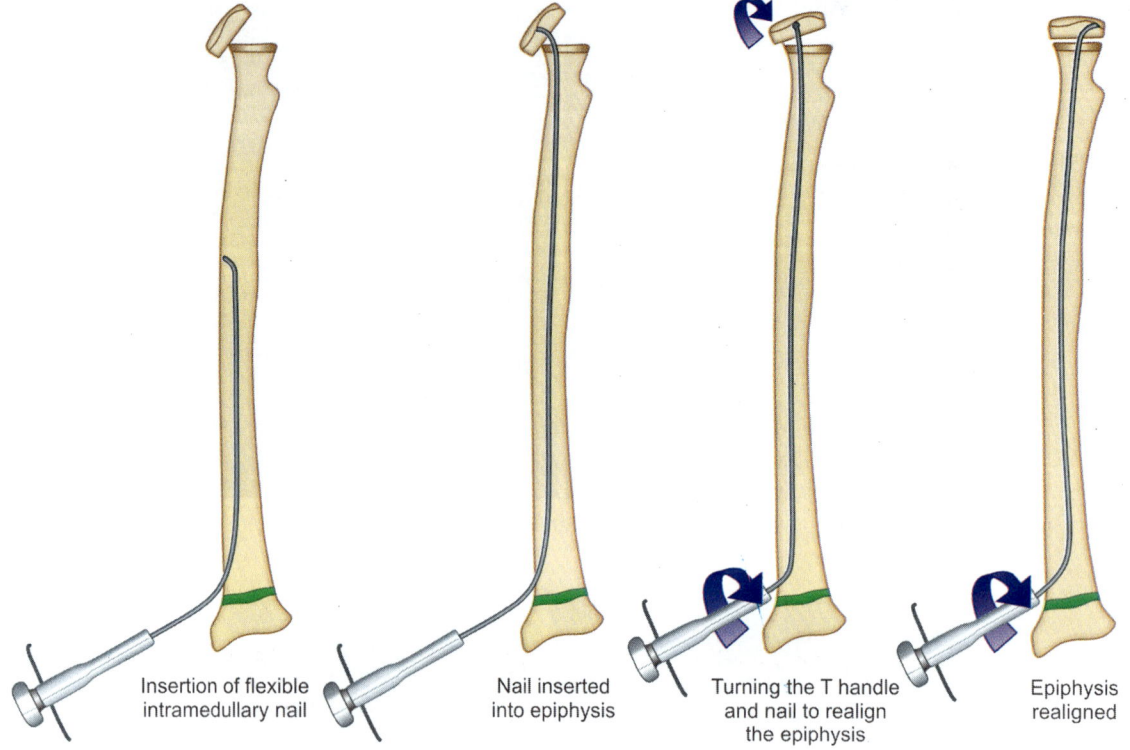

Insertion of flexible intramedullary nail

Nail inserted into epiphysis

Turning the T handle and nail to realign the epiphysis

Epiphysis realigned

Fig. 17.23: Elastic nailing

that it simultaneously allows accurate and stable reduction without disturbing the blood supply (Fig. 17.23).

COMPLICATIONS

Complications include malunion, elbow stiffness, radioulnar synostosis, posterior interosseous nerve palsy, rarely non-union and avascular necrosis.

BIBLIOGRAPHY

- www.wheelessonline.com/ortho/radial_neck_fracture
- www.orthobullets.com/pediatrics/.../radial-head-and-neck-fractures
- http://www.slidesearchengine.com/slide/radial-neck-fractures

OLECRANON FRACTURES IN CHILDREN

Accounts for <5% of all paediatric fractures. Peak age between 5–10 years old.

Olecranon apophyseal fractures in children are uncommon. The bulk of these injuries are non-displaced and, therefore, can be treated non-operatively. Few published reports of children with displaced fractures of the olecranon apophysis exist, and the large majority of reports describe children with osteogenesis imperfecta (Fig. 17.24).

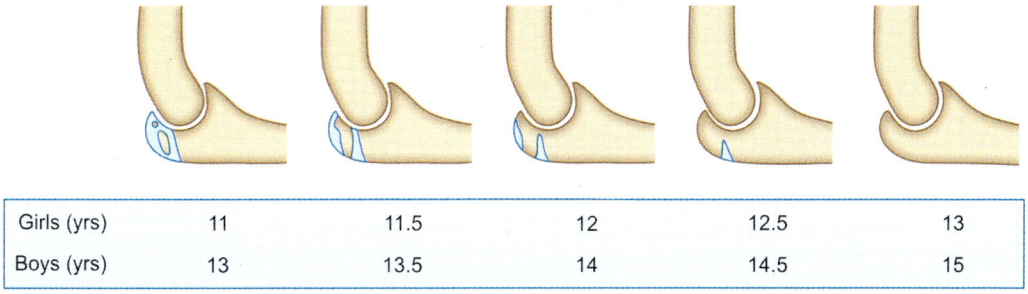

Girls (yrs)	11	11.5	12	12.5	13
Boys (yrs)	13	13.5	14	14.5	15

Fig. 17.24: Olecranon physeal closure pattern

Location of the Fracture (Fig. 17.25)

- Metaphyseal (most common)
- Physeal
- Epiphyseal (apophyseal)
- Intra-articular
- Extra-articular

Treatment (Fig. 17.26)

- *Undisplaced fractures:* Above-elbow plaster slab/cast for 2–3 weeks.

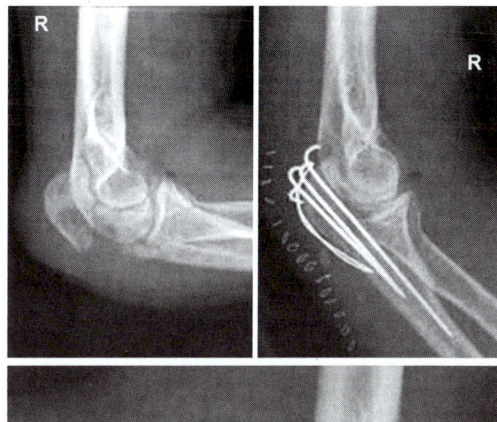

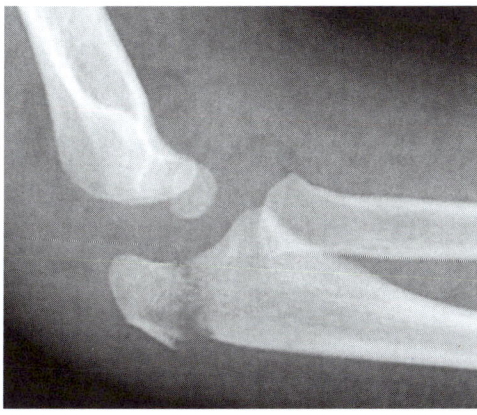

Fig. 17.25: Olecranon fracture

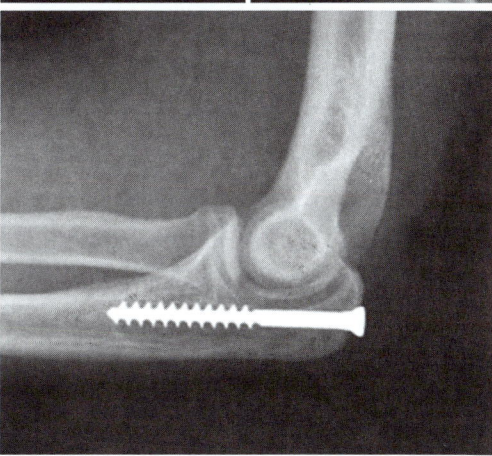

Fig. 17.26: Methods of internal fixation

- *Displaced fractures:* ORIF (Tension band wiring/plate and screws)

Complications

- Non-union
- Delayed union
- Compartment syndrome
- Ulnar nerve neuropraxia due to pseudarthrosis with inadequate fixation

- Loss of reduction
- Elbow stiffness

BIBLIOGRAPHY

- www.orthobullets.com/pediatrics/4010/olecranon-fractures
- https://www.youtube.com/watch?v=c5NQMPkW4ps

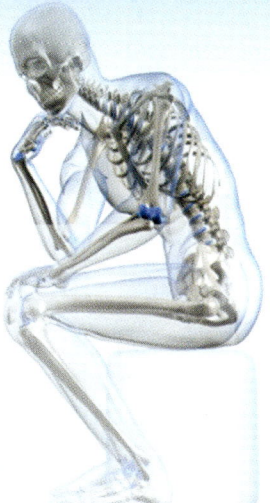

Fracture Both Bones of Forearm

Both bone fractures (Fig. 18.1) can be complicated by acute compartment syndrome of the forearm; this is rare but possible. Signs suggesting compartment syndrome are pain on extension of digits, and marked oedema. The phrase "pain out of proportion to the injury" is difficult to apply when there is a broken bone, but in general, immobilizing a fracture should reduce the patient's distress; if it does not, compartment syndrome should be explicitly ruled out by measuring compartment pressures.

OTA Classification

Radial and ulna diaphyseal fractures
- *Type A:* Simple fracture of ulna (A1), radius (A2), or both bones (A3)
- *Type B:* Wedge fracture of ulna (B1), radius (B2), or both bones (B3)
- *Type C:* Complex fractures

Associated Conditions

- Elbow injuries
  - Evaluate DRUJ and elbow for
  - Galeazzi fractures
  - Monteggia fractures
- Compartment syndrome
  - Evaluate compartment pressures if concern for compartment syndrome

The radial bow and the relations between the proximal and distal radioulnar joints comprise a complex three-dimensional functional unit. Even small deformities caused by fracture malunion can result in significant functional impairment. Unlike fractures in infants and children, fractures of the adult forearm are unstable. Non-unions and malunions of both bone forearm fractures are functionally and cosmetically limiting, with midshaft radius or ulna angulation substantially impeding forearm rotation.

Radiographs of the wrist and elbow must be obtained in isolated radius and ulna fractures to rule out Monteggia and Galeazzi injury patterns.

Treatment objectives for both bone forearm fractures have remained relatively constant, with early extremity range of motion. Non-operative treatment of middle third forearm fractures is reserved for isolated ulnar shaft fractures, better known as nightstick fractures.

Adults with this injury are typically treated with open reduction and internal fixation because of the propensity for malunion of the radius and ulna and the resulting loss of forearm rotation.

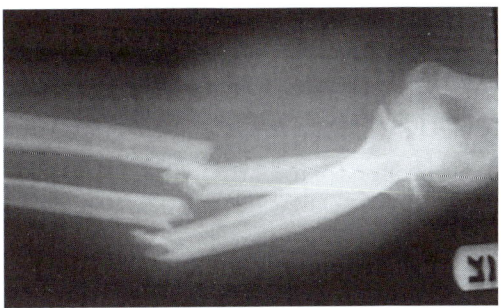

Fig. 18.1: Fracture both bones of forearm

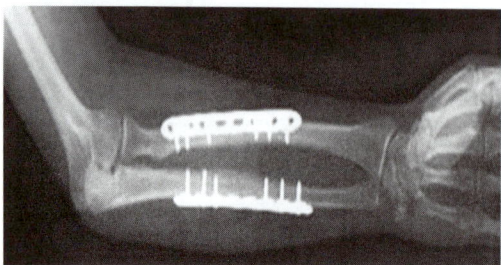

Fig. 18.2: Plating of radius and ulna

Restoration of the radial bow is important to the functional outcome. Failure to restore the radial bow to within 5% of the contralateral side results in a 20% loss of forearm rotation, as well as loss of grip strength.

Forearm shaft fractures in paediatric patients are often treated with elastic nails, whereas adult patients are normally treated with plates. Adolescent patients (close to closure of growth plate) remain subject to individual solutions; some adolescents are similar to paediatric patients, whereas others are closer to adults.

Both bone middle third forearm fractures in adults are unstable injuries that lead to shortening and angulation. The goal of treatment is to achieve a stable anatomic reduction. The literature recommends open reduction and internal fixation (ORIF) for displaced fractures of the middle third of the forearm in adults to restore early forearm motion (Fig. 18.2).

A minimally invasive approach, IM stabilization through nailing is an attractive alternative to formal ORIF, but indications for it are not yet clearly defined. IM fixation may be performed by either open or closed reduction in unstable transverse fractures (Fig. 18.3).

COMPLICATIONS

Complications of forearm fractures include the following:
- Refracture after plate removal
- Non-union

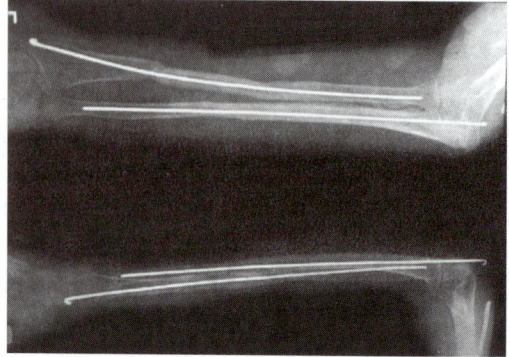

Fig. 18.3: Nailing of radius and ulna

- Malunion
- Infection
- Neurovascular injury
- Compartment syndrome
- Radioulnar synostosis

The incidence of refracture of the forearm after plate removal is unknown but is reportedly 4–25%. Forearm plate removal is not without risk, including infection and nerve injury. The incidence of these complications is 10–20%, and plate removal is not routinely recommended.

The incidence of radioulnar synostosis has been reported to be 0–11% (most commonly, 3%). Risk factors include the following:
- Fracture of the radius and ulna at the same level
- Head injury
- Infection
- High-energy trauma
- Single-incision surgical approach
- Bone graft within the interosseous space
- Screws that are too long
- Delay of 2 weeks in operating

BIBLIOGRAPHY

- https://www.youtube.com/watch?v=cdodDRv9Nms
- https://www.youtube.com/watch?v=gQDebkQEmUE
- https://www2.aofoundation.org

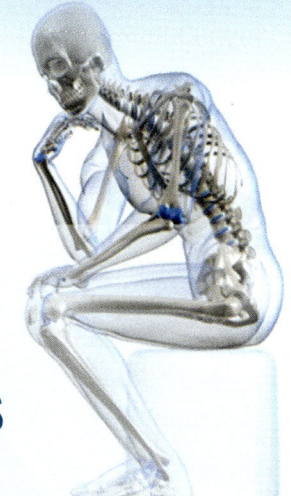

Chapter 19

Monteggia Fractures

Named after Giovanni Battista Monteggia, Italian surgeon (1762–1815), who first described the Bado type I fracture in 1814, a year before his death.

In 1814, Giovanni Battista Monteggia of Milan first described this injury as a fracture of the proximal third of the ulna with associated anterior dislocation of the radial head.

The eponym Monteggia fracture is most precisely used to refer to a dislocation of the proximal radioulnar joint in association with a forearm fracture. These injuries are relatively uncommon, accounting for fewer than 5% of all forearm fractures. The keys to successful diagnosis of a Monteggia fracture are clinical suspicion and radiographs of the entire forearm and elbow. Monteggia fractures constitute less than 5% of forearm fractures, with published literature supporting 1–2%.

Whenever one of the two bones of the forearm fractures with considerable shortening (usually through angulation), then something has to happen to "shorten" the other bone:

- The other bone can also fracture.
- The other bone can dislocate.
- Ligaments are torn.

Galeazzi and Monteggia fractures are both fractures in which there is a fracture with shortening of one of the two bones of the forearm with dislocation of the other bone.

More than 150 years later, in 1967, Bado coined the term Monteggia lesion and classified the injury into the following four types.

CLASSIFICATION (BADO TYPE)

There are four types (depending upon displacement of the radial head) (Figs 19.1 to 19.3):

- Type I: Extension type (60%)—ulna shaft angulates anteriorly (extends) and radial head dislocates anteriorly.

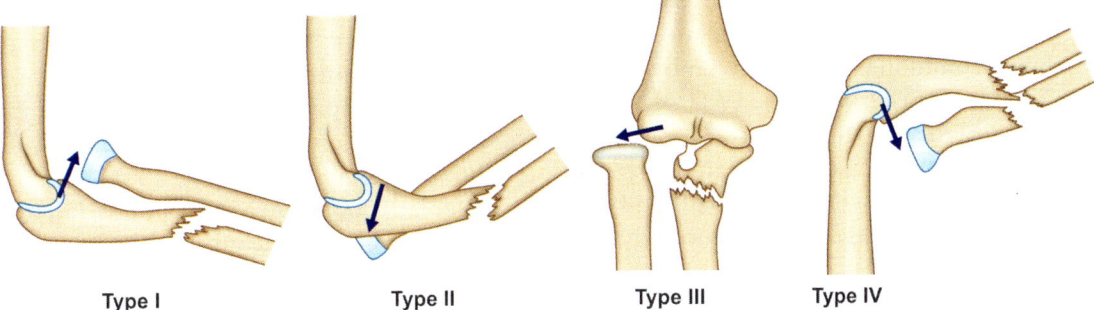

| Type I | Type II | Type III | Type IV |

Fig. 19.1: Bado classification

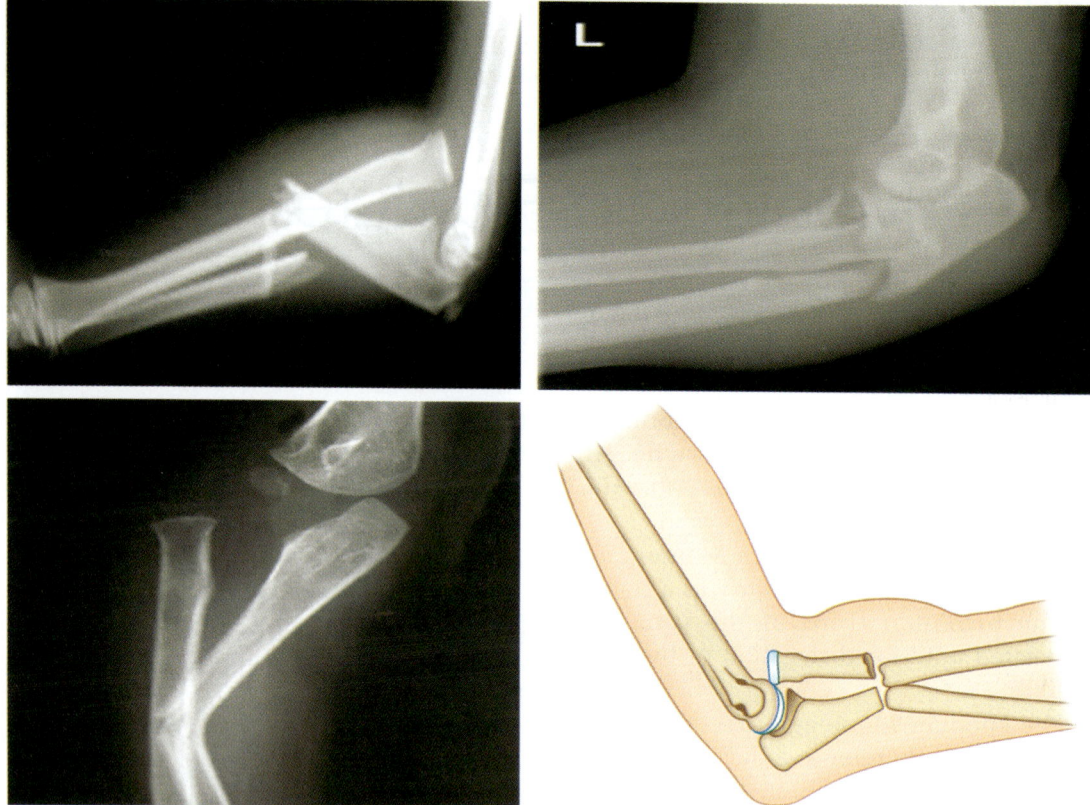

Fig. 19.2: Bado classification: X-rays

- Type II: Flexion type (15%)—ulna shaft angulates posteriorly (flexes) and radial head dislocates posteriorly.
- Type III: Lateral type (20%)—ulna shaft angulates laterally (bent to outside) and radial head dislocates to the side.
- Type IV: Combined type (5%)—ulna shaft and radial shaft are both fractured and radial head is dislocated, typically anteriorly.

Of the Monteggia fractures, Bado type I is the most common (59%), followed by type III (26%), type II (5%), and type IV (1%).

In his classic 1943 text, Watson-Jones stated that "no fracture presents so many problems; no injury is beset with greater difficulty; no treatment is characterized by more general failure".

The posterior interosseous branch of the radial nerve, which courses around the neck of the radius, is especially at risk, particularly in Bado type II injuries.

MANAGEMENT

All Monteggia fracture dislocations require an urgent orthopaedic assessment. Reduction is always required. Delayed or missed diagnosis is the most frequent complication.

Monteggia fractures may be managed conservatively in children with closed reduction (resetting and casting), but due to high risk of displacement causing malunion, open reduction internal fixation is typically performed.

After adequate analgesia and sedation, a closed reduction of the radial head can be performed with distal traction and direct pressure over the radial head. This can be done in the emergency department or in the

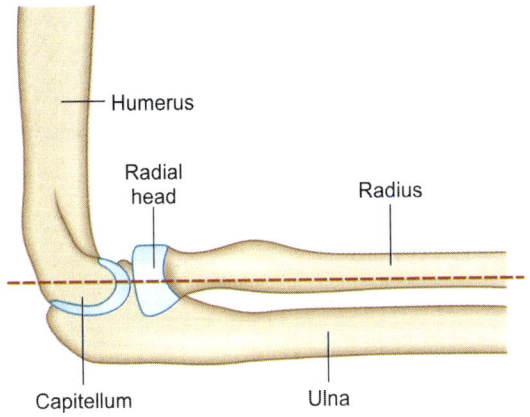

Humerus

Radial head

Radius

Capitellum

Ulna

Fig. 19.3: Radiocapitellar line

operating room. An open technique should be considered, if the radius is fractured or irreducible. Once the radius has been reduced, the ulnar fracture is addressed with rigid internal fixation. In adult Monteggia fracture, fixation with a 3.5 mm dynamic compression (DC) plate or a limited contact dynamic compression (LC-DC) plate is recommended.

Osteosynthesis (open reduction and internal fixation) of the ulnar shaft is considered the standard of care in adults. It promotes stability of the radial head dislocation and allows very early mobilization to prevent stiffness. The elbow joint is particularly susceptible to loss of motion.

Once the ulna is stabilized, the stability of the radial head is assessed using intra-operative fluoroscopy.

Complications of ORIF surgery for Monteggia fractures can include non-union, malunion, nerve palsy and damage, muscle damage, arthritis, tendonitis, infection, stiffness and loss of range of motion, compartment syndrome, audible popping or snapping, deformity, and chronic pain associated with surgical hardware.

Most nerve injuries are neurapraxias, and function usually returns within 1 to 6 months.

APPENDIX
Important consideration in treatment of Monteggia fracture-dislocation

- The keys to successful diagnosis of a Monteggia fracture are clinical suspicion and radiographs of the entire forearm and elbow.
- The Monteggia lesion is most precisely characterized as a forearm fracture in association with dislocation of the proximal radioulnar joint.
- Separate radiographs should be taken of the elbow. The radial head should point towards the capitellum on all radiographs of the elbow.
- A high index of suspicion, therefore, should be maintained with any ulna fracture.
- The forearm structures are intricately related, and any disruption to one of the bones affects the other.
- Typical presentation: Elbow pain, elbow swelling, deformity, crepitus, and paraesthesia or numbness.
- Delay in reduction of the radius is a cause of articular damage and further nerve injury, thus treatment should be timely.

BIBLIOGRAPHY

- http://emedicine.medscape.com/article/1231438-overview#a0199
- http://radiologymasterclass.co.uk/gallery/trauma/x-ray_arm_1/fractures_10.html#top_first_img
- https://www2.aofoundation.org
- https://www.youtube.com/watch?v=yCJhQe3wLYM

Galeazzi Fractures

The Galeazzi fracture is a fracture of the radius with dislocation of the distal radioulnar joint (Fig. 20.1). It classically involves an isolated fracture of the junction of the distal third and middle third of the radius with associated subluxation or dislocation of the distal radioulnar joint; the injury disrupts the forearm axis joint.

The Galeazzi fracture is named after Ricardo Galeazzi (1866–1952), an Italian surgeon at the Instituto de Rachitici in Milan, who described the fracture in 1934. However, it was first described in 1842, by Cooper,

92 years before Galeazzi reported his results. Galeazzie fractures account for 3–7% of all forearm fractures. Galeazzi fractures are primarily encountered in children, with a peak incidence of 9–12 years of age. They are seen most often in males. In 1941, Campbell termed the Galeazzi fracture the "fracture of necessity", because it necessitates surgical treatment.

Galeazzi fractures are classified according to the position of the distal radius:
- Type I: Dorsal displacement
- Type II: Volar displacement

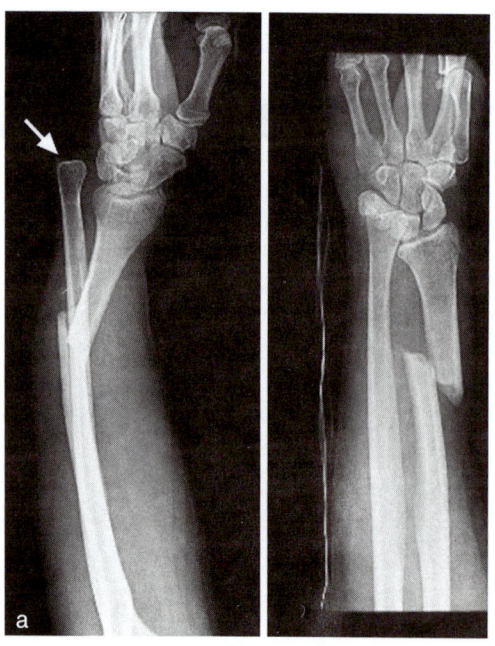
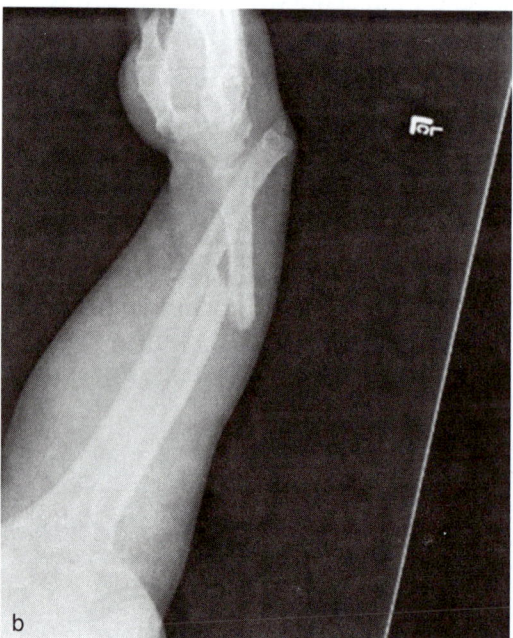

Fig. 20.1a and b: Galeazzi fractures

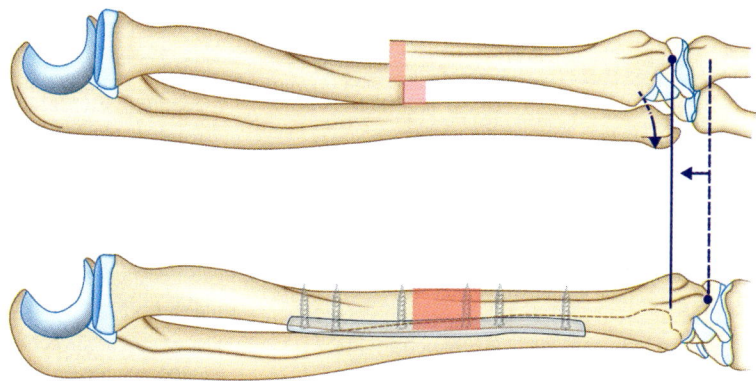

Fig. 20.2: Open reduction

Plain radiographic findings suggestive of injury to the distal radioulnar joint (DRUJ) are as follows:

- Fracture at the ulnar styloid base
- Widening of the DRUJ space on an AP radiograph
- Dislocation of the radius relative to the ulna on a true lateral radiograph, which is obtained with the shoulder abducted 90°.
- Shortening of the radius by more than 5 mm relative to the distal ulna.

These fractures are unstable and operative fixation is usually required to reduce and fix the radial fracture, and the forearm is immobilized in pronation. The exact mode of fixation depends on the location of the radial fracture:

- Diaphysis: Elastic nail
- Metaphyseal-diaphyseal junction: Plate and screw
- Distal radius: K-wire

Intraoperatively, if the DRUJ is stable, specifically evaluate in supination. If reducible and stable in supination, splint in supination for 4 weeks after surgery.

If the DRUJ is reducible in supination but unstable, stabilize the DRUJ in supination by placing 20.045 Kirschner wires (K-wires) from the ulna into the radius, just proximal to the articular surface.

If the DRUJ is unstable and irreducible, perform an open reduction (Fig. 20.2) through a dorsal approach, remove soft tissue from the DRUJ, and stabilize the DRUJ.

Galeazzi fractures in skeletally immature patients are typically treated with closed reduction and casting because of the enhanced viscoelastic nature of paediatric bone, as well as the presence of a stout periosteal sleeve.

COMPLICATIONS

The overall complication rate in the treatment of Galeazzi fractures approaches 40%. Complications include the following:

- Nonunion
- Malunion
- Infection
- Refractories following plate removal
- Posterior interosseous nerve (PIN) injury
- Instability of the DRUJ

Differences between Monteggia fractures and Galeazzi fractures are dipicted in Table 20.1.

Table 20.1: Differences between Monteggia and Galeazzi fractures

Monteggia		Galeazzi
Anterior dislocation of the radial head with a fracture of the ulna, usually angulated dorsally	Description	Fracture of the radius with shortening and dislocation of the distal ulna
Dislocation at the head	Radius	Isolated fracture at the junction of the distal and middle third
Fracture of the proximal third	Ulna	Subluxation or dislocation of the distal radioulnar joint
Fall on an outstretched hand with the forearm in excessive pronation Direct blow on back of upper forearm in sefl-defense (night-stick injury)	Mechanism	Fall on an outstretched arm with elbow flexed
ORIF	Management	Open reduction in adults Closed reduction in children
Non-union	Complications	Malunion/non-union Limitation of pronation or supination
Limitation of motion at elbow		Anterior interosseous nerve palsy
Giovanni Battista Monteggia	Credit goes to...	Ricardo Galeazzi

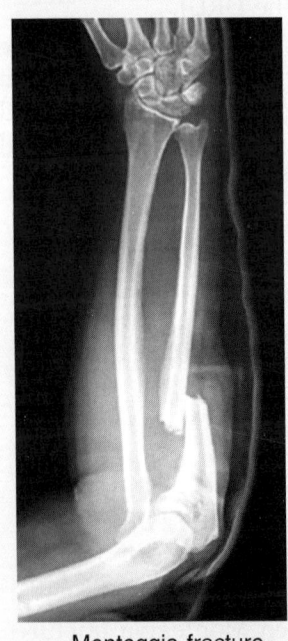

Monteggia fracture

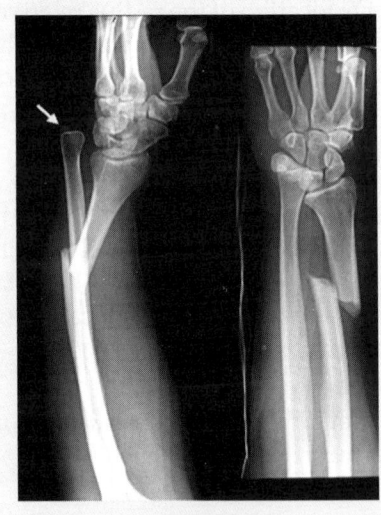

Galeazzi fracture

BIBLIOGRAPHY

- https://www2.aofoundation.org/.../04
- radiopaedia.org/articles/galeazzi-fracture-dislocation
- emedicine.medscape.com/article/1239331-overview
- https://www.youtube.com/watch?v=B-nbxsUrzy8

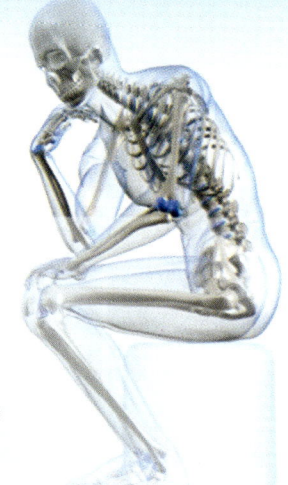

Fractures of Distal Radius

Distal radius fractures (Fig. 21.1) are very common. It is common in the elderly because of the frequent osteopenia and osteoporosis in this age group. A distal radius fracture almost always occurs about 1 inch from the end of the bone. Fractures of the distal radius account for one-sixth of all fractures seen in the emergency department.

In the times of Hippocrates and Galen, distal radius fractures (DRFs) were thought to be wrist dislocations. Pouteau first varied from this tradition when he described a variety of forearm fractures in the French literature, including a DRF. As a result, DRFs are termed Pouteau fractures in the French-speaking world.

One of the most common distal radius fractures is a Colles' fracture, in which the broken fragment of the radius tilts upward. This fracture was first described in 1814 by an Irish surgeon and anatomist, Abraham Colles, hence the name Colles fracture.

Other ways the distal radius can break include:
- Intra-articular fractures
- Extra-articular fractures
- Open fractures
- Comminuted fractures

Specific types of distal radius fractures are Colles' fracture; Smith's fracture; Barton's fracture; and Chauffeur's fracture.

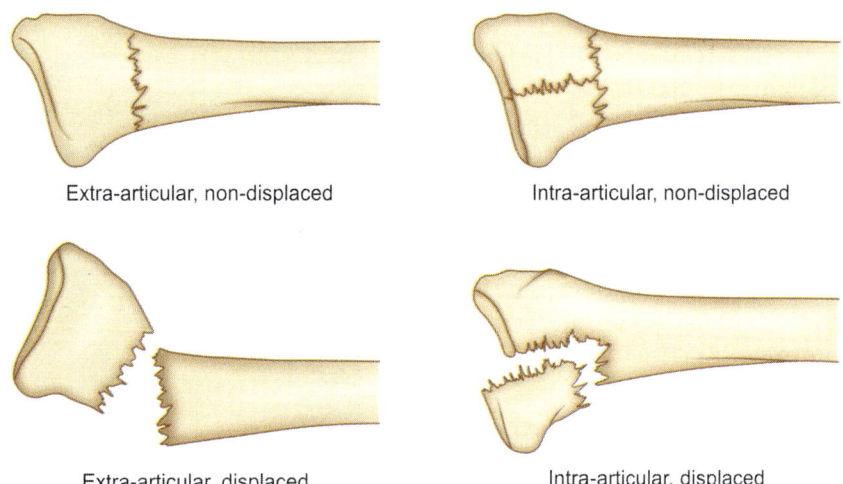

Extra-articular, non-displaced   Intra-articular, non-displaced

Extra-articular, displaced   Intra-articular, displaced

Fig. 21.1: Fractures of distal radius

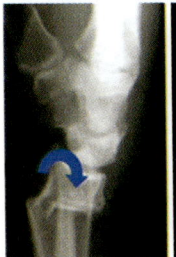 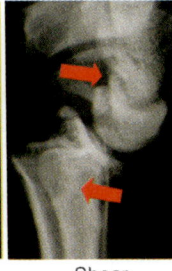 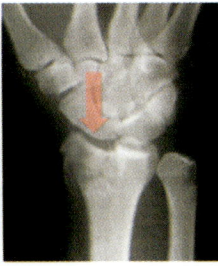 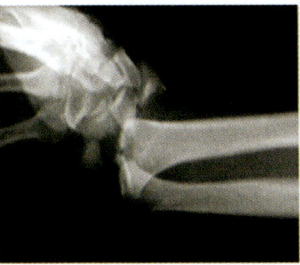 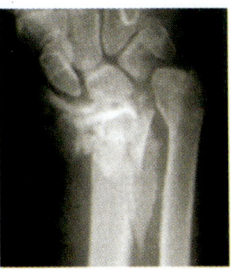

| Bending | Shear | Compression | Fracture dislocation | Complex |

Fig. 21.2: Fernandez classification

In current practice, as a result of greater knowledge of the varieties of fracture configurations, eponyms tend to be avoided, and a direct description of the fracture is preferred.

No consensus has been reached on classification systems, indications for surgery, or a particular choice of surgery.

The classification systems used most frequently are the Frykman, Melone, AO [Arbeitsgemeins chaft für Osteosynthese (Association for the Study of Osteosynthesis)], and Fernandez systems (Fig. 21.2). Their key characteristics are as follows:

- The Frykman classification highlights the injury to the distal radioulnar joint (DRUJ)
- The Melone classification, based on the paper by Scheck, highlights the fragmentation of the articular surface, especially the dorsoulnar corner of the distal radius.
- The AO classification emphasizes the location as extra-articular, partial articular, and completely articular.
- The Fernandez classification is based on the mechanism of injury, deduced from the displacement of the bone and the location of the fracture lines. Five distinct fracture patterns have been described by Fernandez, based on the direction and degree of force applied to the radius in the fall: Bending, shear, compression, fracture dislocation and complex fractures.

The distal radius consists of three columns. They are as follows (Fig. 21.3):

- Lateral column (the radial half of the radius, including the radial styloid and the scaphoid facet, though Medoff differentiates these two)
- Central column (the ulnar half of the radius, including the lunate facet)
- Medial column [the ulna, the triangular fibrocartilage (TFC), and the DRUJ]

The Frykman classification of distal radial fractures is based on the AP appearance and encompasses the eponymous entities of Colles' fracture, Smith fracture, Barton fracture, Chauffeur fracture, etc. (Fig. 21.5a to e).

- Type I: Transverse metaphyseal fracture: This includes both a Colles and Smith fracture as angulation is not a feature.
- Type II: Type I + ulnar styloid fracture

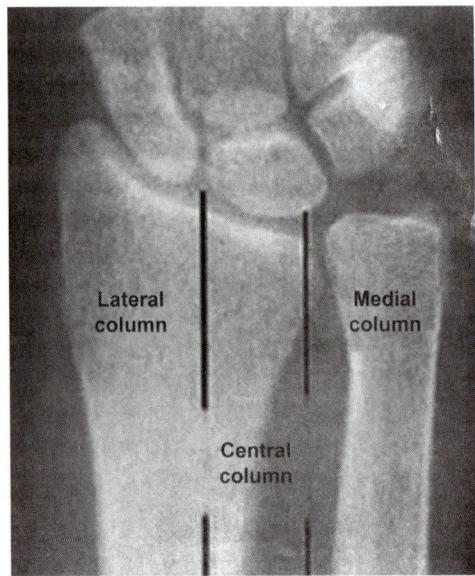

Fig. 21.3: Three columns

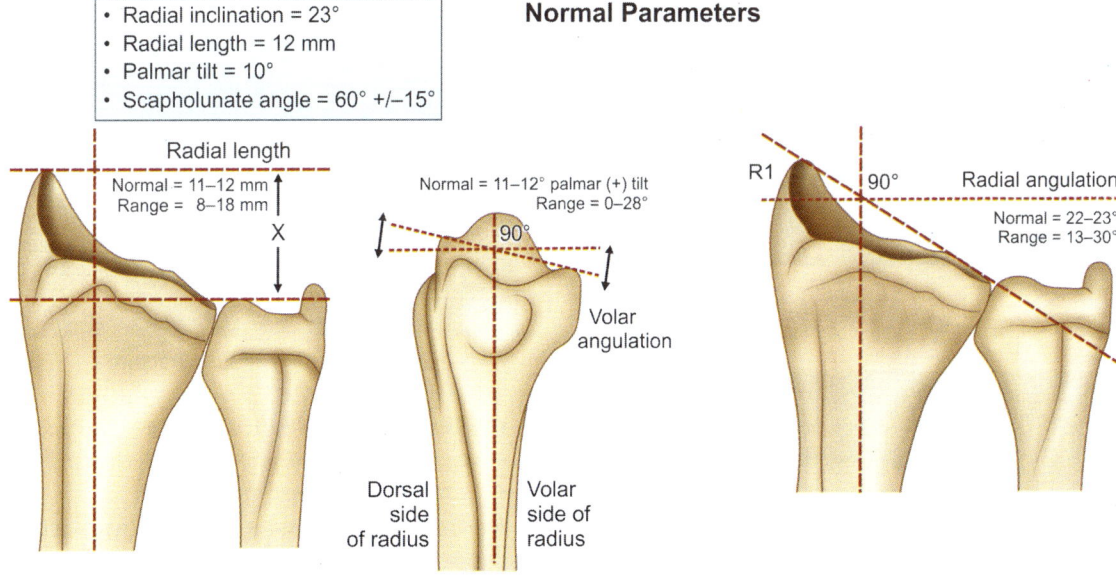

- Radial inclination = 23°
- Radial length = 12 mm
- Palmar tilt = 10°
- Scapholunate angle = 60° +/–15°

Normal Parameters

Radial length

Normal = 11–12 mm
Range = 8–18 mm

X

Normal = 11–12° palmar (+) tilt
Range = 0–28°

90°

Volar
angulation

Dorsal
side
of radius

Volar
side of
radius

R1   90°   Radial angulation

Normal = 22–23°
Range = 13–30°

Fig. 21.4: Radiological parameters

- Type III: Fracture involves the radiocarpal joint. This includes both a Barton and reverse Barton fractures.
- Type IV: Type III + ulnar styloid fracture
- Type V: Transverse fracture involves distal radioulnar joint.
- Type VI: Type V + ulnar styloid fracture.
- Type VII: Comminuted fracture with involvement of both the radiocarpal and radioulnar joints.
- Type VIII: Type VII + ulnar styloid fracture

Fracture description (Fig. 21.4)
Location: Extra-articular or intra-articular

Configuration Simple: Transverse or oblique or comminutive

Displacement:
- Radial tilt
- Radial length
- Radial angle
- Intra-articular incongruity—offset of 2 mm in any plane

Ulna/DRUJ: Fracture at the tip, midportion or base, subluxation or instability—compare to non-involved side

DRFs have a bimodal distribution, with a peak in younger persons (aged 18–25 years) and a second peak in older persons (aged >65 years). The median nerve is always compressed after a fall on the palmar aspect of the hand that results in a distal radius fracture (DRF), and the chart note should specifically document the quality (not just the presence or absence) of median nerve function.

Fracture treatment depends on
- Fracture type and characteristics
- Age of the patient
- Activity level
- Quality of the bone

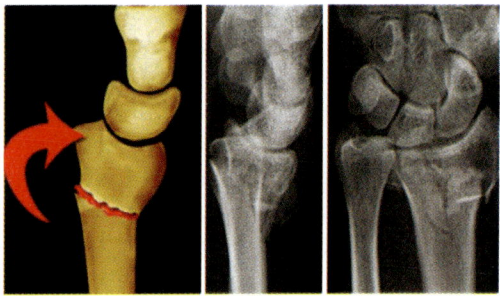

Fig. 21.5a: Colles' fracture

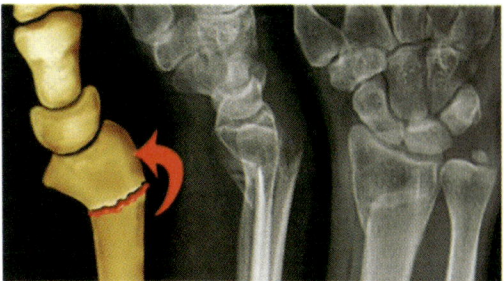

Fig. 21.5b: Smith's fracture

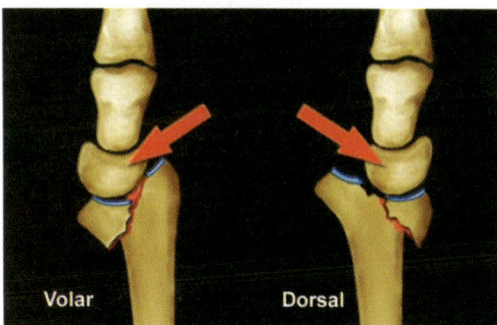

Fig. 21.5c: Barton's fracture

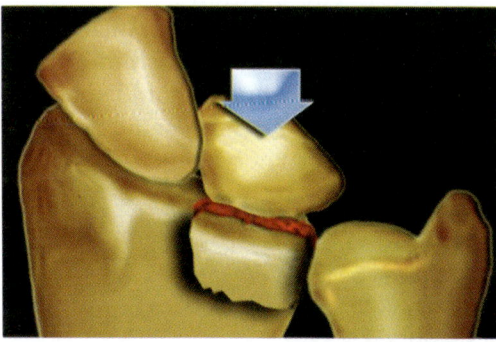

Fig. 21.5d: Die-punch fracture

Most authors would recommend anatomic reduction in a patient who is active in recreation. Usually, three parameters are relevant:

- *Intra-articular step off:* Most authors would accept less than 1 mm of intra-articular step off but not more than 2 mm.
- *Dorsal tilt:* Most authors would accept neutral dorsal tilt but not more than 10° (the

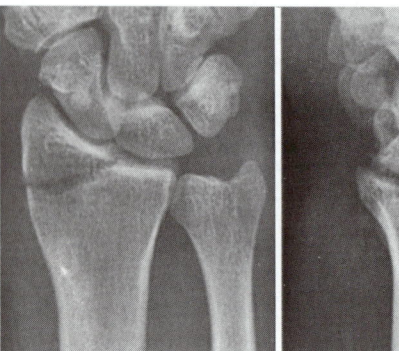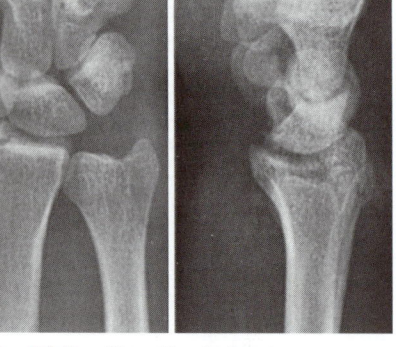

Fig. 21.5e: Chauffeur's fracture

range is quite large in the literature, with some authors not accepting more than neutral).

- *Radial length:* Most authors would accept 2 mm of radial shortening but not more than 5 mm.
- *Radial tilt* is generally considered a less important parameter.
- *Distal radius acceptable reduction*
  - <2 mm articular step off
  - <5 mm shortening
  - <10° dorsal tilt
- *Surgical indications:* Radial shortening >3 mm, dorsal tilt >10°, intra-articular displacement or step-off >2 mm. (AAOS Clinical Practice Guideline, 2011)

Traditionally, surgical treatment has been reserved for displaced, irreducible DRFs or reducible but unstable DRFs.

Indications of instability
- >10° loss of angulation
- >5 mm of axial radial shortening
- >2 mm of articular incongruity
- Comminution of cortex across the midaxial line on lateral X-ray
- Comminution of dorsal and palmar cortices
- Irreducible fracture
- Loss of reduction at follow up

Operative (Fig. 21.6)

Surgical fixation (CRPP, external fixation, ORIF)

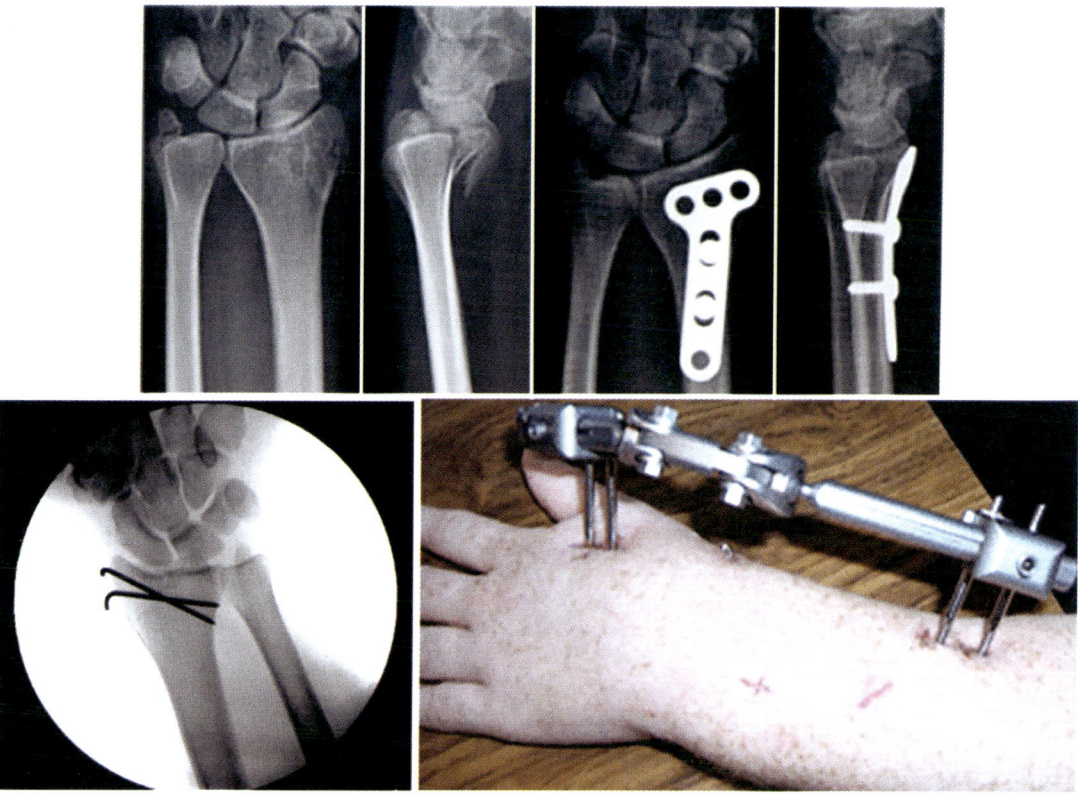

Fig. 21.6: Surgical techniques

Indications for Surgery

- Radiographic findings indicating instability (pre-reduction radiographs best predictor of stability)
- Displaced intra-articular fractures
- Volar or dorsal comminution
- Articular margin fractures
- Severe osteoporosis
- Dorsal angulation >5° or >20° of contralateral distal radius
- >5 mm radial shortening
- Comminuted and displaced extra-articular fractures (Smith's fracture).
- Progressive loss of volar tilt and loss of radial length following closed reduction and casting.
- Associated ulnar styloid fractures do not require fixation.

Complications

- Malunion = typically loss of radial height, ulnar and volar inclination less commonly intra-articular incongruity.
- *Non-union:* Uncommon except with volar and dorsal plating with extensive subperiosteal stripping.
- Distal radioulnar joint injury
- Contracture
- Neurologic injury
- Complex regional pain syndrome (CRPS) (2–20%)
- Hardware failure
- Painful hardware
- Risks of surgery

Summary

Fractures of the distal radius are very common, and are treated using either casting or surgical techniques such as internal and external fixation.

There are nearly as many ways to treat a distal radius fracture as there are distal radius fractures.

In other words, there is no one treatment that is effective for all types of fractures. Each fracture requires individual treatment customized to deal with the specific characteristics of the fracture.

"An important consideration when treating a fracture of the distal radius is to assess its 'personality' and customize one's treatment to best match its personality".

BIBLIOGRAPHY

- https://www2.aofoundation.org/
- http://www.radiologyassistant.nl/
- https://www.youtube.com/watch?v=ZibbMiX5BYo
- https://www.youtube.com/watch?v=lHD4jY28vRY
- https://www.youtube.com/watch?v=Xfuq5b7QNRY

Scaphoid Fractures

Fractures of the scaphoid bone mainly occur in young adults and constitute 2–7% of all fractures. Scaphoid fractures account for 70–80% of all carpal bone fractures. A fracture of the scaphoid, though a relatively frequent wrist injury, is often ignored, overlooked, or mistakenly attributed to a wrist sprain.

A scaphoid fracture is usually caused by a fall on an outstretched hand, with the weight landing on the palm. Fractures of the scaphoid occur in people of all ages, including children. The injury often happens during sports activities or a motor vehicle accident. Men aged 20 to 30 years are most likely to experience this injury. Scaphoid fractures usually cause pain and sensitivity to palpation in the anatomic snuffbox at the base of the thumb accompanied by swelling in the same area. Classically there can be pain in anatomical snuffbox which is thought to have a sensitivity of ~90% and a specificity ~40%.

Scaphoid fractures are significant because a delay in diagnosis can lead to a variety of adverse outcomes that include non-union, delayed union, decreased grip strength, decreased range of motion, and osteoarthritis of the radiocarpal joint. Timely diagnosis, appropriate immobilization, and referral when indicated can decrease the likelihood of adverse outcomes.

Scaphoid fractures (Fig. 22.1) are often diagnosed by X-rays. However, not all fractures are apparent initially. Therefore, people with tenderness over the scaphoid

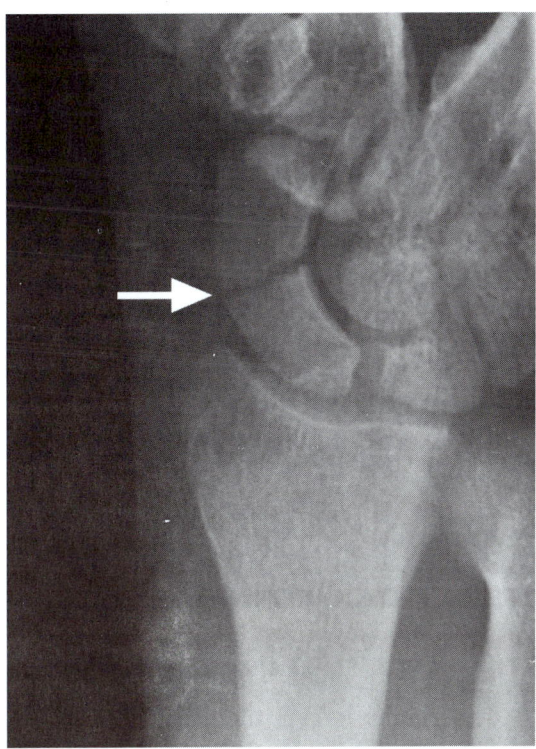

Fig. 22.1: Fracture of scaphoid

(those who exhibit pain to pressure in the anatomic snuffbox) are often casted for 7–10 days at which point a second set of X-rays is taken. If there was a hairline fracture, healing will now be apparent. Even then a fracture may not be apparent. A CT scan can then be used to evaluate the scaphoid with greater resolution.

The scaphoid receives its blood supply primarily from lateral and distal branches of the radial artery. Blood flows from the top/

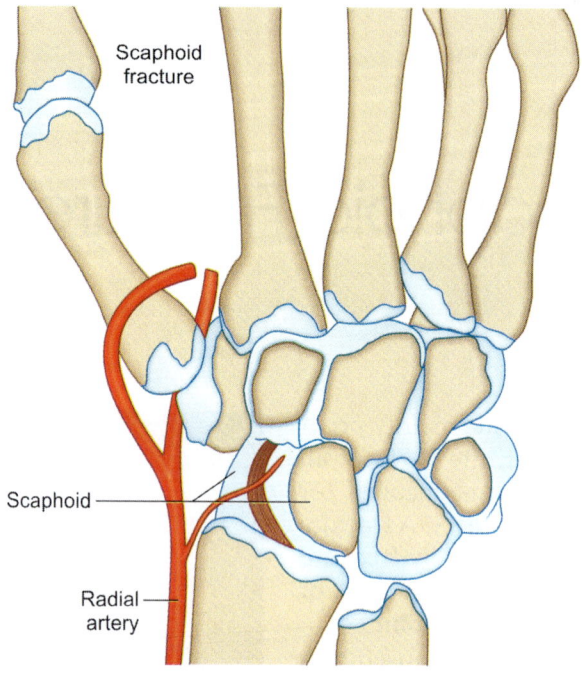

Scaphoid
fracture

Scaphoid

Radial
artery

Fig. 22.2: Carpal bones

distal end of the bone in a retrograde fashion down to the proximal pole; if this blood flow is disrupted by a fracture, the bone may not heal (Fig. 22.2).

There are no reliable clinical tests to confirm or rule out the diagnosis of a scaphoid fracture.

SPECIAL PROVOCATION MANOEUVRES

Watson (Scaphoid Shift) Test

- The patient sits with the forearm pronated. The examiner takes the patient's wrist into full ulnar deviation and extension. The examiner presses the patient's thumb with his/her other hand and then begins radial deviation and flexion of the patient's hand.
- If the scaphoid and lunate are unstable, the dorsal pole of the scaphoid subluxes over the dorsal rim of the radius and the patient complains of pain, indicating a positive test.

Scaphoid Stress Test

- The patient sits while the examiner holds the patient's wrist with one hand, with the

examiner applying pressure with his/her thumb over the patient's distal scaphoid. The patient then attempts radial deviation of the wrist.
- If excessive laxity is present, the scaphoid is forced dorsally out of the scaphoid fossa of the radius with a resulting audible clunk and pain, indicating a positive test.

CLASSIFICATION

Herbert Classification

The Herbert classification is based on the stability of the fracture. Unstable fractures are fractures with a dislocation of more than 1 mm or an angulation of more than 15° between the fragments. Additional fractures, transscaphoid-perilunate dislocations, multifragment fractures and proximal pole fractures are also classified as unstable.

Mayo Classification

The Mayo classification divides scaphoid fractures into proximal (10%), middle (70%)

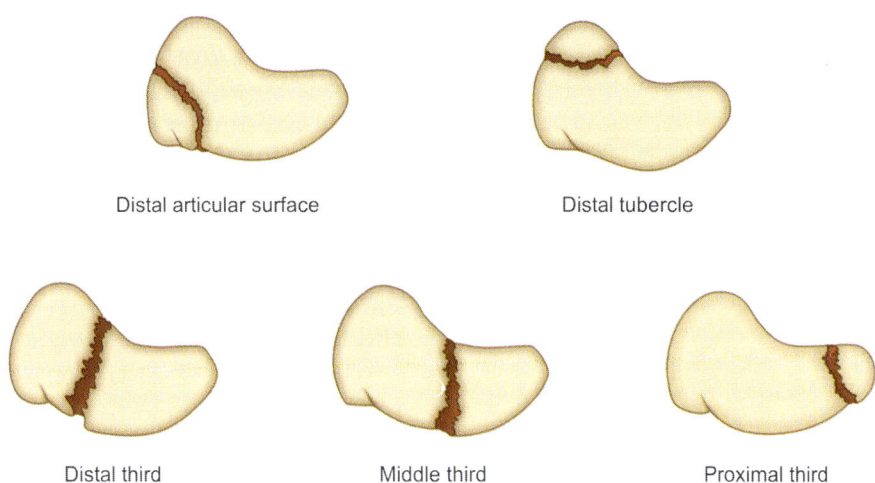

Distal articular surface

Distal tubercle

Distal third

Middle third

Proximal third

Fig. 22.3: Mayo classification of scaphoid fractures

and distal (20%) fractures. Within the distal third, distinction is made between the distal articular surface and the distal tubercle (Fig. 22.3).

Russe Classification

The anatomic classification according to Russe predicts the tendency of the fracture to heal. The classification distinguishes among horizontal oblique, transverse or vertical oblique fracture lines. The vertical oblique fracture is unstable, whereas the horizontal oblique and the transverse fractures are more stable fractures.

RADIOGRAPHY

Anteroposterior, lateral, and oblique radiographic views are required for evaluation of a suspected scaphoid fracture. Occasionally, a special radiograph called a scaphoid view may be helpful; the wrist is ulnarly deviated and extended while the film is shot from a dorsovolar angle. Plain radiographs of the wrist, including dedicated scaphoid views are the initial imaging modality of choice. It should, however, be noted that initial radiograph can miss from 5–20% of fractures in the acute setting.

X-ray features include:
- Visualization of the fracture +/- displacement
- Soft tissue swelling and lateral displacement of the adjacent fat pads
  - *Scaphoid fat pad sign:* Formation of a straight/convex line adjacent to the concave aspect of the scaphoid.
- Associated scapholunate ligament disruption (Terry Thomas sign) which can be accentuated with a clenched fist view.

For therapeutic decision making, the scaphoid is divided into three anatomic sections: Proximal, medial, and distal. Fractures are further subdivided into displaced and non-displaced types. Fractures of the proximal third of the scaphoid account for 20% of scaphoid fractures, those of the middle portion account for 60%, and fractures of the distal part make up the remaining 20%. Almost 100% of proximal pole fractures result in aseptic necrosis. Displaced scaphoid fractures have a non-union rate of 55–90%.

TREATMENT (Flowchart 22.1)

Non-Displaced Fractures

- Initially, non-displaced fractures are treated with a long-arm thumb spica cast with the

Flowchart 22.1: Treatment of scaphoid fractures

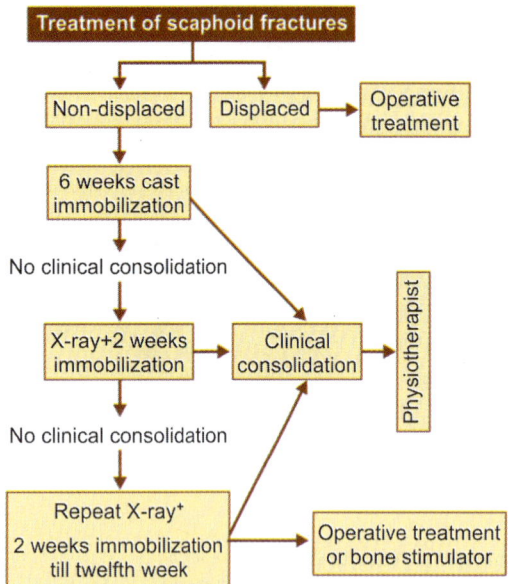

wrist in neutral position for 6 weeks, followed by a short-arm spica cast for an additional 6 weeks, until roentgenographic union is evident. If there is a displacement or widening of the fracture line after 6 weeks, the patient should be referred for surgical evaluation.

- After immobilization, active ROM exercises to the forearm, wrist, and thumb should be performed 6–8 times daily.
- A wrist-and-thumb static splint with the wrist in neutral should be worn between exercise sessions and at night.

The more proximal the fracture, the longer the healing time:

- Distal 1/3rd: 6–8 weeks
- Middle 1/3rd: 8–12 weeks
- Proximal 1/3rd: 12–23 weeks

Treatment of scaphoid fractures is guided by the location in the bone of the fracture (proximal, waist, distal), displacement (or instability) of the fracture, and patient tolerance for cast immobilization.

Displaced or unstable fractures require percutaneous pin fixation or compression screw fixation to prevent malunion. Internal fixation is accomplished with either smooth Kirschner wires or a Herbert screw (Fig. 22.4).

COMPLICATIONS

Avascular necrosis (AVN) is a common complication of a scaphoid fracture. Risk

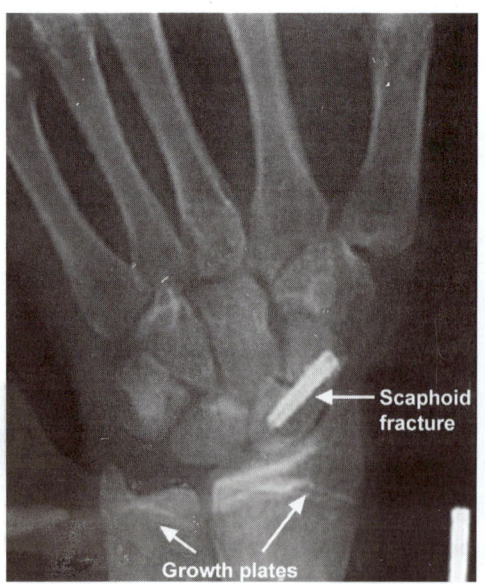

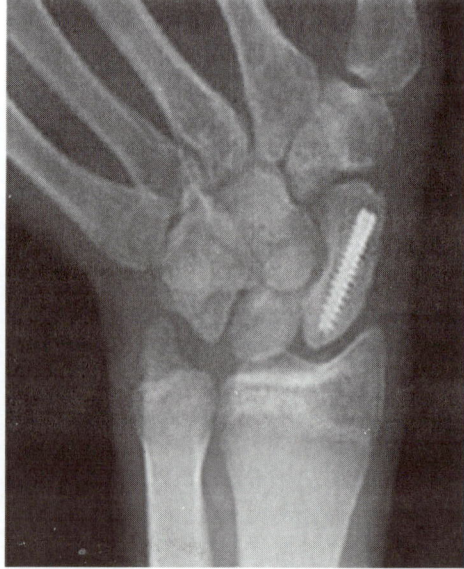

Fig. 22.4: Herbert screw

of AVN depends on the location of the fracture.

- Fractures in the proximal 1/3rd have a high incidence of AVN (~30%)
- Waist fracture in the middle 1/3rd is the most frequent fracture site and has moderate risk of AVN.
- Fractures in the distal 1/3rd are rarely complicated by AVN.
- Non-union can also occur from undiagnosed or undertreated scaphoid fractures. Arterial flow to the scaphoid enters via the distal pole and travels to the proximal pole. This blood supply is tenuous, increasing the risk of non-union, particularly with fractures at the wrist and proximal end. If not treated correctly, non-union of the scaphoid fracture can lead to wrist osteoarthritis. This complication is influenced by delayed diagnosis, gross displacement, associated injuries of the carpus, and impaired blood supply. Of these fractures, 40% are undiagnosed at the time of original injury. Non-union is 20% more common in smokers.

Non-unions of the scaphoid are treated in one of the following ways:

- Radial styloidectomy
- Excision of the proximal fragment
- Proximal row carpectomy

- Traditional bone grafting
- Total or partial arthrodesis of the wrist

The Matti-Russe procedure involves treatment of non-displaced fractures by excavation of the scaphoid and placement of a volar corticocancellous bone graft.

A silicone carpal implant is no longer recommended.

Scapholunate disassociation is a well-known complication of scaphoid fracture.

Key Points

1. Occult fracture rate = 20% (7% scaphoid).
2. ED decision = Wait and see vs day 1 CT/MRI.
3. Simple removable wrist splint appropriate for low-index-of-suspicion cases.
4. Simple Colles' cast probably as good and less disabling as a scaphoid cast.
5. Consider long arm casting in waist and proximal third fractures.
6. Early surgery becoming more common place.

BIBLIOGRAPHY

- http://emedicine.medscape.com/article/397230-overview
- http://emedicine.medscape.com/article/397230-overview
- https://www.youtube.com/watch?v=CalS5MKGD-A
- https://www.youtube.com/watch?v=dptkvsAvL-A

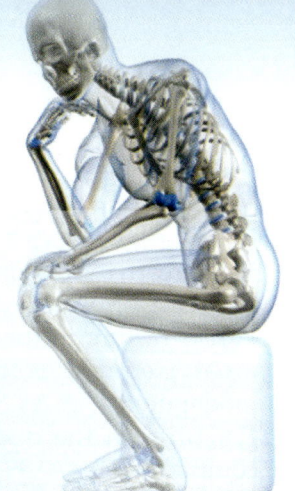

Carpal Instability

Motion and stability of the carpus provide the critical foundation for maximum hand function from precise fine motor control to power grip activities. When the normal mechanics of the wrist are disrupted, the instability of the carpal bones results in weakness, stiffness, chronic pain, and often arthritis, if not treated appropriately. Linscheid et al described traumatic carpal instability in 1972 (Fig. 23.1).

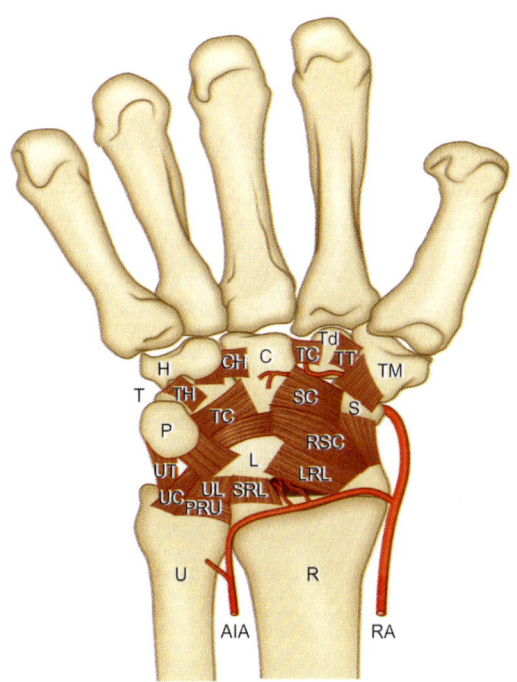

Fig. 23.1: Anatomy of wrist, showing the carpal bones and intercrpal ligaments

VOLAR CARPAL LIGAMENTS

Carpal ligament instability is defined as any malalignment of the carpus. This may be evident on plain radiography as a static deformity; alternatively, the situation may be a dynamic one, which becomes evident only when external forces are placed on the wrist. The malalignment may appear after a single traumatic event or may be secondary to chronic attenuation of supporting ligaments after a traumatic event or secondary to an underlying disease process (e.g. rheumatoid arthritis, pseudogout).

Carpal ligament instability results from an injury to one or more ligamentous or bony constraints in the wrist. Depending on the force, rate, and point of impact and on the position of the wrist, a fall on an outstretched wrist can result in a range of injuries. This spectrum includes wrist sprains, distal radius fractures, and fractures to the scaphoid and other carpal bones.

The carpal bones are said to be "intercalated". That term technically means "layered", but the key concept is that the bones are linked to each other via ligaments, and as such, when a ligament is injured the bones do not move in concert, as they should. Two patterns of disruption are common enough to warrant their own name:

- Dorsal intercalated segmental instability (DISI), in which the scapholunate ligament is injured, and

- Volar intercalated segment instability (VISI) caused by rupture of the lunotriquetral ligament and dorsal radiocarpal ligament.

Using a cadaveric trauma model, Mayfield et al observed progressive injury patterns when the wrist was loaded in extension, ulnar deviation, and carpal supination. This perilunar instability is divided into 4 stages:

Stage I refers to injury to the scapholunate interosseous ligament (SLIL). Further trauma results in dorsal subluxation of the capitate relative to the lunate, or stage II. As the load increases, the lunotriquetral interosseous ligament (LTIL) is injured, causing a perilunate dislocation in stage III. Finally, stage IV is characterized by dislocation of the lunate from the radiolunate fossa (Fig. 23.2).

However, if the carpus is pronated and the hypothenar area is struck first, an ulnar traumatic pattern may be observed. Specifically, disruption of the ulnotriquetral ligament complex and the LTIL occurs. As the triquetrum no longer holds the lunate, it falls into a flexed position because of pressure from the capitate and its connection with the scaphoid. With attenuation or injury to the dorsal intercarpal ligament, a volar intercalated segment instability (VISI) pattern ensues; this can be visualized on lateral radiography. An LTIL tear most commonly results in a VISI deformity.

In addition to a direct loading type of trauma, rotational force to the wrist can also result in ligamentous injuries, e.g. the forces that occur when holding a power drill while the drill bit is jammed. This type of trauma can result in injuries to the LTIL and ulnar-triquetral ligament complex and result in the lunotriquetral instability.

The scaphoid acts like a bridge between the proximal and distal rows and protects the link from collapsing. The wrist is a simple link between the proximal and distal rows. The pivot point is at the centre of rotation of the capitate and lunate. This joint, without other supporting structures, is stable only in tension. It is unstable in compression, as Fig. 23.2 depicts, and tends to collapse.

Perilunate instability classification (carpal dislocations) describes carpal ligament injuries.

Instability has been divided into four stages:
- *Stage I:* Scapholunate dissociation (rotatory subluxation of the scaphoid)
  - Disruption of scapholunate ligament with resultant Terry Thomas sign.
  - Exacerbated in clenched fist views.
- *Stage II:* Perilunate dislocation
  - The lunate remains normally aligned with the distal radius, and the remaining carpal bones are dislocated (almost always dorsally).
  - Capitolunate joint is disrupted, and the lunate projects through the space of Poirier.
  - 60% are associated with scaphoid fractures.
- *Stage III:* Midcarpal dislocation
  - Triquetrolunate interosseous ligament disruption or triquetral fracture

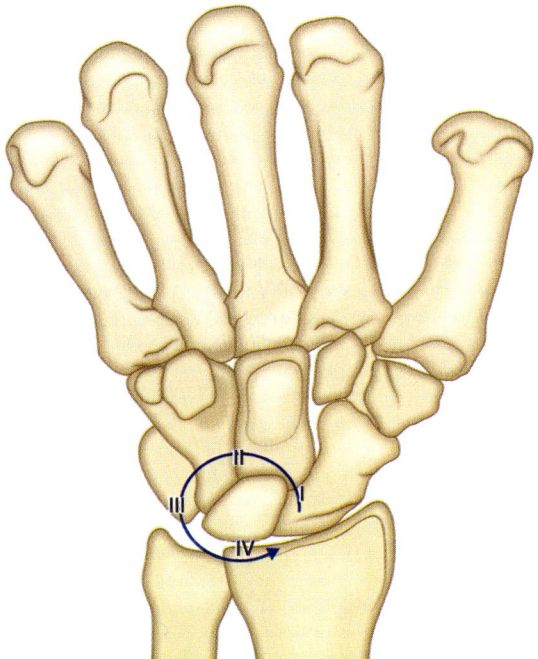

Fig. 23.2: Mayfield perilunate instability pattern

- – Neither the capitate nor the lunate is aligned with the distal radius.
- *Stage IV:* Lunate dislocation
  - – Dorsal radiolunate ligament injury
  - – Dislocation of the lunate in a palmar direction

CLINICAL TESTS

Scaphoid Shift Test (Watson) (Fig. 23.3)

In this test, the examiner's thumb is placed on the scaphoid tuberosity of the volar aspect of the wrist. Pressure is applied to the tuberosity as the wrist is passively brought from ulnar to radial deviation. This pressure attempts to block normal scaphoid flexion. In theory, if the SLIL is torn and scapholunate instability is present. The proximal scaphoid subluxates dorsally over the rim of the radius. A positive result is when a painful "clunk" is elicited as the scaphoid reduces back into the radial scaphoid fossa as the thumb pressure is released.

MANOEUVRES TO DIAGNOSE LUNOTRIQUETRAL INSTABILITY

Kleinman Shear Test (Fig. 23.4)

It is performed with the wrist in neutral position. The examiner's contralateral thumb is placed over the dorsal lunate while the ipsilateral thumb loads the pisotriquetral joint with a dorsally directed force. A shear force is created across the lunotriquetral joint. A positive result is when this manoeuvre produces pain.

Reagan Shuck Test (Fig. 23.5)

A similar test, except the examiner's thumb and index finger grasp the whole pisotriquetral unit. The contralateral thumb and index finger hold the lunate. The lunotriquetral joint is stressed by applying dorsally directed force with one hand and volarly directed force with the other hand. This force is switched in the opposite directions in both hands. This creates a shear stress at the lunotriquetral joint, and if painful, the result is positive.

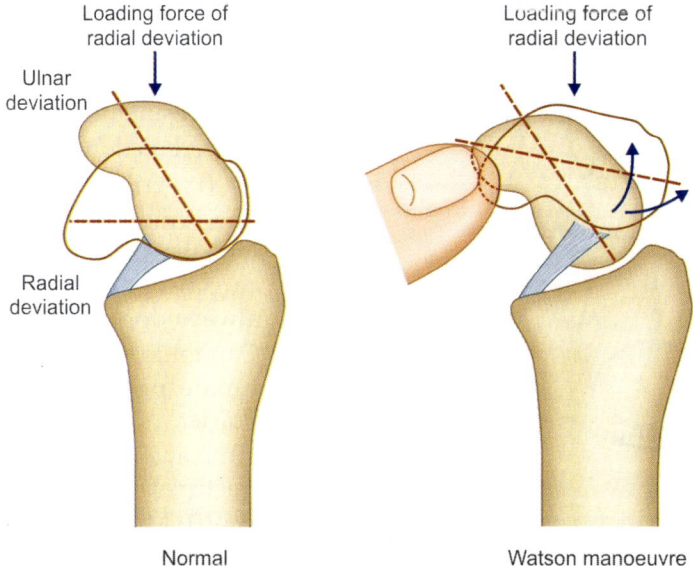

Normal　　　　　　　　　　Watson manoeuvre

Fig. 23.3: Watson's test

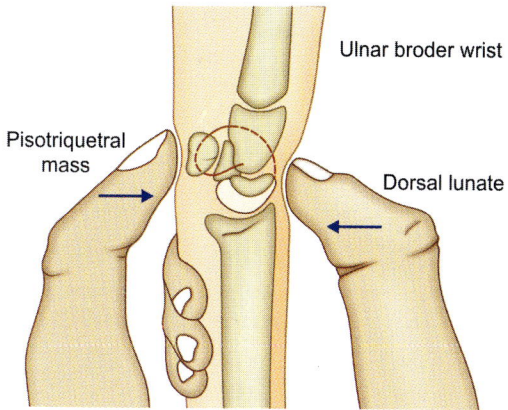

Ulnar broder wrist

Pisotriquetral mass

Dorsal lunate

Fig. 23.4: Kleinman shear test

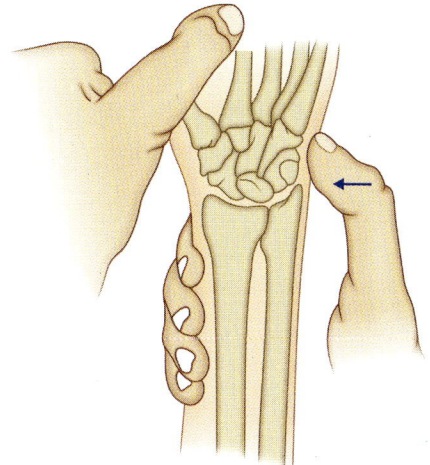

Fig. 23.6: Linscheid test

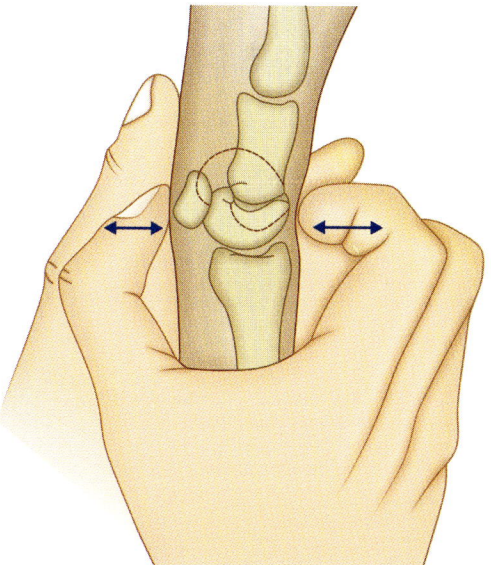

Fig. 23.5: Reagan shuck test

Linscheid Test (Fig. 23.6)

Lichtman et al described a pivot shift test for midcarpal instability. This manoeuvre is a combination ulnar deviation, axial compression, and pronation of the wrist. A positive result is when this manoeuvre results in a painful wrist click.

X-RAYS

Standard radiographic examination of the wrist should include a posteroanterior (PA) view in neutral rotation and also lateral views. To determine scapholunate dissociation, the scapholunate gap can be measured on PA and PA grip radiographs.

> **Wrist Analysis**
> *Radiography:* Proper positioning?
> *Joint spaces:* Look for parallelism
> *Carpal arches:* Disruption indicates fracture or ligament tear
> **Shape:** Lunate and scaphoid
> *Axis:* Normal, DISI or VISI

The three carpal arcs: Smooth curves joining the surfaces of the carpal bones as shown on the left (Fig. 23.7).

The first arc is a smooth curve outlining the proximal convexities of the scaphoid, lunate and triquetrum.

The second arc traces the distal concave surfaces of the same bones, and the third arc follows the main proximal curvatures of the capitate and hamate.

The amount of gap that is diagnostic of scapholunate dissociation is not agreed upon. Many authors define the gap to be pathologic, if it is greater than 3 mm.

If the lunate is dorsiflexed more than 15° than the capitate on lateral radiography, a diagnosis of a DISI deformity is confirmed.

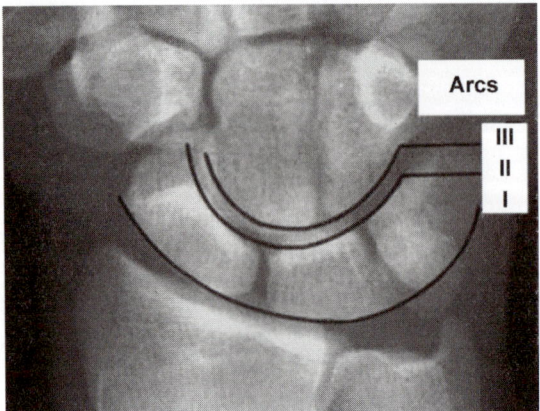

Fig. 23.7: Carpal arcs

Conversely, VISI is defined, if the lunate is volarly flexed more than 15 °.

A DISI deformity is associated with scapholunate instability, while a VISI deformity is associated with lunotriquetral instability.

In lunotriquetral instability, the lunate is usually palmarly flexed, and the scapholunate angle can be less than 30°.

LUNATE VS PERILUNATE DISLOCATION

Common dislocations of the wrist are the lunate and perilunate dislocations. The key to differentiation between both is what is centred over the radius. If the capitate is centred over the radius and the lunate is tilted out, it is a lunate dislocation. If, however, the lunate centres over the distal radius and the capitate is dorsal, we are dealing with a perilunate dislocation (Figs 23.8 and 23.9).

Other studies include fluoroscopy, wrist arthrography, CT scanning, MRI, and ultrasonography.

A static instability is one that can be clearly recognized on routine radiography by a loss of the normal alignment. A dynamic instability is any instability that requires external forces placed on the carpus to elicit an instability pattern. Therefore, the diagnosis of dynamic instability relies on other means, such as dynamic radiography, physical examination

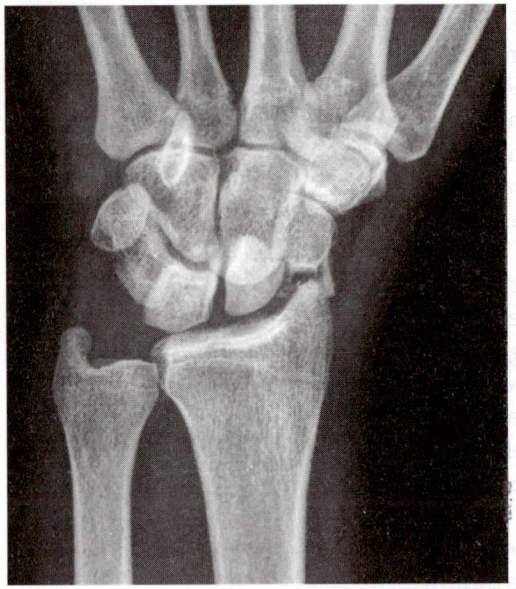

Fig. 23.8: Trans-scaphoid perilunate dislocation

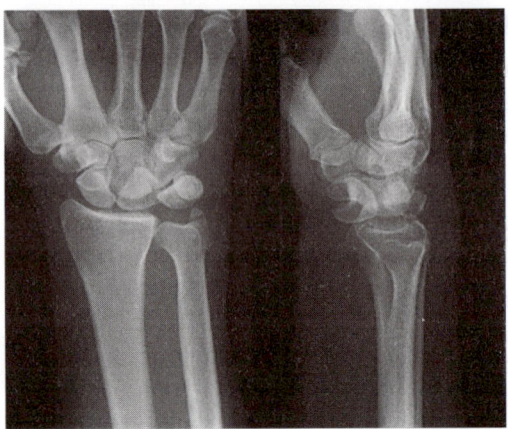

Fig. 23.9: Lunate dislocation

with provocative manoeuvres, and/or arthroscopic evaluation.

Treatment of carpal instability is complex and usually specific to the type of instability and is certainly controversial.

SCAPHOLUNATE INSTABILITY

There is no consensus on the appropriate treatment of scapholunate instability. The treatment is usually specific to the different stages or degree of injury. Partial tears of the

SLIL are thought to represent occult or predynamic instability. For these injuries, most recommend an initial trial of splinting and/or casting. Arthroscopic debridement with or without pinning can be an option in these patients in whom initial conservative treatment is unsuccessful.

In patients with unrepairable SLIL but with a reducible scapholunate interval and without degenerative changes, an indirect or direct ligament reconstruction has been advocated. Indirect ligament reconstruction is based on stabilizing the scaphoid to prevent the rotatory subluxation that often occurs in scapholunate instability (Fig. 23.10).

Fusions that have been described involve the scaphocapitolunate, the scaphotrapezial trapezoid, the scaphocapitate, and the scapholunate.

LUNOTRIQUETRAL INSTABILITY

There is no consensus on the appropriate treatment of lunotriquetral instability. Treatment algorithm can probably be based on the type and age of the injury. For patients in whom conservative treatment fails, lunotriquetral dissociation direct repair with or without augmentation has been advocated. For patients who present late after their initial injury, surgical management includes techniques of capsulodesis, ligament reconstruction, arthrodesis, or ulnar shortening.

MIDCARPAL INSTABILITY

Tightening the radiocapitate ligament and midcarpal arthrodesis are the recommended procedures.

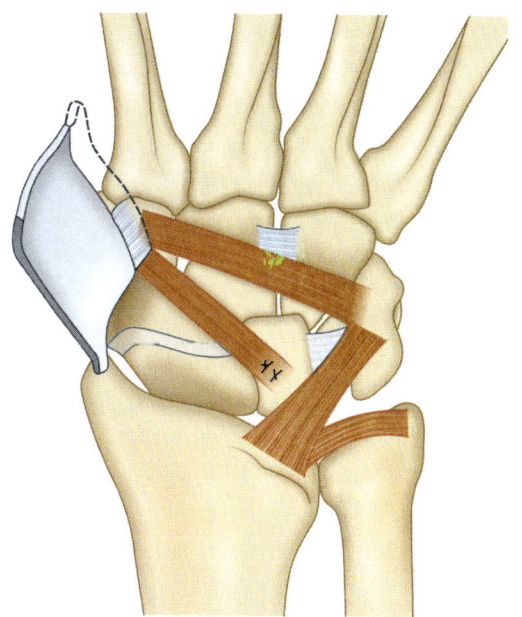

Fig. 23.10: Mayo dorsal intercarpal (DIC) capsulodesis

ULNAR TRANSLOCATION

In the rheumatoid wrist, ulnar translocation is usually effectively treated with radiolunate fusion. Significant arthritis at the radio-scaphoid joint may also require radioscaphoid fusion. Total wrist fusion is probably the best option significant midcarpal arthrosis is present as well.

BIBLIOGRAPHY

- http://www.radiologyassistant.nl/en/p42a29ec06b9e8/wrist-carpal-instability.html
- emedicine.medscape.com/article/1241610-overview
- https://www.youtube.com/watch?v=Je70cejEsLo

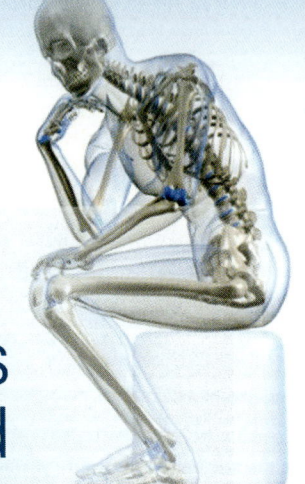

Chapter
24

Bony and Joint Injuries
of the Hand

Trauma to the hand is common, with resultant fracture of the metacarpals and phalanges comprising approximately 10% of all fractures. Most of these injuries are treated with splinting followed by early motion. However, certain fractures and dislocations require intervention to ensure optimal restoration of function.

Metacarpal fractures account for 30–40% of all hand fractures; fractures of the first and fifth metacarpals are the most frequent. Fractures of the fifth metacarpal neck (boxer fractures) alone account for 10% of all fractures of the hand.

CARPOMETACARPAL DISLOCATIONS AND FRACTURES

A dislocation and fracture at the base of a single metacarpal should signal the examiner to look for fractures or dislocations of the adjacent metacarpals. Fracture-dislocation of the base of the fifth metacarpal is a common intra-articular injury (Reverse Bennett's fracture).

Other commonly seen base fractures include the Bennett and Rolando patterns (Fig. 24.1); each of these is classically described for the first metacarpal. Both may develop as fracture dislocations of the first metacarpal because of extrinsic and intrinsic muscular forces acting on the fragments.

Bennett fracture is a fracture of the base of the first metacarpal bone which extends into

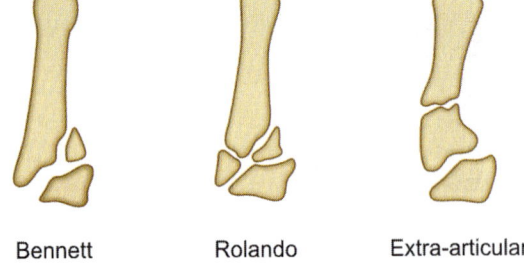

| Bennett | Rolando | Extra-articular |

Fig. 24.1: Fracture at base of 1st metacarpal

the carpometacarpal (CMC) joint. This intra-articular fracture is the most common type of fracture of the thumb, and is nearly always accompanied by some degree of subluxation or frank dislocation of the carpometacarpal joint (Fig. 24.2).

Tension from the abductor pollicis longus and adductor pollicis muscles frequently leads to displacement of the fracture fragments, even in cases where the fracture fragments are initially in their proper anatomic position.

Bennett fractures nearly always require some form of intervention to ensure healing in the correct anatomical position and restoration of proper function of the thumb CMC joint.

- For Bennett fractures where there is between 1 and 3 mm of displacement at the trapeziometacarpal joint, closed reduction and percutaneous pin fixation with Kirschner wires is often sufficient to ensure a satisfactory functional outcome. The wires are not employed to connect the two

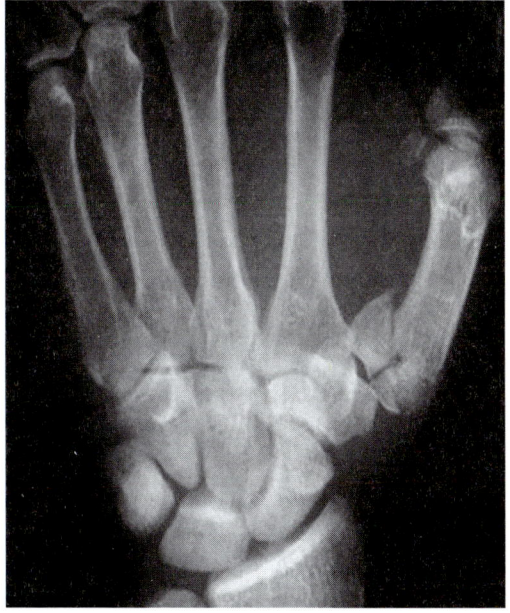

Fig. 24.2: Bennett's fracture

fractures are appropriately described by location, fracture pattern, and displacement. Transverse, oblique, and spiral are the accepted terms used to describe the patterns most commonly seen.

Fractures of the metacarpal neck are among the most frequent fractures of the hand; in these fractures, the fifth metacarpal is most likely to be fractured. Such fractures are usually caused by striking a solid object with a closed fist and have been commonly named boxer fractures.

Metacarpal Head Injuries

These fractures are rare, they are intra-articular and, if displaced, usually require open reduction and internal fixation (ORIF).

MCP DISLOCATIONS

Almost all MCP dislocations occur with the proximal phalanx displaced dorsally on the metacarpal head. Simple dislocations can be reduced without operative intervention under local anaesthesia or a combination of local anaesthesia and sedation.

Volar plate or, in the case of the thumb, sesamoid, interposition into the MCP may prevent reduction. Index and small finger MCP dislocation reductions, in particular, may be inhibited by MCP entrapment of lumbrical and flexor tendons. They warrant open reduction.

fracture fragments together, but rather to secure the first or second metacarpal to the trapezium. When there is more than 3 mm of displacement at the trapezio-metacarpal joint, open reduction and internal fixation (ORIF) is typically recommended (Fig. 24.3).

Metacarpal Shaft/Neck Fractures

Axial loading, direct blow, or torsional loading can cause metacarpal shaft fractures. These

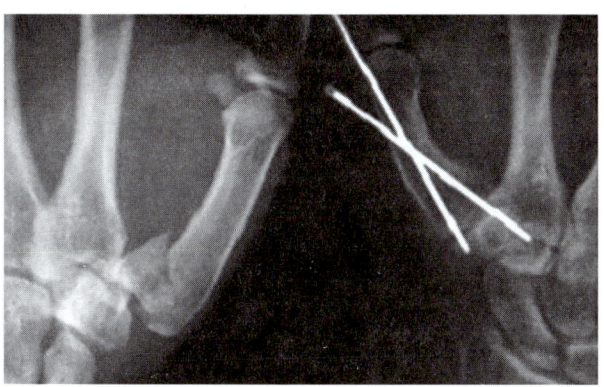

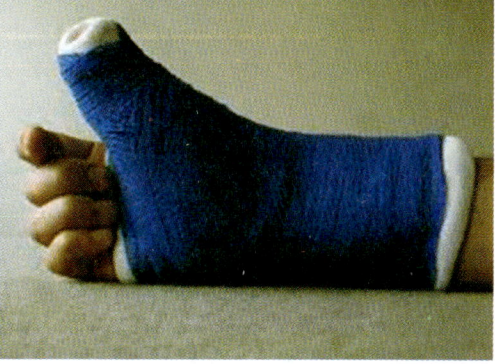

Fig. 24.3: Surgical management of Bennett's fracture

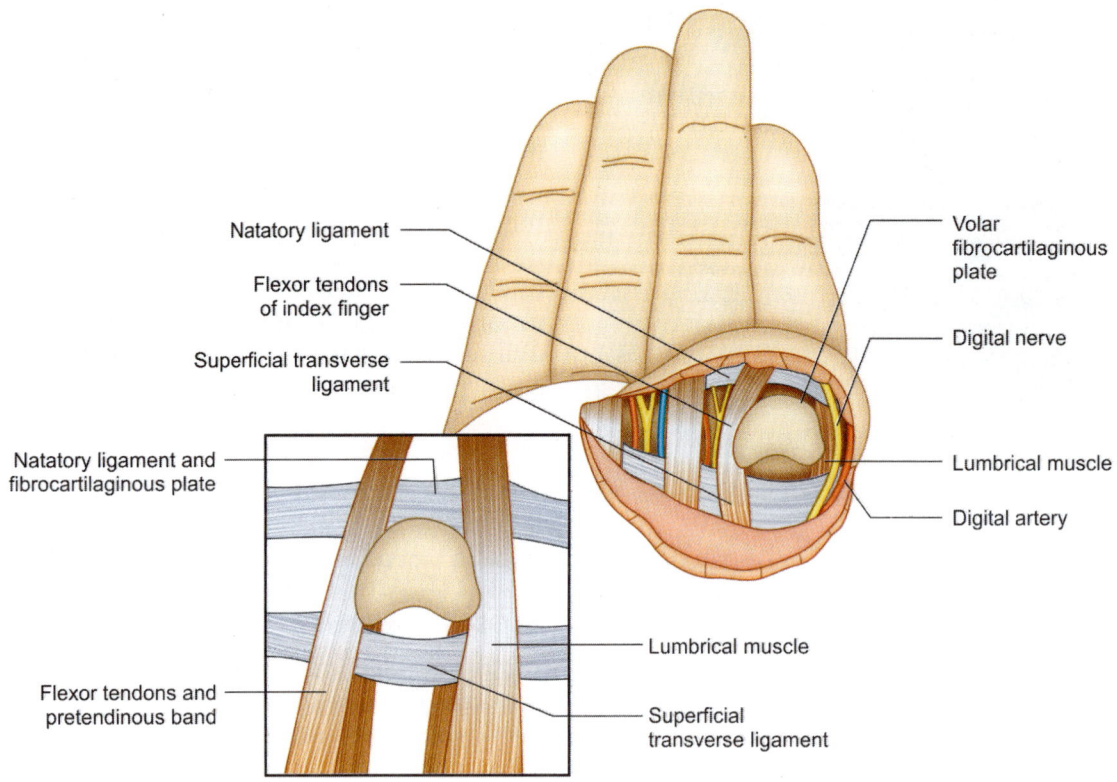

Natatory ligament

Flexor tendons of index finger

Superficial transverse ligament

Natatory ligament and fibrocartilaginous plate

Flexor tendons and pretendinous band

Volar fibrocartilaginous plate

Digital nerve

Lumbrical muscle

Digital artery

Lumbrical muscle

Superficial transverse ligament

Fig. 24.4: Kaplan lesion

- Dislocation of the metacarpophalangeal joint of the index is rare (Kaplan's lesion).
- Kaplan's lesion (Fig. 24.4)
  - Most common in index finger
  - Complex dorsal dislocation of finger, irreducible
  - Metacarpal head buttonholes into palm (volarly)
  - Volar plate is interposed between base of proximal phalanx and metacarpal head
  - Complete dislocation is almost always irreducible by the closed method and requires open reduction.

MANAGEMENT

Most injuries to the metacarpal are managed with closed reduction and external splint immobilization. Indications for operative treatment include failure to achieve or maintain acceptable reduction, open fractures, multiple fractures in the hand, complex injuries, displaced intra-articular injuries, and fractures with serious soft tissue injury requiring stable skeletal support.

Only a small amount of angulation (<10°) is acceptable in the second and third metacarpals because of their limited CMC motion. The fourth and fifth finger metacarpals are much more mobile, and volar angulations of 30° and 40° can be accepted, respectively. The more proximal the fracture, the less angulation should be tolerated by the treating physician.

Minifragment AO plates are useful for multiple metacarpal fractures in the same hand and in "combined" injuries where there is damage to the skin, tendon, and bone (Figs 24.5–24.7).

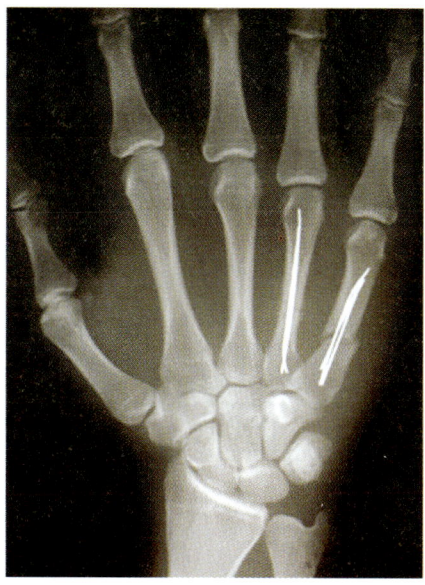

Fig. 24.5: Intramedullary pinning

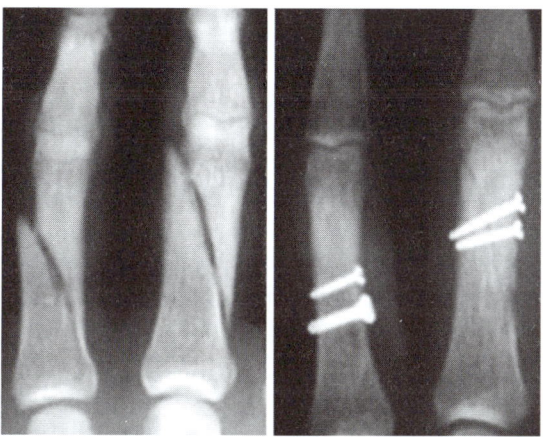

Fig. 24.6: Screw fixation

Metacarpal neck fractures usually can be managed closed without operative intervention. Although the degree of angulation acceptable is controversial, higher degrees of angulation can be accepted with little or no functional deficits in fractures of the neck, especially in the fourth and fifth digits.

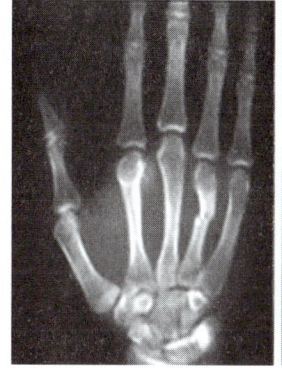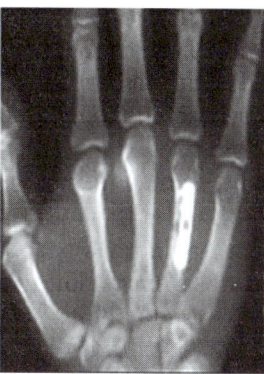

Fig. 24.7: Minifragment plating

Displacement of a metacarpal head fracture should be treated with ORIF to ensure a stable, anatomic reduction and allow for early motion.

Most MCP dislocations are easily reducible but may require open reduction, if they are complex or are associated with unstable fractures.

Most MCP joint injuries should be partially immobilized with a dorsal blocking splint, which prevents movement that might permit recurrence.

Recommended treatment is closed reduction and pin fixation to stabilize the CMC joint. Pin placement can either transit the CMC joint or secure the reduced metacarpal to the adjacent metacarpal shaft. Patients are splinted postoperatively for 3 weeks, after which they are encouraged to begin movement. The pins should be removed at 6 weeks.

BIBLIOGRAPHY

- http://radiologymasterclass.co.uk/tutorials/musculoskeletal/
- https://www.youtube.com/watch?v=uWQtpqXRx-w
- https://www.youtube.com/watch?v=iX8Jb0iPoEI
- https://www.youtube.com/watch?v=ltR-K-XPU8M

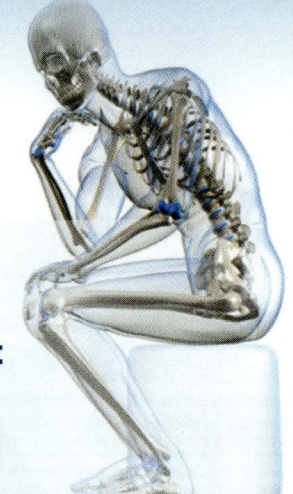

Chapter

25

Tendon Injuries of the Hand

Tendon injuries are the second most common injuries of the hand. Most injuries are open injuries to the flexor or extensor tendons, but less frequent injuries, e.g. damage to the functional system tendon sheath and pulley or dull avulsions, also need to be considered. The hand is always exposed to injuries and overuse. On average, hand injuries count for 14 to 30% of all treated patients in emergency care. Even though only 2% of the patients are hospitalized, hand injuries, especially tendon lesions, play a key role in orthopaedic and traumatic treatment.

The long fingers hold 4 common extensor tendons, namely extensor digitorum communis, and additionally the extensor indices for the index finger and the extensor digiti minimi for the little finger. The system of flexor tendons is not looked at individually but as a functional unit of tendons, tendon sheath and pulleys. The annular ligaments and cruciate ligaments are seen as a re-enforcement system of the flexor tendons along the osteofibrous channels of the fingers and hereby are fixed to the phalanges. Four to 5 annular (A1–A5) and 3 weaker crucial ligaments (C1–C3) are distinguished (Fig. 25.1).

The A2 crucial ligament plays the most important role in guidance of the flexor tendons, whereas opinions concerning the A3 and A4 vary considerably.

Injury patterns are differentiated into open or closed, sharp or blunt, traumatic or degenerative lesions, as well as injury to the dorsal or palmar part (Figs 25.2 and 25.3).

MANAGEMENT

Extensor Tendon Injury

In open injuries, the wound itself should be used as a surgical approach and extended Z-shaped. Due to the diameter of the tendon, several U-shaped sutures should be used, optionally combined with fine adaptation sutures using PDS (5-0, 6-0). In treatment of the extensor tendon injury at PIP and DIP joint, the suture should be secondarily stabilized with a temporary K-wire arthrodesis (diameter 0.8–1.0 mm) (6 weeks immobilization in a neutral position). Extensor tendon injuries of the hand require immobilization using the intrinsic plus position (Fig. 25.4).

Flexor Tendon Injury

Open flexor tendon injuries require a surgical procedure using magnifying glasses. A palmar Bruner's incision is followed by a modified (Zechner) Kessler suture with non-absorbable 4-0 suture material. For fine adaptation, "running-sutures" (a monofil 6-0) is used, either absorbable or non-absorbable (e.g. PDS). Extensive retracted proximal tendon stumps can be produced and refixed, using an additional incision to insert a flexible catheter through the tendon sheath-pulley system and fix the tendon stump to it, to pull

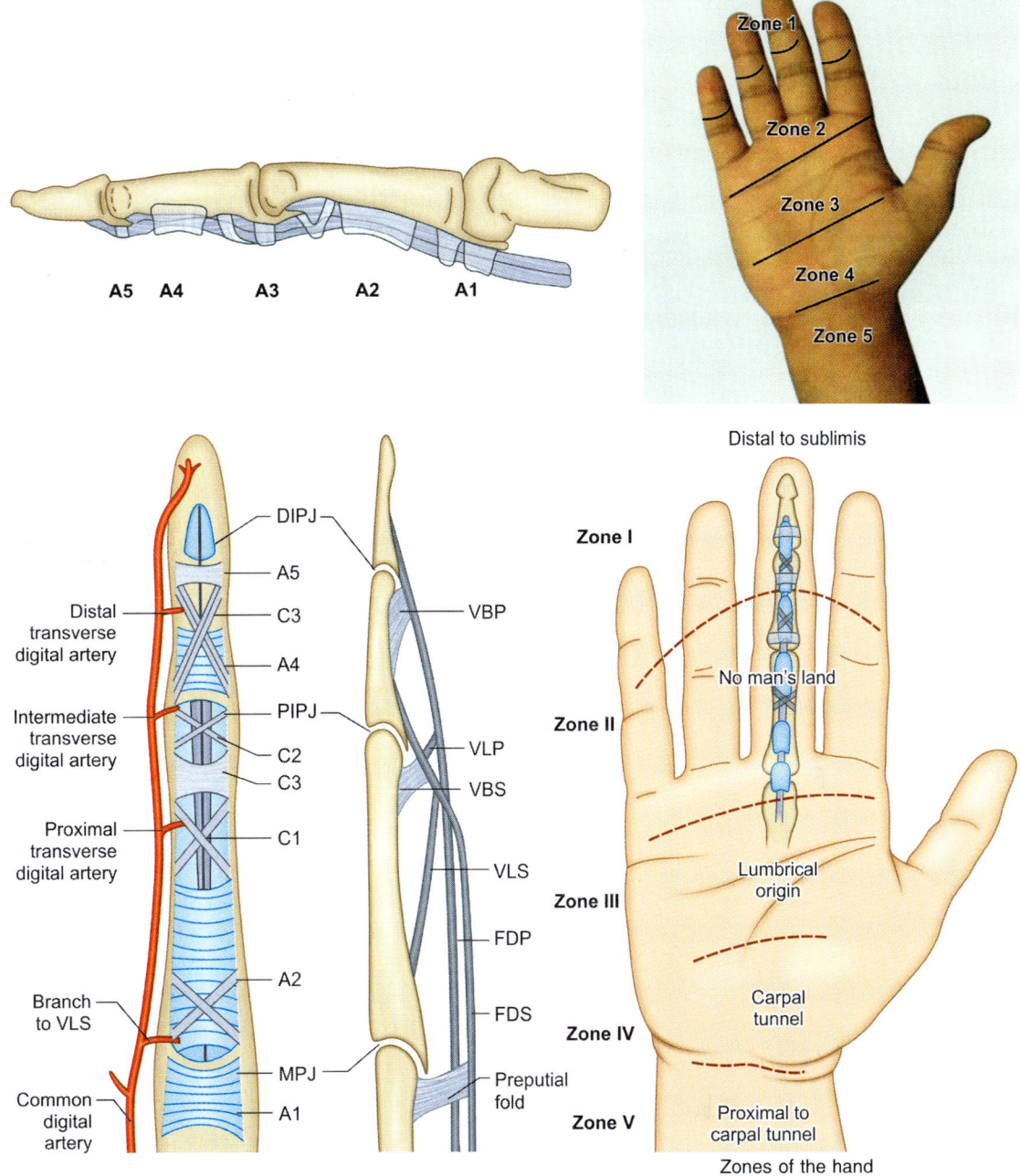

Fig. 25.1: Anatomy of flexor tendons

the tendon further distally. Blunt flexor tendon disruptions are sutured; osseous avulsions are refixed transosseous (using a periosteal flap, if necessary). Incisions should always cross flexion creases transversely or obliquely to avoid contractures (never longitudinal). A2 and A4 pulleys should be preserved to prevent bowstringing and flexion deformity (Fig. 25.5).

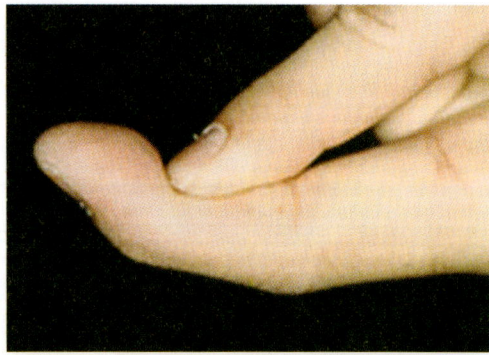

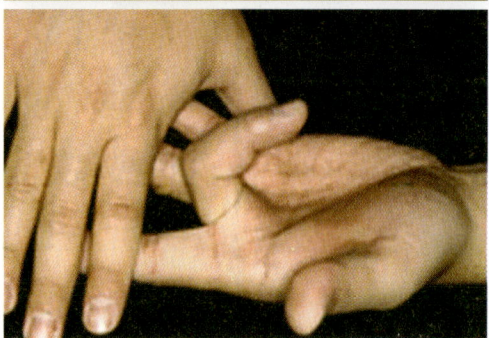

Fig. 25.2: Flexor tendon testing

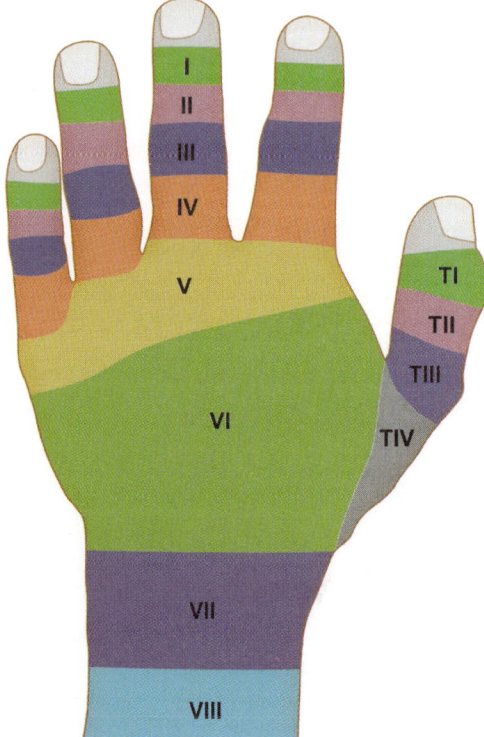

Fig. 25.3: Extensor tendons

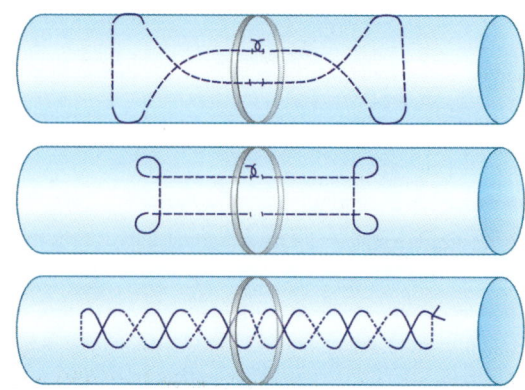

Fig. 25.4: Methods of extensor tendon repair: Modified Bunnell, modified Kessler, and modified Becker

POSTOPERATIVE CARE

Extensor tendon injuries require immobilization transfixation or an "intrinsic plus" cast. Aftercare of flexor tendon injuries should follow the scheme of dynamic early mobilization, as proposed by Kleinert, which allows passive flexion, carried out by a rubber string and active extension.

Early Passive Motion Protocols

- *Duran protocol*
  - Low force and low excursion
  - Active finger extension with patient-assisted passive finger flexion
- *Kleinert protocol*
  - Low force and low excursion
  - Active finger extension, dynamic splint-assisted passive finger flexion
- *Mayo synergistic splint* (Fig. 25.6)
  - Low force and high tendon excursion
  - Adds active wrist motion which increases flexor tendon excursion the most
- Immobilize children and non-compliant patients

COMPLICATIONS

- *Tendon adhesions:* Most common complication following flexor tendon repair

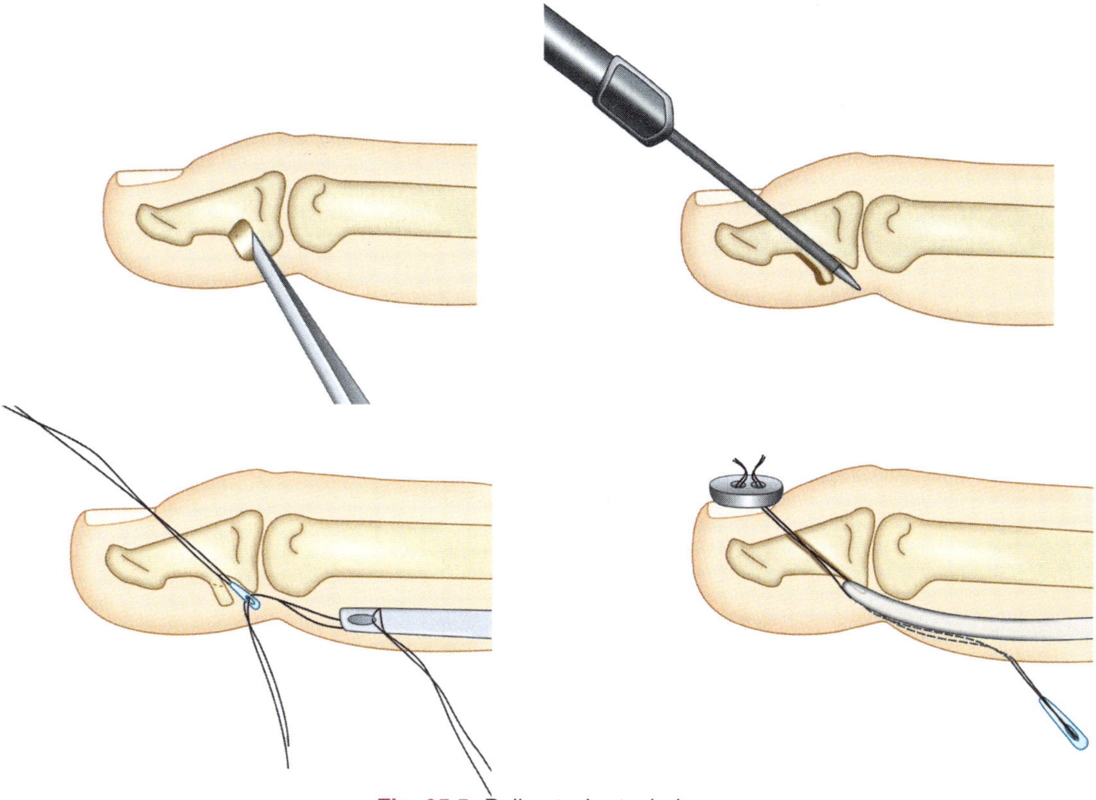

Fig. 25.5: Pull out wire technique

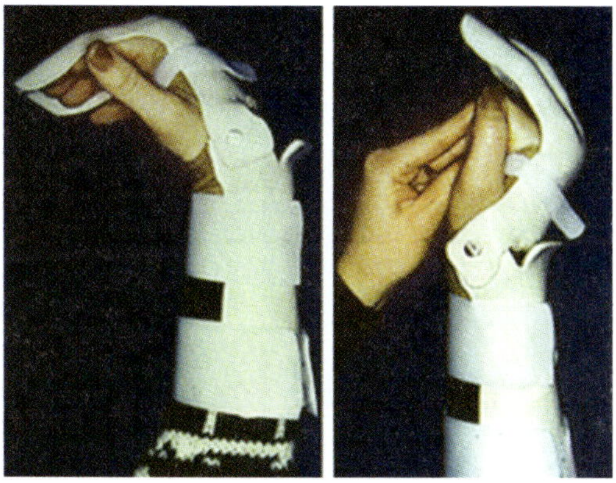

Fig. 25.6: Postoperative splinting

- *Rerupture*
  - 15–25% rerupture rate
  - Treatment
    - If <1 cm of scar is present, resect the scar and perform primary repair

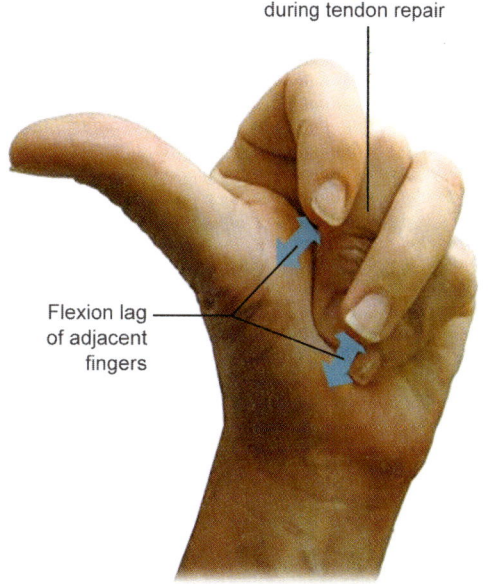

Over-advancement of the FDP during tendon repair

Flexion lag of adjacent fingers

Fig. 25.7: Quadrigia effect

- If >1 cm of scar is present, perform tendon graft
  - If the sheath is intact and allows passage of a pediatric urethral catheter or vascular dilator, perform primary tendon grafting.
  - If the sheath is collapsed, place Hunter rod and perform staged grafting.
- *Joint contracture:* Rates as high as 17%.
- Swan-neck deformity

- Trigger finger
- Lumbrical plus finger
- Quadrigia (Fig. 25.7)

BIBLIOGRAPHY

- http://www.ncbi.nlm.nih.gov/pmc/articles/PMC3377907/
- https://www.youtube.com/watch?v=1z8BdDzdd88
- http://www.orthobullets.com/video/view?id=859

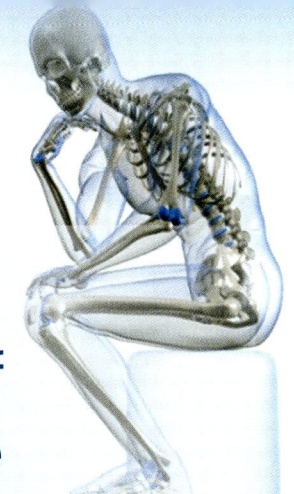

Injuries of the Cervical Spine

Approximately 5–10% of unconscious patients who present to the ED as the result of a motor vehicle accident or fall have a major injury to the cervical spine. Most cervical spine fractures occur predominantly at 2 levels. One-third of injuries occur at the level of C2, and one-half of injuries occur at the level of C6 or C7. Most fatal cervical spine injuries occur in upper cervical levels, either at craniocervical junction C1 or C2.

Cervical spine injuries cause an estimated 6000 deaths and 5000 new cases of quadriplegia each year. Male-to-female ratio is 4:1. Most patients with a cervical spine injury are in their prime and leading an active lifestyle prior to injury. Approximately 80% of patients are aged 18–25 years.

Cervical spine injuries are best classified according to several mechanisms of injury. These include flexion, flexion-rotation, extension, extension-rotation, vertical compression, lateral flexion, and imprecisely understood mechanisms that may result in odontoid fractures and atlanto-occipital dislocation (Fig. 26.1).

FLEXION INJURIES

Common injuries associated with a flexion mechanism include the following:

- *Simple wedge compression fracture without posterior disruption:* The posterior column remains intact, making this a stable fracture that requires only use of a cervical orthosis for treatment.

- *Flexion teardrop fracture:* A flexion teardrop fracture occurs when flexion of the spine, along with vertical axial compression, causes a fracture of the anteroinferior aspect of the vertebral body. A flexion teardrop fracture occurs when flexion of the spine, along with vertical axial compression, causes a fracture of the anteroinferior aspect of the vertebral body (Fig. 26.2).

- *Anterior subluxation:* Posterior ligamentous complexes (nuchal ligament, capsular ligaments, ligamenta flava, posterior longitudinal ligament) rupture. Since the anterior columns remain intact, this fracture is considered mechanically stable by definition.

- *Bilateral facet dislocation:* This injury involves the annulus fibrosus, anterior longitudinal ligament and posterior ligamentous complex. Radiographically, this is seen as a displacement of more than half of the anteroposterior diameter of the vertebral body in the lateral view (Fig. 26.3).

- *Clay-shoveler fracture:* Abrupt flexion of the neck, combined with a heavy upper body and lower neck muscular contraction, results in an oblique fracture of the base of the spinous process, which is avulsed by the intact and powerful supraspinous ligament. Since injury involves only the spinous process, this fracture is considered stable, and it is not associated with neurologic impairment. Management involves only cervical immobilization with an orthotic device for comfort.

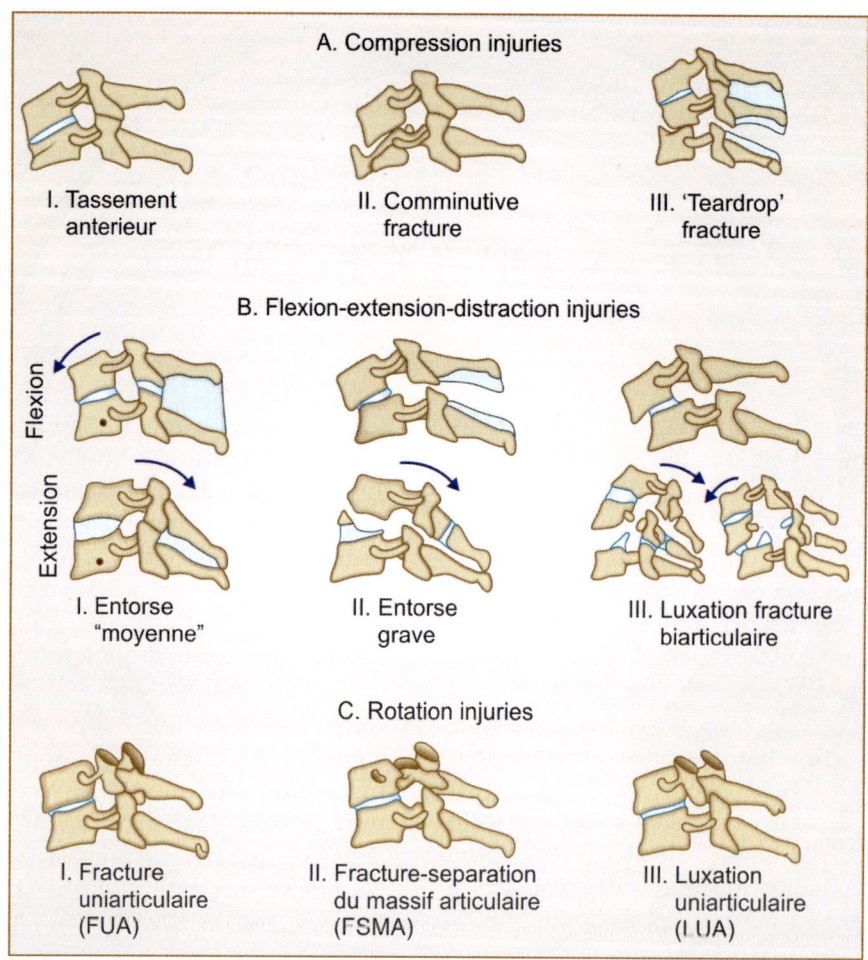

Fig. 26.1: Classification of lower cervical spine injuries

ANTERIOR ATLANTOAXIAL DISLOCATION

Flexion-Rotation Injuries

Common injuries associated with a flexion-rotation mechanism include unilateral facet dislocation and rotary atlantoaxial dislocation. The injury seldom is associated with neurologic deficits. The orthopedic consultant performs initial management, applying cervical traction to attempt closed reduction.

Extension Injuries

Common injuries associated with an extension mechanism include hangman's fracture, extension teardrop fracture, fracture of the posterior arch of C1 (posterior neural arch fracture of C1) and posterior atlantoaxial dislocation (Fig. 26.4).

Hangman's fracture: The name of this injury is derived from the typical fracture that occurs after hangings. Presently, it commonly is caused by motor vehicle collisions and entails bilateral fractures through the pedicles of C2 due to hyperextension. Although considered an unstable fracture, it seldom is associated with spinal injury, since the anteroposterior diameter of the spinal canal is the greatest at this level, and the fractured pedicles allow decompression (Fig. 26.5).

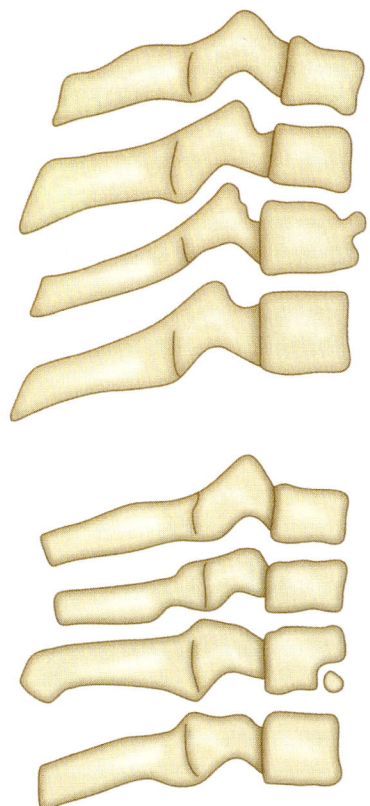

Fig. 26.2: Wedge compression fracture and teardrop fracture

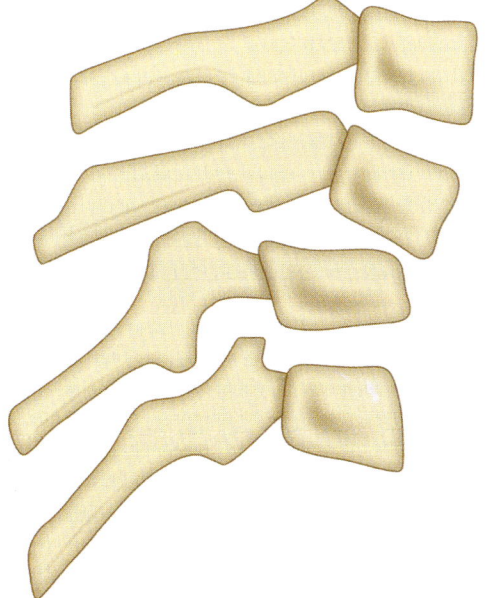

Fig. 26.3: Bilateral facet dislocation

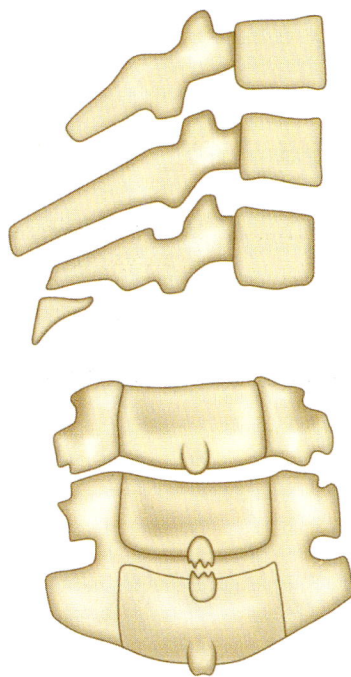

Fig. 26.4: Clay-shoveler's fracture

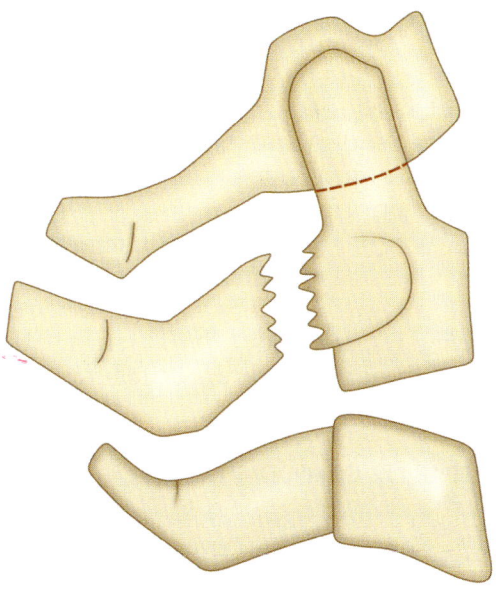

Fig. 26.5: Hangman's fracture

VERTICAL (AXIAL) COMPRESSION INJURY

Common injuries associated with a vertical compression mechanism include Jefferson

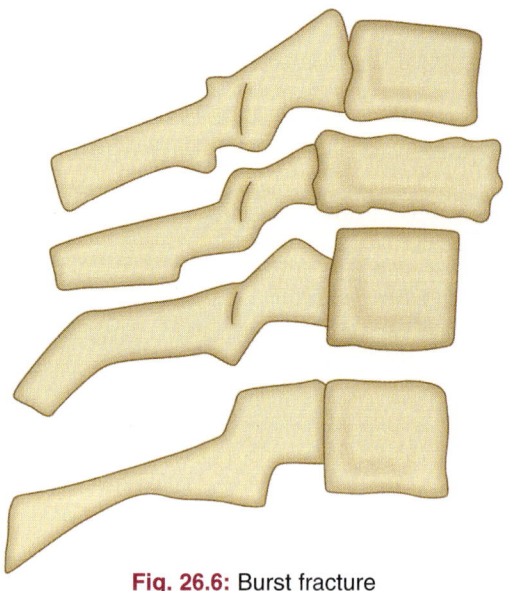

Fig. 26.6: Burst fracture

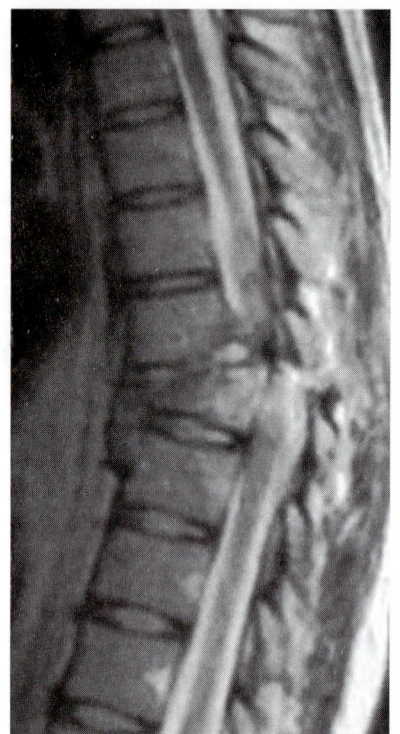

Fig. 26.7: Burst fracture—MRI scan

fracture (burst fracture of the ring of C1), burst fracture (dispersion, axial loading), atlas fracture, and isolated fracture of the lateral mass of C1 (pillar fracture) (Fig. 26.6).

Posterior protrusion of the middle column may extend into the spinal canal and can be associated with anterior cord syndrome. Burst fractures always require an axial CT scan or MRI to document amount of middle column retropulsion (Fig. 26.7).

Initial management of burst fractures with a loss in height of more than 25%, retropulsion, or neurologic deficit is accomplished by applying traction with cervical tongs. When none of those problems exists, the fracture is considered stable.

MULTIPLE OR COMPLEX INJURIES

Common injuries associated with multiple or complex mechanisms include odontoid fracture, fracture of the transverse process of C2 (lateral flexion), atlanto-occipital dislocation (flexion or extension with a shearing component), and occipital condyle fracture (vertical compression with lateral bending).

UPPER CERVICAL SPINE (OCCIPUT TO C2) INJURIES

Injuries at the upper cervical level are considered unstable because of their location. Nevertheless, since the diameter of the spinal canal is the greatest at the level of C2, spinal cord injury from compression is the exception rather than the rule. Common injuries include fracture of the atlas, atlantoaxial subluxation, odontoid fracture, and hangman's fracture. Less common injuries include occipital condyle fracture, atlanto-occipital dislocation, atlantoaxial rotary subluxation (see Flexion-rotation injury above), and C2 lateral mass fracture.

ODONTOID PROCESS FRACTURES

The three types of odontoid process fractures are classified based on the anatomic level at which the fracture occurs (Fig. 26.8):
- *Type I odontoid fracture* is an avulsion of the tip of the dens at the insertion site of

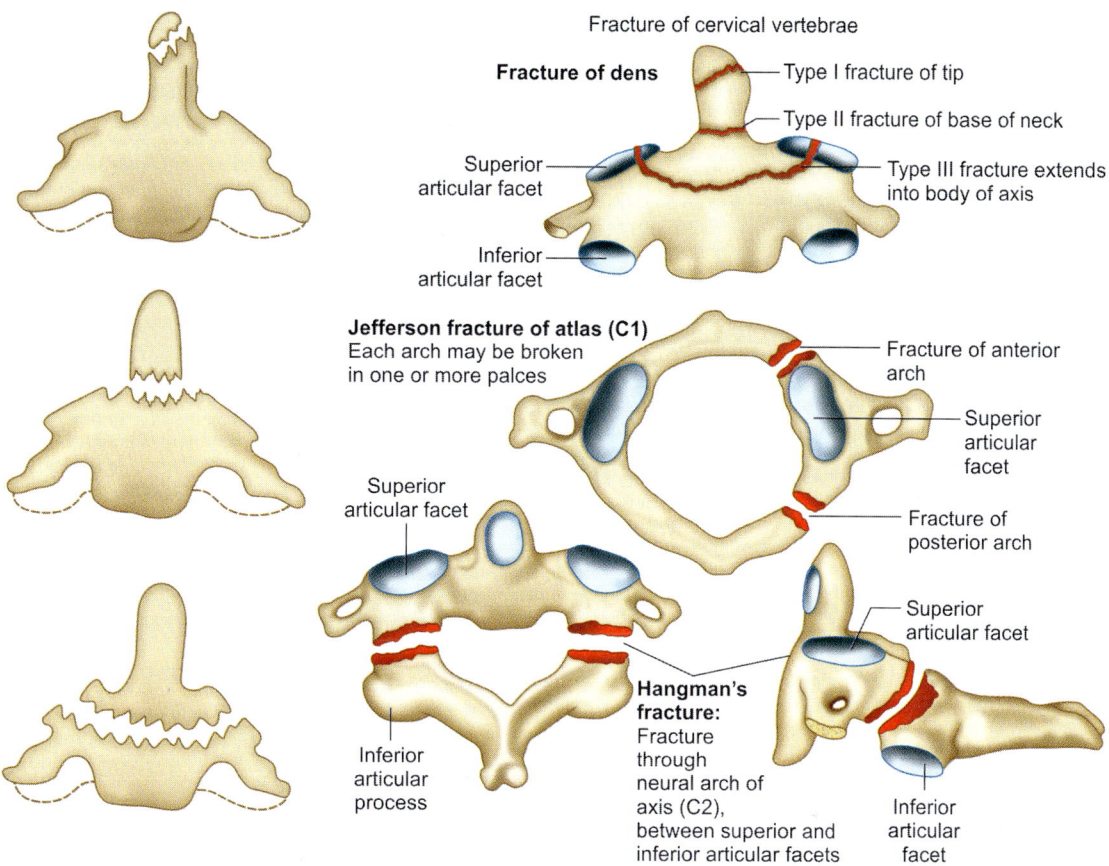

Fracture of cervical vertebrae

Fracture of dens

Type I fracture of tip

Type II fracture of base of neck

Superior articular facet

Type III fracture extends into body of axis

Inferior articular facet

Jefferson fracture of atlas (C1)
Each arch may be broken in one or more palces

Fracture of anterior arch

Superior articular facet

Superior articular facet

Fracture of posterior arch

Superior articular facet

Hangman's fracture:
Fracture through neural arch of axis (C2), between superior and inferior articular facets

Inferior articular process

Inferior articular facet

Fig. 26.8: Types of odontoid fracture

the alar ligament. Although a type I fracture is mechanically stable, it often is seen in association with atlanto-occipital dislocation and must be ruled out because of this potentially life-threatening complication.

- *Type II fractures* occur at the base of the dens and are the most common odontoid fractures. This type is associated with a high prevalence of non-union due to the limited vascular supply and small area of cancellous bone.
- *Type III odontoid fracture* occurs when the fracture line extends into the body of the axis. Non-union is not a major problem with these injuries because of a good blood supply and the greater amount of cancellous bone.

Common findings on physical examination in cervical spine injury include:

- Spinal shock
  - Flaccidity
  - Areflexia
  - Loss of anal sphincter tone
  - Fecal incontinence
  - Priapism
  - Loss of bulbocavernosus reflex
- Neurogenic shock
  - Hypotension
  - Paradoxical bradycardia
  - Flushed, dry, and warm peripheral skin
- Autonomic dysfunction
  - Ileus
  - Urinary retention
  - Poikilothermia

Radiographic evaluation is indicated in the following:

- Patients who exhibit neurologic deficits consistent with a cord lesion.
- Patients with an altered sensorium from head injury or intoxication.
- Patients who complain about neck pain or tenderness.
- Patients who do not complain about neck pain or tenderness but have significant distracting injuries.

A standard trauma series is composed of 5 views: Cross-table lateral, swimmer's, oblique, odontoid, and anteroposterior. Check alignment of cervical spine by following three imaginary contour lines (Fig. 26.9):

1. The first line connects the anterior margins of all the vertebrae and is referred to as the anterior contour line.
2. The second line should connect the posterior aspect of all vertebrae in a similar way and is referred to as the posterior contour line.
3. The third line should connect the bases of the spinous processes and is referred to as the spinolaminar contour line.

Each of these lines should form a smooth lordotic curve. Suspect bony or ligamentous injury, if disruption is seen in the contour lines.

The American College of Orthopaedic Surgeons now recommends routine cervical spine screening via CT scan instead of plain radiography.

MANAGEMENT

The main goal in spinal cord injury treatment is to keep the highest level of function possible. Treatment is also aimed at preventing complications and further injury. Treatment may be non-surgical and/or surgical.

Prehospital Care

When a cervical spine injury is suspected, minimize neck movement during transport to the treating facility. Ideally, transport the patient on a backboard with a semirigid collar, with the neck stabilized on the sides of the head with sand bags or foam blocks taped from side-to-side (of the board), across the forehead (Fig. 26.10).

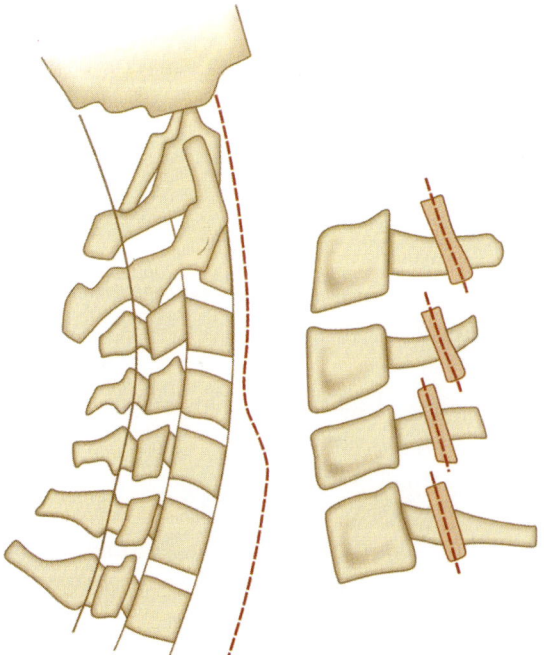

Fig. 26.9: Anterior, posterior and spinolaminar lines

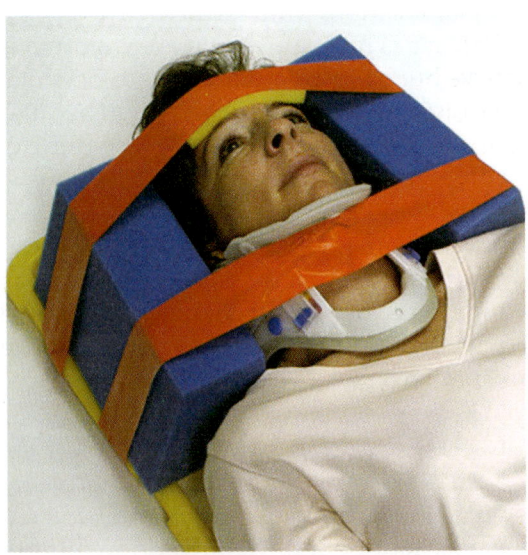

Fig. 26.10: Splinting of injured neck

Emergency Department Care

If spinal malalignment is identified, place the patient in skeletal traction with tongs as soon as possible (with very few exceptions), even if no evidence of neurologic deficit exists.

Administer steroids to any patient with blunt cervical spine injury and associated neurologic symptoms of less than 8 hours in onset.

- *Load:* Methylprednisolone 30 mg/kg IV over 15 minutes.
- *Infusion* (begin 45 minutes after bolus)
  - *Within 0–3 hours of injury:* Methylprednisolone 5.4 mg/kg/hr IV for 23 hours.
  - *Within 3–8 hours of injury:* Methylprednisolone 5.4 mg/kg/hr IV for 47 hours.
- All patients receiving steroids must also have the following ordered: Pepcid 20 mg IV/PO/FT Q12 or prevacid 30 mg PO/FT daily.
- Routine finger stick blood sugar monitoring is indicated.

Neurogenic Shock

Neurogenic shock is spinal shock that causes vasomotor instability because of loss of sympathetic tone.

Patients with neurogenic shock are hypotensive but have paradoxical bradycardia.

Flushed, dry, and warm peripheral skin (in contrast to findings with hypovolemic or cardiogenic shock) may be present. Other signs of autonomic dysfunction include ileus, urinary retention, and poikilothermia.

Loss of anal sphincter tone with fecal incontinence and priapism suggest spinal shock. Return of bulbocavernosus reflex heralds resolution of spinal shock. Besides spinal shock, complete and incomplete spinal cord syndromes may occur.

Spinal shock mimics a complete spinal cord lesion. Emergency physicians should wait until spinal shock resolves to make an accurate estimate of the patient's prognosis.

Incomplete cord syndromes are described and include anterior spinal cord syndrome, central spinal cord syndrome, Brown-Séquard syndrome, and less frequent, cord syndromes at high cervical levels (i.e. Horner syndrome, posteroinferior cerebellar artery syndrome).

Surgical Treatment

If the injury primarily involves the anterior column, a Smith-Robinson or standard anterior approach to the spine is used to allow anterior decompression and reconstruction with either allograft or autograft iliac crest or fibula, followed by stabilization with anterior locking plates.

The posterior approach is indicated when the pathoanatomy involves the posterior elements and is the basic midline approach with muscle retraction off the cervical spine to the lateral aspect of the facet joints bilaterally.

Occasionally, a dual approach is necessary to remove an offending disk fragment anteriorly prior to reduction, followed by posterior stabilization with anterior reconstruction. These global injuries are usually quite unstable, and they benefit from both anterior and posterior reconstruction.

WHIPLASH INJURY (Fig. 26.11)

Whiplash is a non-medical term describing a range of injuries to the neck caused by or related to a sudden distortion of the neck associated with extension, although the exact injury mechanism(s) remain unknown. Whiplash is commonly associated with motor vehicle accidents, usually when the vehicle has been hit in the rear; however, the injury can be sustained in many other ways, including head banging, bungee jumping and falls. It is one of the main injuries covered by insurance. Before the invention of the car, whiplash injuries were called "railway spine" as they were noted mostly in connection with train collisions.

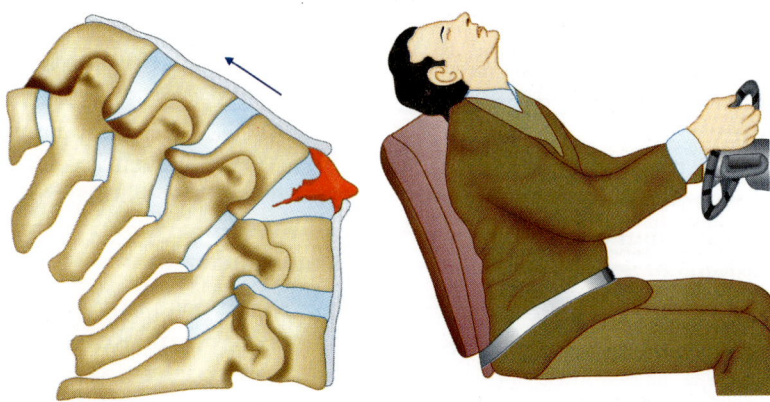

Tear of intervertebral disc and anterior longitudinal ligament may cause persistent neck, scapular and shoulder pain, necessitating disc removal and inerbody fusion

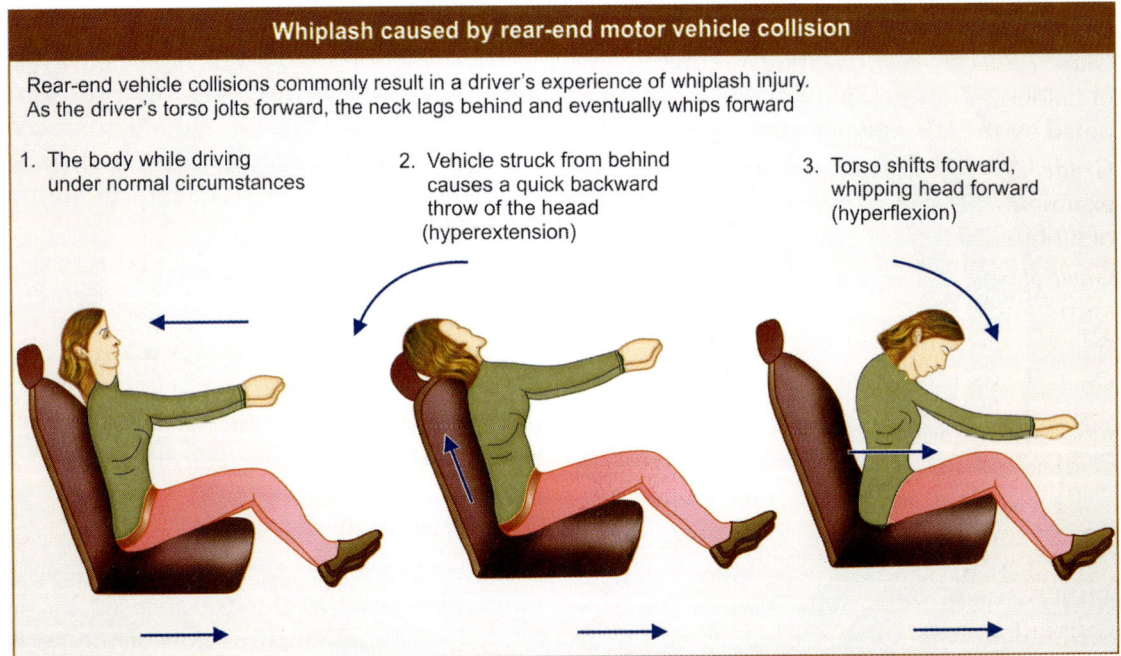

Fig. 26.11: Whiplash injury

Whiplash can be described as a sudden strain to the muscles, bones and nerves in the neck. There are four phases that occur during "whiplash": Initial position (before the collision), retraction, extension and rebound. In the initial position, there is no force on the neck, it is stable due to inertia. Anterior longitudinal ligament injuries in whiplash may lead to cervical instability. They explain that during the retraction phase that is when the actual "whiplash" occurs, since there is an unusual loading of soft tissues. The next phase is the extension, the whole neck and head switches to extension, and it is stopped or limited by the head restraint. The rebound phase transpires as a result of the phases that are mentioned.

During the retraction phase, the spine forms an S-shaped curve, caused by the flexion in the upper planes and hyperextension at the lower planes, and this exceeds their physiological limits. In this phase, the injuries occur to the lower cervical vertebrae. At the extension phase, all cervical vertebrae and the head are fully extended, but do not surpass their physiological limits. Most of the injuries happen in C5 and C6.

The Québec Task Force (QTF) has divided whiplash-associated disorders into five grades:

- *Grade 0:* No neck pain, stiffness, or any physical signs are noticed.
- *Grade 1:* Neck complaints of pain, stiffness or tenderness only but no physical signs are noted by the examining physician.
- *Grade 2:* Neck complaints and the examining physician finds decreased range of motion and point tenderness in the neck.
- *Grade 3:* Neck complaints plus neurological signs such as decreased deep tendon reflexes, weakness and sensory deficits.
- *Grade 4:* Neck complaints and fracture or dislocation, or injury to the spinal cord.

Symptoms remaining more than six months after trauma is labelled whiplash syndrome. The main purpose with early rehabilitation is to reduce the risk for development of whiplash syndrome.

Current research supports that active mobilization rather than a soft collar results in a more prompt recovery both in the short- and long-term perspective. Furthermore, Schnabel and colleagues stated that the soft collar is not a suitable medium for rehabilitation, and the best way of recovery is to include an active rehabilitation program that includes physical therapy exercises and postural modifications.

GUIDELINES FOR THE TREATMENT OF CERVICAL FRACTURES WITH OR WITHOUT SPINAL CORD INJURY

Admission Guidelines

All patients with the following clinical conditions MUST be admitted to the ICU for close respiratory and neurological monitoring. The pre-printed Spinal Cord Injury Orders will be used on all patients.

- Radiographic evidence of unstable cervical fracture or dislocation (i.e. atlanto-occippital dislocation, bilateral subaxial facet dislocation,..) and/or
- Clinical or radiographic evidence of spinal cord injury
- All field collars should be changed out to a permanent rigid collar (Aspen or Miami-J) within 6 hours of admission.

Admission location and monitoring criteria for patients with documented cervical fractures without radiographic evidence of dislocation (i.e. transverse foramen fractures, spinous process fractures, ...) and without clinical or radiographic evidence of spinal cord injury is left to the discretion of the admitting attending physician.

Immobilization Guidelines

Unstable cervical fracture or dislocation, with/without spinal cord injury:

- All patients will be maintained in a rigid cervical collar with strict cervical and log roll precautions until temporary stabilization using halo traction or halo vest is applied. (Note: If the patient will be maintained in halo traction for >24 hours, he/she should be placed on a rotorest bed to promote respiratory toileting, to be discontinued after surgical fixation.)
- Definitive operative stabilization of such fracture dislocations should occur within the first 24–48 hours of hospitalization

Stable cervical fracture without dislocation, without spinal cord injury:

- All patients will be maintained in a rigid cervical collar, unless otherwise determined by the attending physician.
- Log roll precautions, operative intervention and length of collar use to be determined by the attending physician.

Neurological Examination

- Every 1–2 hours until definitive stabilization is achieved and for at least 24 hours postoperatively, unless otherwise determined by the attending physician.
- After 24 hours, the frequency of neurological examination may be progressively weaned as determined by the attending physician.
- Evaluation should be based upon the ASIA scoring system, unless otherwise determined by the attending physician.

Steroids Administration

- Steroids can be administered in all patients with evidence of spinal cord injury (excluding penetrating injury and/or nerve root injury) unless contraindicated by co-morbidities or injuries as determined by the attending physician.
- *Load:* Methylprednisolone 30 mg/kg IV over 15 minutes
- *Infusion* (begin 45 minutes after bolus):
  - *Within 0–3 hours of injury:* Methylprednisolone 5.4 mg/kg/hr IV for 23 hours.
  - *Within 3–8 hours of injury:* Methylprednisolone 5.4 mg/kg/hr IV for 47 hours.
- All patients receiving steroids must also have the following ordered:
  - Pepcid 20 mg IV/PO/FT Q12 or prevacid 30 mg PO/FT daily
- Routine finger stick blood sugar monitoring is needed.

Blood Pressure Management

- To promote spinal cord perfusion, MAPs will be maintained >85 mm Hg for 7 days post injury.
- Pressures should be maintained using the following:
  - Dopamine 2–10 µg/kg/min IV
  - Phenylephrine 5–200 µg/min IV
- When able to take POs institute one of the following oral agents and begin weaning glucose tolerance test.
  - Ephedrine 25 mg PO Q6 (maximum dose 150 mg/24 hours)
  - NaCl tablets 1–2 g PO TID (maximum dose 4 g TID
  - Florinef 0.2 mg PO daily (maximum 1 mg/24 hours)
  - Midodrine 10 mg 30 min before sitting up or TID (do not use in combination with ephedrine)
- Institute abdominal binding and elastic (ACE) bandages to lower extremities when placed in the sitting position or cleared for OOB activity.

Respiratory Management

- All patients must receive continuous oxygen saturation monitoring (maintain a low threshold for intubation in high cervical injury C5 or above).
- Initiate quad cough and suctioning Q2 hours when appropriate.
- Incentive spirometer Q2 hours when appropriate.
- Albuterol 2.5 mg in 3cc NS per nebulizer, every 6 hours in the intubated and high cervical (C5 or above) non-intubated patients.

DVT Prophylaxis

- Upon admit, all patients will receive SCS with antiembolic stockings unless contra-indicated by lower extremity injuries.

- Non-operative cases will receive enoxaparin 30 mg SQ BID within 48 hours of admission, unless otherwise determined by the attending physician.
- Operative cases will have enoxaparin 30 mg SQ BID started within 48 hours of surgery regardless of drain placement.
- DVT prophylaxis in patients with traumatic brain injury, in addition to their spinal injury, will be evaluated on a case by case basis by the attending neurosurgeon.

Additional Treatment Guidelines

- All patients not on a rotorest bed will be turned every 2 hours.
- All patients will initially receive an indwelling Foley catheter with Q2 I&O monitoring.
- The patient will initially be allowed an attempt at self-evacuation, this will be followed up with a bladder scan or straight catheterization, if results provide proof of retention (>100 cc unless history significant for BPH then may liberalize to 150 cc) a routine catheterization program will be instituted.
- I&O catheterization will begin once urine output is <2 liters in 24 hours and will be ordered in the following manner:
  - I&O catheterization Q6 hours, if >400cc change frequency to Q4 hours

- All patients will have the following consults within 48 hours of admission unless contraindicated secondary to instability (emphasis on early mobilization:
  - Physical therapy
  - Occupational therapy
  - Speech therapy for swallow evaluation
  - If unable to pass or participate in swallow evaluation, a feeding tube will be placed and nutritional support initiated within 48 hours of admission
  - Physical medicine and rehabilitation
- All patients with evidence of altered rectal tone, perineal sensation, or with evidence of lack of bowel function will be started on the following bowel regimen within 24–48 hours of admission
  - Colace 100 mg PO/FT BID
  - Bisacodyl suppository 10 mg PR with digital stimulation administered at the same time daily.

BIBLIOGRAPHY

- emedicine.medscape.com/article/824380-overview
- http://www.spinalinjury101.org/
- http://www.racgp.org.au/
- http://www.ncbi.nlm.nih.gov/
- http://www.radiologyassistant.nl/
- http://orthosurg.ucsf.edu/
- https://www.youtube.com/watch?v=U9CnRFj3rWE

Injuries of Thoracic Spine

Fractures of the thoracic and lumbar spine may result from high-energy trauma, such as:

- Car or motorcycle crash
- Fall from height
- Sports accident
- Violent act, such as a gunshot wound

The initial evaluation of a patient with a thoracic spinal fracture should account for a possible multisystem trauma pattern (polytrauma). In such cases, possible cranial, abdominal, pelvic, and extremity injuries must be managed (Figs 27.1 to 27.3).

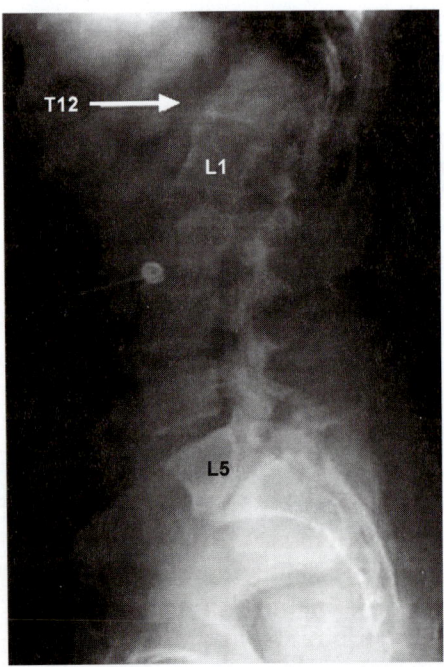

Fig. 27.1: Thoracic spine injury

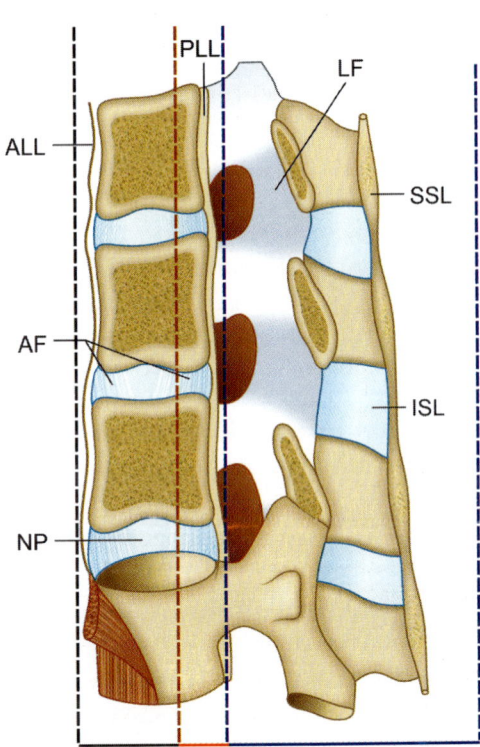

Fig. 27.2: Three columns of spine

TREATMENT

Treatment for a fracture of the thoracic or lumbar spine will depend on:

- Other injuries and their treatment
- The particular fracture pattern

Once the trauma team has stabilized all other life-threatening injuries, the doctor will evaluate the spinal fracture pattern and decide whether spine surgery is needed.

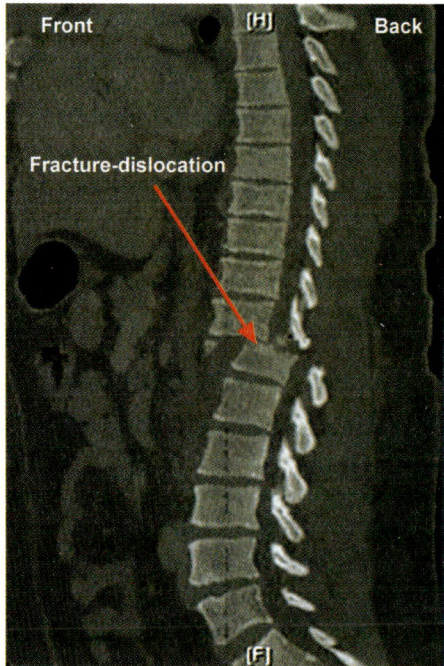

Fig. 27.3: Fracture dislocation

Flexion Fracture Pattern

Non-surgical treatment: Most flexion injuries, including stable burst fractures and osteoporotic compression fractures, can be treated with bracing for 6 to 12 weeks. By gradually increasing physical activity and doing rehabilitation exercises, most patients avoid post-injury problems.

Surgical treatment: Surgery is typically required for unstable burst fractures that have:
- Significant comminution (multiple bone fragments)
- Severe loss of vertebral body height
- Excessive forward bending or angulation at the injury site
- Significant nerve injury due to parts of the vertebral body or disc pinching the spinal cord

These fractures should be treated surgically with decompression of the spinal canal and stabilization of the fracture. The procedure to decompress the spine is called laminectomy.

In a laminectomy, the doctor removes the bony arch that forms the backside of the spinal canal (lamina), along with any bone or other structures that are pressing on the spinal cord. Laminectomy relieves pressure on the spinal cord by providing extra space for it to drift backward.

To perform the laminectomy, your doctor will access your spine with an incision either on your side or on your back. Both approaches allow for safe removal of the structures compressing the spinal cord, while preventing further injury.

Extension Fracture Pattern

Treatment for extension injuries will depend on:
- Where the spine fails.
- Whether the bones can be fit together again (reduction) using a brace or cast.

Non-surgical treatment: Extension fractures that occur only through the vertebral body can typically be treated without surgery. These fractures should be observed closely while the patient wears a brace or cast for 12 weeks.

Surgical treatment: Surgery is usually necessary, if there is an injury to the posterior (back) ligaments of the spine. In addition, if the fracture falls through the discs of the spine, surgery should be performed to stabilize the fracture.

Rotation Fracture Pattern

Non-surgical treatment: Transverse process fractures are predominantly treated with gradual increase in motion, with or without bracing, based on comfort level.

Surgical treatment: Fracture-dislocations of the thoracic and lumbar spine are caused by very high-energy trauma. They can be extremely unstable injuries that often result in serious spinal cord or nerve damage. These injuries require stabilization through surgery. The ideal timing of surgery can often be complicated. Surgery is sometimes delayed because of other serious, life-threatening injuries.

Surgical Procedure

The ultimate goals of surgery are to:
- Achieve adequate reduction (return the bones into their proper position)
- Relieve pressure on the spinal cord and nerves
- Allow for early movement

BIBLIOGRAPHY

- http://orthoinfo.aaos.org
- https://www.youtube.com/watch?v=14gFn_yn5k8
- https://www.youtube.com/watch?v=3Ia5L78UKHI

Injuries of Lumbar Spine

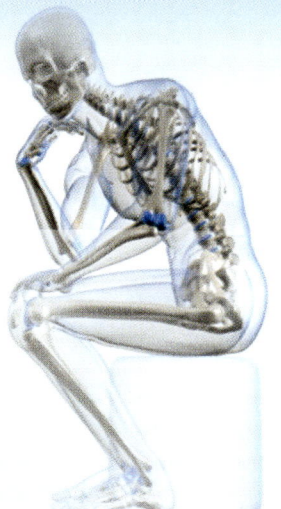

Studies document that 7–13% of all sports injuries in intercollegiate athletes are low back injuries. The most common back injuries are muscle strains (60%) followed by disc injuries (7%).

A lumbar spine injury may take the form of a muscle strain, in which the muscles are stretched or torn; or a lumbar sprain may occur in which the ligaments are torn. Strains are defined as tears, either partial or complete, of the muscle-tendon unit. All major ligaments (i.e. anterior longitudinal, posterior longitudinal, yellow, intertransversal, capsular, interspinosus, supraspinatus) can sustain sprains; however, the posterior ligaments are more prone to injury.

Majority of thoracic and lumbar injuries occur within the region between T11 and L1. Neurologic deficit reportedly occurs in approximately 15 to 20% of thoracolumbar fractures and dislocations.

Fractures of the thoracic and lumbar spine may result from high-energy trauma, such as:
- Car or motorcycle crash
- Fall from height
- Sports accident
- Violent act, such as a gunshot wound

Many times, these patients have additional serious injuries that require rapid treatment. The spinal cord may also be injured, depending on the severity of the fracture. Spinal fractures may also be caused by bone insufficiency. For example, people with osteoporosis, tumors, or other underlying conditions that weaken the bone can fracture a vertebra even during low-impact activities.

The three major types of spine fracture patterns are (Fig. 28.1):
- Flexion
- Extension
- Rotation

Unstable vertebral injuries are those in which bony and ligamentous integrity is

American Spinal Injury Association Impairment Scale (AIS) (Fig. 28.2)

Classification	Description
A	*Complete:* No motor or sensory function is preserved below the level of injury, including the sacral segments S4–S5
B	*Incomplete:* Sensory, but not motor, function is preserved below the neurologic level and some sensation in the sacral segments S4–S5
C	*Incomplete:* Motor function is preserved below the neurologic level, however, more than half of key muscles below the neurologic level have a muscle grade less than 3 (i.e. not strong enough to move against gravity)
D	*Incomplete:* Motor function is preserved below the neurologic level, and at least half of key muscles below the neurologic level have a muscle grade of 3 or more (i.e. joints can be moved against gravity)
E	*Normal:* Motor and sensory functions are normal

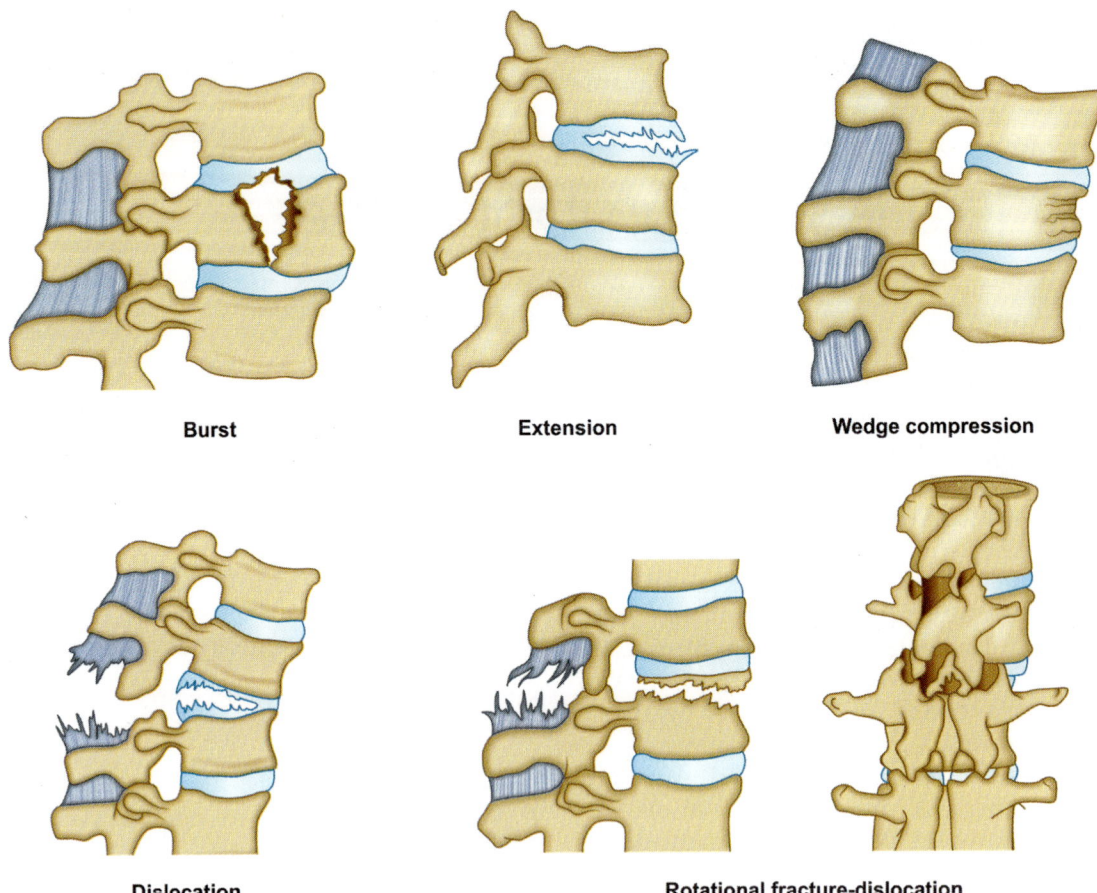

Burst   **Extension**   **Wedge compression**

Dislocation   **Rotational fracture-dislocation**

Fig. 28.1: Types of lumbar spine fracture

disrupted sufficiently that free movement can occur, potentially compressing the spinal cord or its vascular supply and resulting in marked pain and potential worsening of neurologic function. Such vertebral movement may occur even with a shift in patient position (e.g. for ambulance transport, during initial evaluation). Stable fractures are able to resist such movement.

FLEXION FRACTURE PATTERN

- *Compression fracture:* While the front (anterior) of the vertebra breaks and loses height, the back (posterior) part of it does not. This type of fracture is usually stable (the bones have not moved out of place) and

is rarely associated with neurologic problems. Compression fractures commonly occur in patients with osteoporosis.

- *Axial burst fracture:* In this type of fracture, the vertebra loses height on both the front and back sides. It is often caused by landing on the feet after falling from a significant height (Fig. 28.3).

EXTENSION FRACTURE PATTERN

Flexion/distraction (chance) fracture: The vertebra is literally pulled apart (distraction). This type of fracture can occur in a head-on car collision when the upper body is thrown forward while the pelvis is stabilized by a lap seat belt.

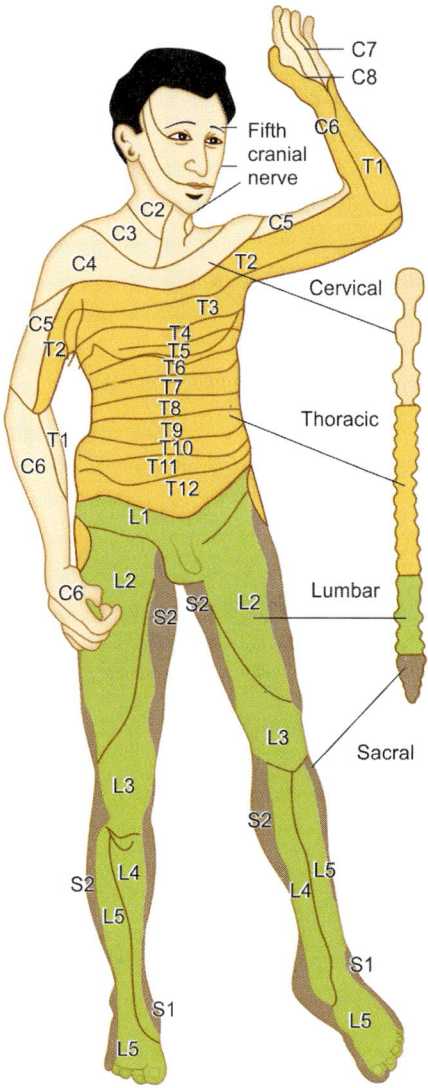

Fig. 28.2: Dermatomes

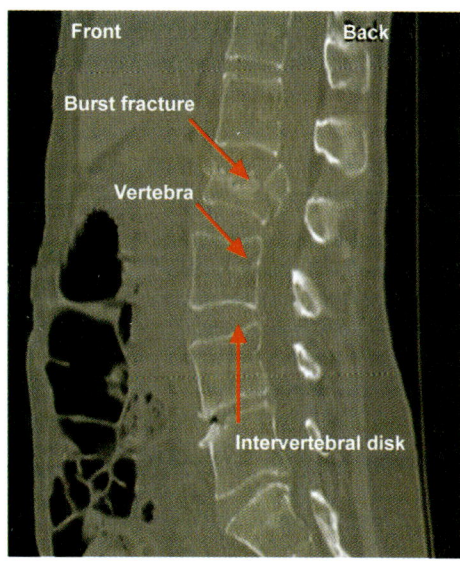

Fig. 28.3: Burst fracture

ROTATION FRACTURE PATTERN

- *Transverse process fracture:* This uncommon fracture results from rotation or extreme sideways (lateral) bending. It does not usually affect stability.
- *Fracture-dislocation:* This is an unstable injury involving bone and/or soft tissue in which a vertebra moves off an adjacent vertebra (displacement). These injuries frequently cause serious spinal cord compression.

TREATMENT

- Immobilization
- Maintenance of oxygenation and spinal cord perfusion
- Supportive care
- Surgical stabilization when appropriate (Fig. 28.4)
- Long-term symptomatic care and rehabilitation

The therapeutic goal for neurogenic shock is adequate perfusion with the following parameters:

- A systolic blood pressure (BP) of 90–100 mm Hg should be achieved; systolic BPs in this range are typical for patients with complete cord lesions. Compelling animal and human studies recommend maintenance of systolic BP above 90 mm Hg and to avoid any hypotensive episodes.
- The most important treatment consideration is to maintain adequate oxygenation and perfusion of the injured spinal cord; supplemental oxygenation and/or mechanical ventilation may be required.
- Heart rate should be 60–100 beats per minute (bpm) in normal sinus rhythm.

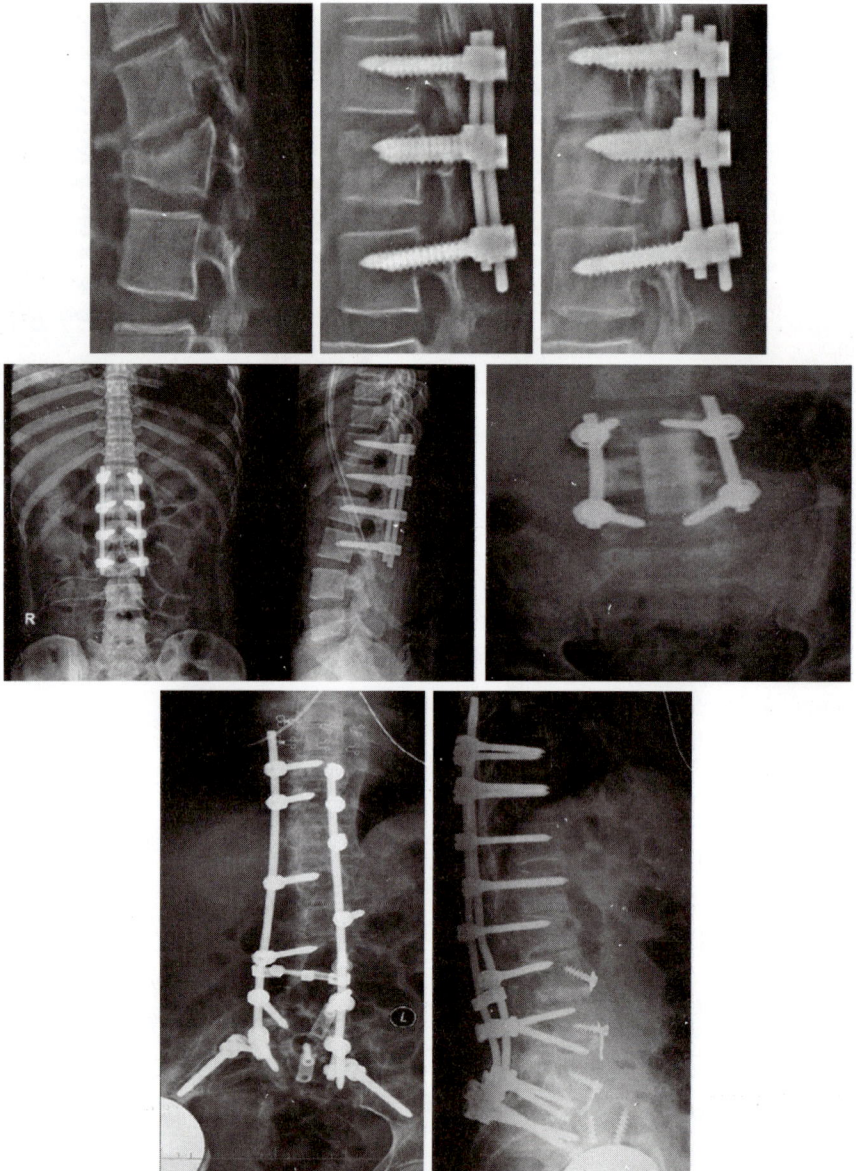

Fig. 28.4: Surgical stabilization

- Haemodynamically significant bradycardia may be treated with atropine.
- Urine output should be more than 30 ml/h; placement of a Foley catheter to monitor urine output and to decompress the neurogenic bladder is essential.
- Rarely, inotropic support with dopamine or norepinephrine is required; this should be reserved for patients who have decreased urinary output despite adequate fluid resuscitation; usually, low doses of dopamine in the 2 to 5 µg/kg/min range are sufficient.
- Prevent hypothermia
- Overall, the benefit from steroids is considered modest at best, but for patients

with complete or incomplete quadriplegia, a small improvement in motor strength in one or more muscles can provide important functional gains.

- The administration of steroids remains an institutional and physician preference in spinal cord injury. Nevertheless, the administration of high-dose steroids within 8 hours of injury for all patients with acute spinal cord injury is practiced by most physicians.
- The current recommendation is to treat all patients with spinal cord injury according to the local/regional protocol. If steroids are recommended, they should be initiated within 8 hours of injury with the following steroid protocol: Methylprednisolone 30 mg/kg bolus over 15 minutes and an infusion of methylprednisolone at 5.4 mg/kg/h for 23 hours beginning 45 minutes after the bolus.

Current research is focused on advancing our understanding of four key principles of spinal cord repair:

- *Neuroprotection*—protecting surviving nerve cells from further damage.
- *Regeneration*—stimulating the regrowth of axons and targeting their connections appropriately.
- *Cell replacement*—replacing damaged nerve or glial cells.
- Retraining CNS circuits and plasticity to restore body functions.

Studies in animals have shown that a transplantation of stem cells or stem-cell-derived cells may contribute to spinal cord repair by:

- Replacing the nerve cells that have died as a result of the injury.
- Generating new supporting cells that will reform the insulating nerve sheath (myelin)

and act as a bridge across the injury to stimulate re-growth of damaged axons.

- Protecting the cells at the injury site from further damage by releasing protective substances such as growth factors, and soaking up toxins such as free radicals, when introduced into the spinal cord shortly after injury.
- Preventing spread of the injury by suppressing the damaging inflammation that can occur after injury.

Technological developments over the last two centuries have advanced the spinal surgeon's capability to service the needs of the spinal cord injured person. While the role that surgery can play in shortening hospitalization for tetraplegics has yet to be proven, it does play a much needed role in the correction of instability and prevention of deformity when the possibility of these conditions exist. Surgical intervention for purposes of neural decompression has yet to be proven as justifiable in view of the risks involved. All surgical procedures must be undertaken only after due consideration of the patients' general medical condition, including coexisting trauma, the potential for and actual instability and deformity of the spine, and the neurological level and degree of incompleteness of the patient.

Currently, there are no defined standards existing regarding the timing of decompression and stabilization in spinal cord injury. The role of immediate surgical intervention is limited.

BIBLIOGRAPHY

- http://www.radiologyassistant.nl
- http://www.disabled-world.com
- http://z0mbie.host.sk
- http://boneandspine.com
- http://www.facingdisability.com
- http://www.ninds.nih.gov

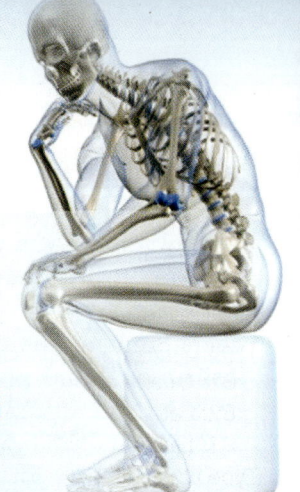

Chapter 29

Pelvic Fractures

Pelvic fracture is a disruption of the bony structure of the pelvis, including the hip bone, sacrum and coccyx. A pelvic fracture is a break in 1 or more of the 5 pelvic (hip) bones. This also includes a fracture of the acetabulum. The most common cause in elderly is a fall, but the most significant fractures involve high-energy forces such as a motor vehicle accident. Most pelvic fractures result from trauma:

- Motor vehicle collision (~50%)
- Pedestrian vs. motor vehicle (~30%)
- Fall from height (~10%)
- Motorbike collisions (~4%)
- Others, e.g. sports injury, low-energy fall

Pelvic fractures carry a significant risk of uncontrolled pelvic bleeding and exsanguination from pelvic fractures is a real possibility. This may result in pelvic, thigh and/or retroperitoneal haemorrhage.

Emergency treatment consists of advanced trauma life support management. After stabilization, the pelvis may be surgically reconstructed.

TILE'S CLASSIFICATION OF PELVIC INJURIES
(Mechanism of Injury)

Four main forces have been described in high-energy blunt force trauma that result in unstable pelvic fractures:

- *Anteroposterior compression:* Result in open book or sprung pelvis fractures.
- *Lateral compression:* Result in a windswept pelvis.
- *Vertical shear:* Results in Malgaigne fracture or bucket handle fracture.

- *Combined mechanical:* Occur when two different force vectors are involved and results in a complex fracture pattern.

Isolated stable pelvic fractures can also occur in the context of lower energy mechanisms or sporting injuries:

- Acetabular fracture
- Pubic ramus fracture
- Iliac wing fracture (Duverney fracture)
- Avulsion fractures (e.g. ASIS, iliac crest, ischial tuberosity).

Two of the most prominent are the Tile classification (Table 29.1) and the Young and Burgess classification (Table 29.2).

TILE'S CLASSIFICATION (Details of Fractures)

Type A

- *Stable injuries* include avulsion fractures, isolated pubic ramus fractures, iliac wing fractures or single stable fractures elsewhere in the pelvic ring.
- Avulsion fractures occur at the point of attachment of muscles (Fig. 29.1).
- *Anterior inferior iliac spine:* Tectus femoris; often resulting from a mis-kick into the ground.
- Anterior superior iliac spine: Sartorius.
- Ischial tuberosity: Hamstrings.

Type B

- Rotationally unstable but vertically stable.
- B1: 'Open book' anteroposterior compression fractures (Fig. 29.2), causing

Table 29.1: Tile classification of pelvic ring fractures (Fig. 29.4)

Type A: Pelvic ring stable
  A1: Fracture not involving the ring (i.e. avulsions, iliac wing or crest fractures)
  A2: Stable minimally displaced fractures of the pelvic ring
Type B: Pelvic ring rotationally unstable, vertically stable
  B1: Open book
  B2: Lateral compression, ipsilateral
  B3: Lateral compression, contralateral or bucket handle-type injury
Type C: Pelvic ring rotationally and vertically unstable
  C1: Unilateral
  C2: Bilateral
  C3: Associated with acetabular fracture

Table 29.2: Young and Burgess classification

	Grade I	Grade II	Grade III
Anterior posterior compression	Symphyseal diastasis—slight widening ± sacroiliac joint. Intact anterior and posterior ligaments	Symphyseal diastasis—widening of SU, anterior ligaments disrupted, posterior ligaments intact	Complete hemipelvis separation without vertical displacement. Symphyseal disruption and complete disruption of sacroiliac joint, anterior and posterior ligaments
Lateral compression (Fig. 29.3)	Anterior transverse fracture of pubic rami plus ipsilateral sacral compression	Plus—crescent (iliac wing) fracture	Plus—contralateral anterior posterior compression injury
Vertical shear (Fig. 29.3)	Vertical displacement, anterior and posterior through sacroiliac joint		
Combined mechanical injuries	Combination of other injury patterns: Lateral compression/vertical shear or lateral compression/anterior posterior compression		

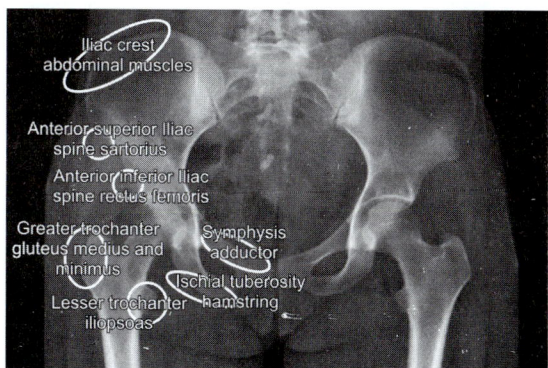

Fig. 29.1: Sites of avulsion fractures in pelvis

separation of the pubic symphysis and widening of one or both sacroiliac joints.
- *B2:* Ipsilateral compression causing the pubic bones to fracture and override.
- *B3:* Contralateral compression injury resulting in pubic rami fractures on one side and compression sacroiliac injury on the other side.

Type C
- Rotationally and vertically unstable.
- The pelvic ring is completely disrupted or displaced at two or more points.

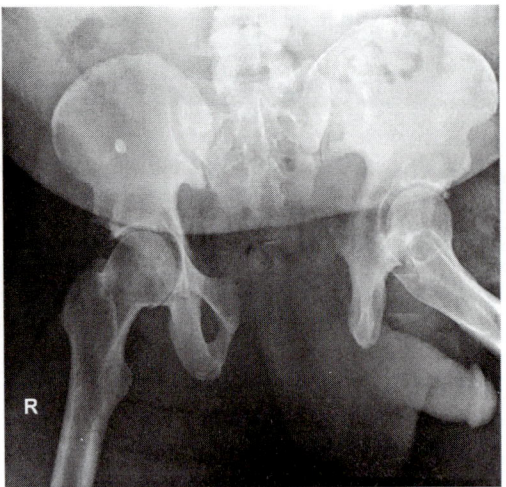

Fig. 29.2: Open book injury

- Associated with massive blood loss and a very high mortality.
- Subdivided into:
  - C1: Unilateral.
  - C2: Bilateral.
  - C3: Involving acetabular fracture.

Disruption of the anterior pelvic ligaments creates rotational instability, whereas posterior ligamentous injury creates both rotational and vertical instability. The pubic symphysis is important for pelvic support, but disruption of the symphysis by itself does not make the pelvis unstable.

Advanced Trauma Life Support guidelines recommend an anteroposterior pelvic radiograph for all patients with multiple trauma. On radiographs, a normal pubic symphysis is less than 5 mm wide and has less than 3 mm of vertical offset. Overlap is abnormal. The greater detail and multiple views with CT scanning are especially useful for evaluating sacral, sacroiliac, posterior arch, and acetabular injuries, and CT scans also allow visualization of retroperitoneal hematomas.

MANAGEMENT

When pelvic fracture is accompanied by head, chest, or extremity injury, management follows trauma guidelines in a fairly straightforward manner, blending specific responses to the associated injuries with the specific management of the pelvic fracture.

Current trauma management guidelines recommend that early external pelvic stabilization be considered in hypotensive patients with unstable pelvic fractures and that external fixation precede laparotomy incision, if that operation is performed. Anterior external fixation provides adequate rotational stability and reduces bleeding by reapproximating bleeding bony surfaces and preventing clot disruption. It may provide an advantageous reduction in pelvic volume (Fig. 29.5).

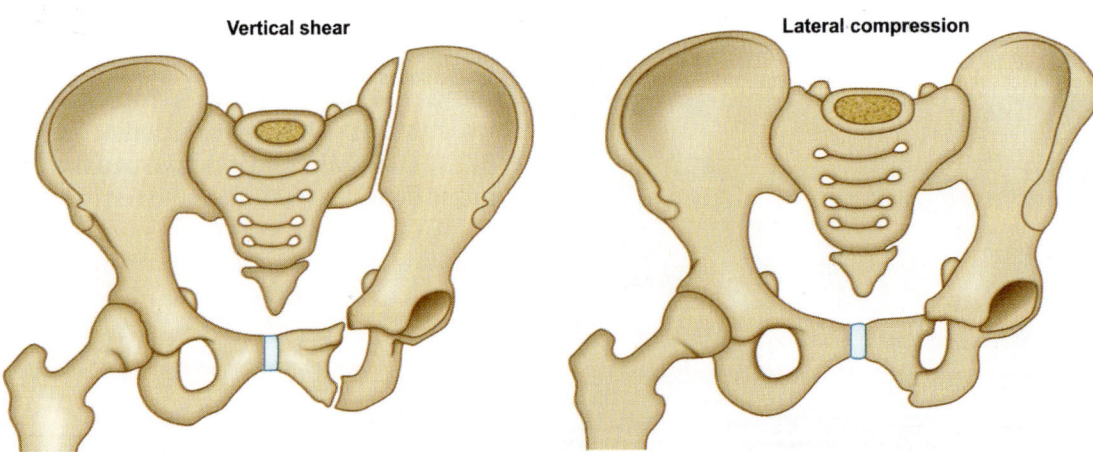

Fig. 29.3: Vertical shear and lateral compression injury

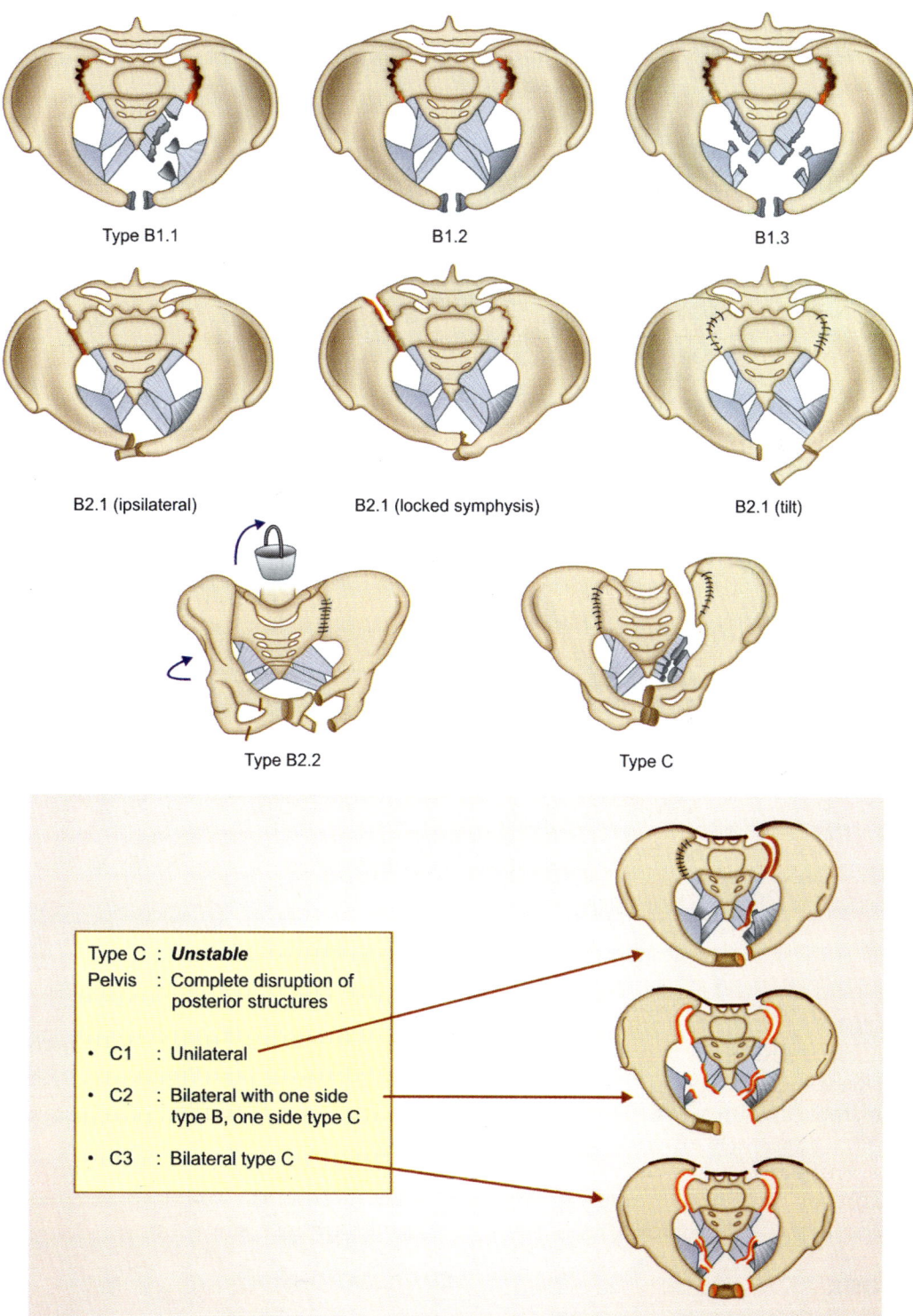

Fig. 29.4: Tile's classification system/unstable pelvic fractures

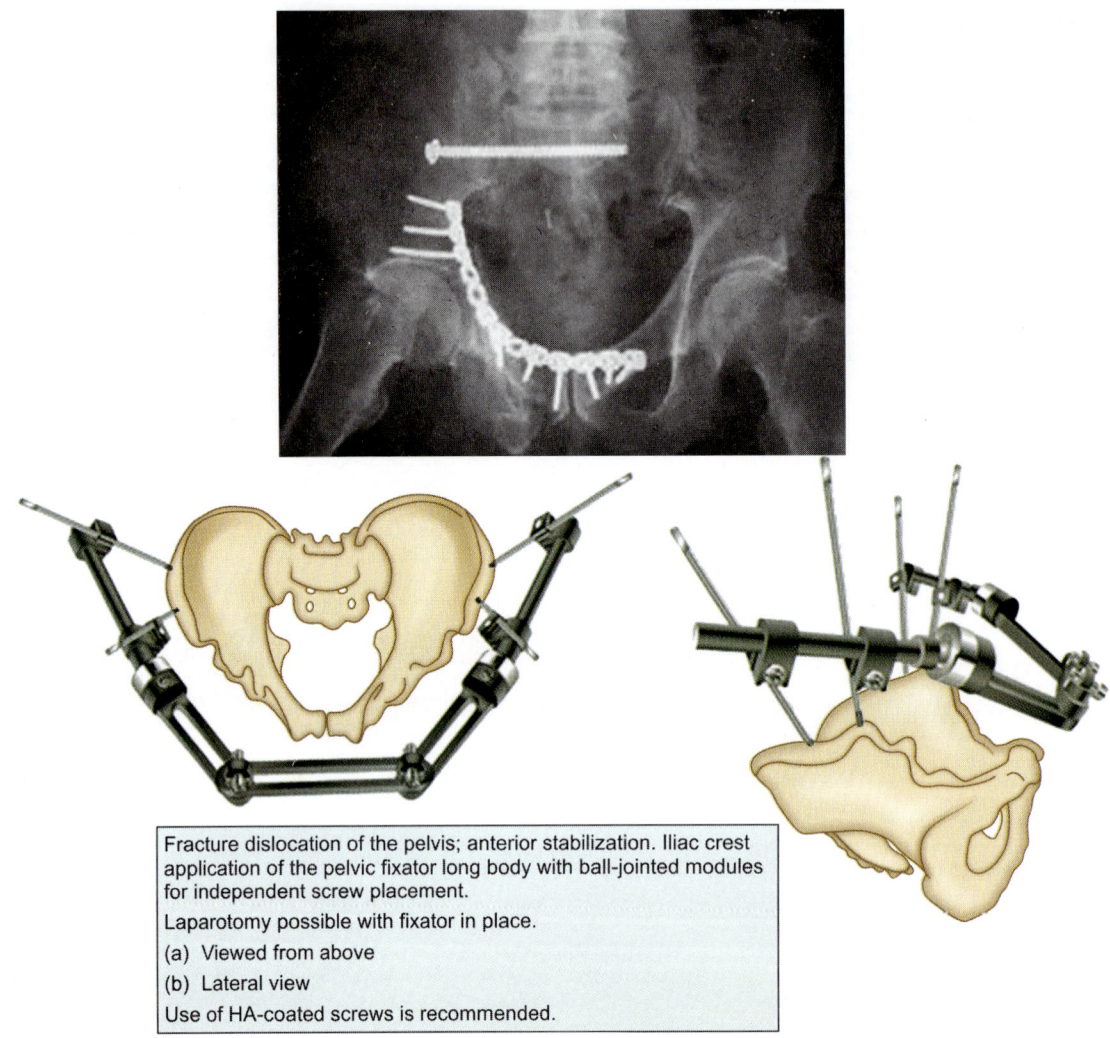

Fracture dislocation of the pelvis; anterior stabilization. Iliac crest application of the pelvic fixator long body with ball-jointed modules for independent screw placement.

Laparotomy possible with fixator in place.

(a) Viewed from above

(b) Lateral view

Use of HA-coated screws is recommended.

Fig. 29.5: Anterior stabilization of pelvis

Treatment (Figs 29.6 and 29.7)

- For stable fractures, usually only symptomatic treatment.
- For unstable fractures, external fixation, or open reduction and internal fixation (ORIF).
- For significant hemorrhage, external fixation or sometimes angiographic embolization or pelvic packing.

PROGNOSIS

Survival is worse for patients with open pelvic fractures and for pedestrians struck by cars.

Mortality rate is 15–25% for closed fractures, as much as 50% for open fractures. Increased mortality is associated with:

- Systolic BP <90 on presentation
- Age >60 years
- Increased Injury Severity Score (ISS) or Revised Trauma Score (RTS)
- Need for transfusion >4 units

COMPLICATIONS

- Increased incidence of thrombophlebitis.
- Intrapelvic compartment syndrome.

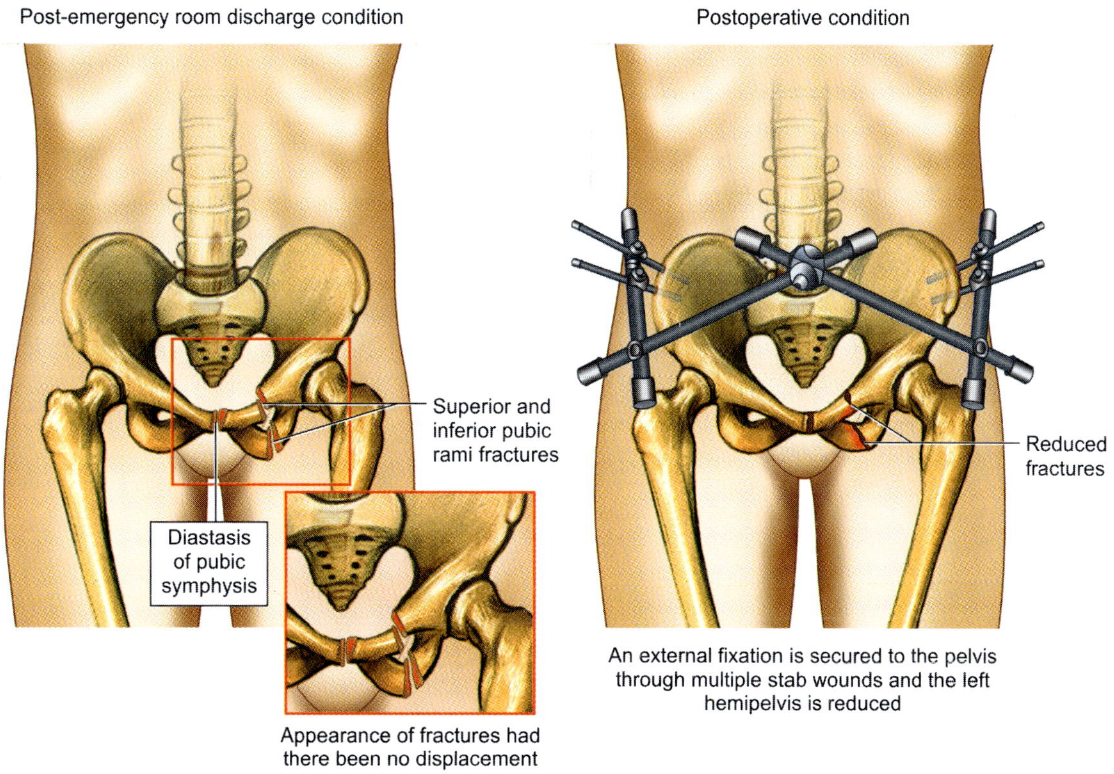

Post-emergency room discharge condition
Postoperative condition
Superior and inferior pubic rami fractures
Diastasis of pubic symphysis
Reduced fractures
Appearance of fractures had there been no displacement
An external fixation is secured to the pelvis through multiple stab wounds and the left hemipelvis is reduced

Fig. 29.6: Displaced pelvic fractures with surgical repair

Unstable pelvic fx and unstable patient
Ultrasound
or
DPL
+
Positive aspirate
Laparotomy
Candidate for external fixation
Apply external fixation in OR
Patient stabilizes?
No
Yes
Systolic BP <80?
Yes
Apply MAST if possible
No
Angiography and embolization
–
–
Positive by laboratory analysis
Candidate for external fixation
Yes
No
Apply external fixation in ED
Patient stabilizes?
No
Systolic BP <80?
Yes
Apply MAST
No
Angiography and embolization
Yes
CT abd (chest and head prn)
To SICU

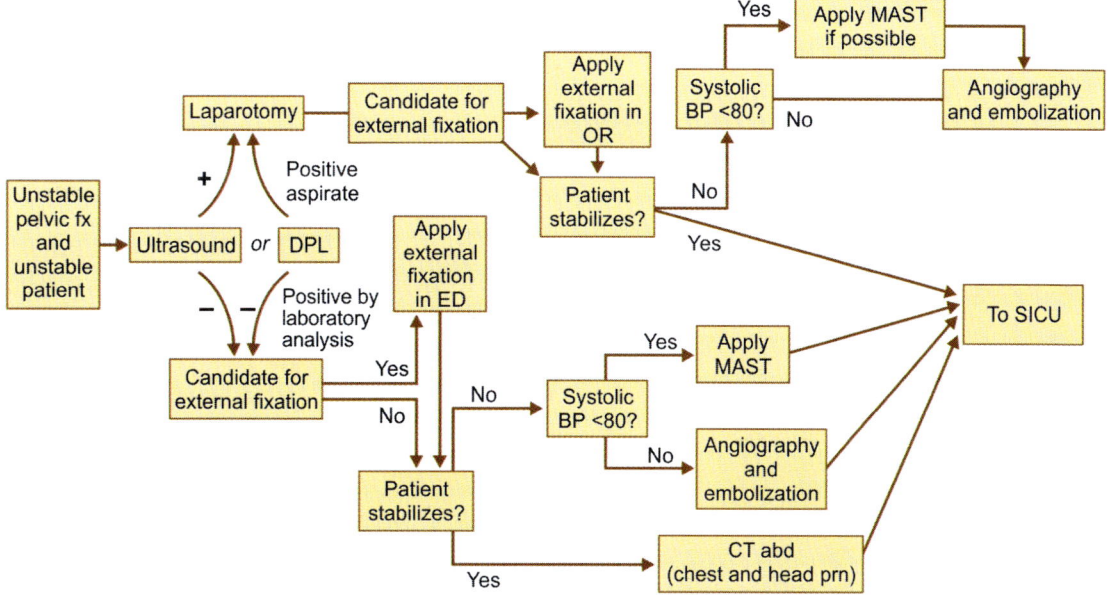

Fig. 29.7: Algorithm of treatment of pelvic fractures

- Continued bleeding from fracture or injury to pelvic blood vessels.
- Associated bladder, urethral prostate or vaginal damage is common.
- Associated thoracic and abdominal injuries occur in 10–20%; massive internal hemorrhage may occur.
- Sexual dysfunction may be a long-term problem.

Summary

Pelvic fractures can range from simple, stable injuries to a component of injury in severe multisystem trauma. Recovery from pelvic fracture is a long-term process and can include multisystem complications. Good basic, critical care, and trauma nursing skills and an understanding of the nature of pelvic injuries are important. Unstable pelvic fractures and dislocations are complex and potentially devastating injuries. Early surgical realignment and stabilization of pelvic fractures decreases related bleeding provides patient comfort and facilitates patient mobility. Serious pelvic fractures due to high-energy injuries are often associated with GU and vascular injuries.

BIBLIOGRAPHY

- http://orthoinfo.aaos.org/topic.cfm?topic=A00520
- http://emedicine.medscape.com/article/1247913-overview
- https://www.youtube.com/watch?v=Ty4eibxAG3U
- https://www.youtube.com/watch?v=nvgp4K9OmpQ

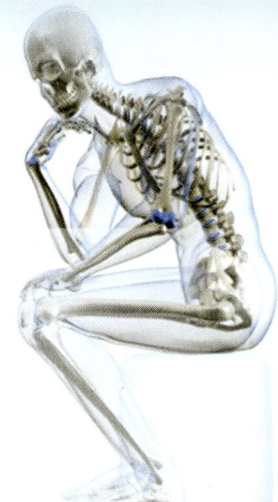

Hip Dislocation

Hip dislocations in younger individuals are relatively rare, with only 5% of cases occurring in patients younger than 14 years. Up to 70% of all hip dislocations are due to motor vehicle accidents. In order to cause a posterior dislocation, a large force is required to strike the flexed knee with the hip flexed, adducted, and internally rotated.

Assessing the neurovascular status of the injured leg is extremely important. Nerve injury, particularly neuropraxia, is not uncommon. The sciatic nerve and the common peroneal division of the sciatic nerve are most often injured in posterior dislocations. Studies of motor vehicle accidents have shown hip dislocations are commonly associated with knee injuries such as fractures, dislocations, and ligamentous damage.

Incidence

- Common in young men
- Posterior/anterior = 9:1

Posterior hip dislocations are the most common (Fig. 30.1). The usual cause is a motor vehicle accident with the passenger's knee hitting the dashboard and forcing the femoral head out of the acetabulum posteriorly. The limb is shortened, and the hip flexed, the foot is in internal rotation.

Associated Injuries

50–95% have other injuries like:
- Acetabular fracture

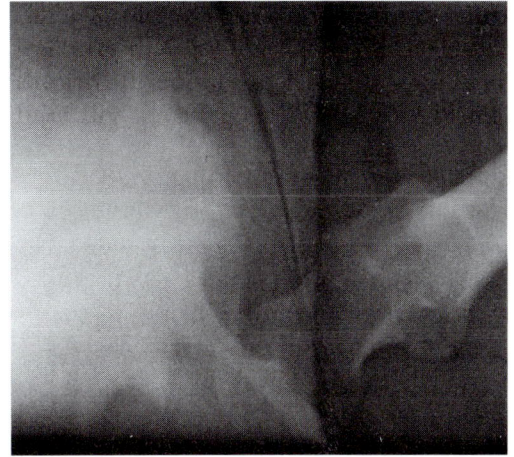

Fig. 30.1: Posterior hip dislocation

- Femoral head fracture/pipkin fracture
- Sciatic nerve (10% of cases) in posterior dislocation
- Patella fracture
- PCL injury
- Femoral artery injury in anterior dislocation
- Femoral shaft fracture

Several classification systems are used to describe posterior hip dislocations.

1. *The Thompson-Epstein classification* is based on radiographic findings.
   - *Type 1:* With or without minor fracture
   - *Type 2:* With large, single fracture of posterior acetabular rim
   - *Type 3:* With comminution of rim of acetabulum, with or without major fragments (Fig. 30.2)

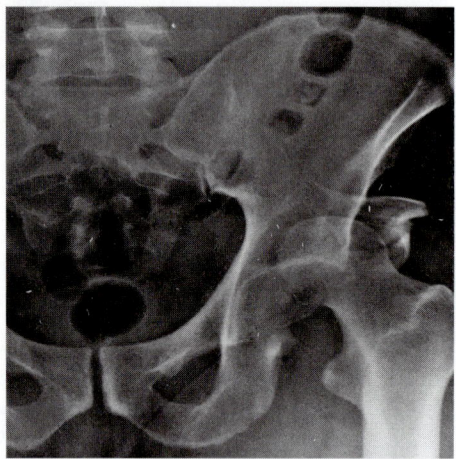

Fig. 30.2: Fracture of posterior wall of acetabulum

- *Type 4:* With fracture of the acetabular floor
- *Type 5:* With fracture of the femoral head
2. *The Steward and Milford classification* is based on functional hip stability.
   - *Type 1:* No fracture or insignificant fracture.

- *Type 2:* Associated with a single or comminuted posterior wall fragment, but the hip remains stable through a functional range of motion.
- *Type 3:* Associated with gross instability of the hip joint secondary to loss of structural support.
- *Type 4:* Associated with femoral head fracture.

MANAGEMENT

Closed Reduction (Fig. 30.3)

Numerous studies have shown that closed reduction should be attempted as soon as possible after a hip dislocation and certainly within the first 6 hours after injury to minimize long-term joint damage.

The following are methods of closed reduction of a dislocated hip:

- The *Allis maneuver*, the most widely performed method, involves having an

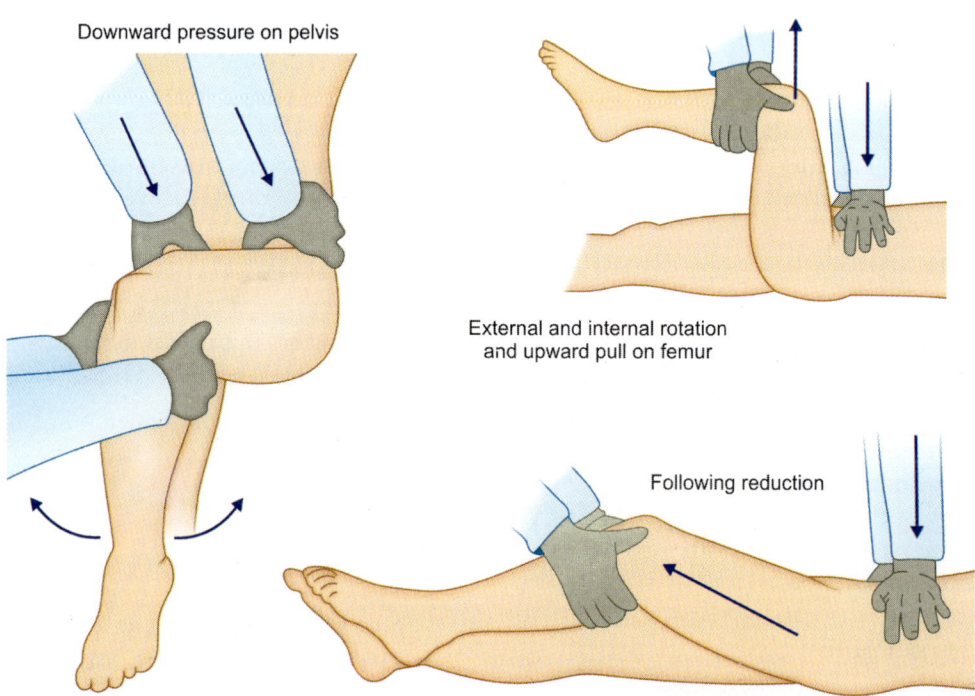

Downward pressure on pelvis

External and internal rotation and upward pull on femur

Following reduction

Fig. 30.3: Closed reduction

assistant bilaterally stabilize the anterior superior iliac spines while the patient is supine. First, the knee of the affected side is flexed, and then the hip is flexed, with traction being placed below the knee pulling upward. The leg is internally and externally rotated until the femoral head is rearticulated with the acetabulum.

- The *Stimson maneuver* places the patient in the prone position and is the least traumatic of the closed reduction methods. An assistant provides pressure on the patient's lower back for stability, while the injured leg is allowed to hang from the side of the bed with the knee and hip fully flexed. Traction is applied along with the force of gravity behind the knee, while internal and external rotation is applied to pop the femoral head back into place. Note: This technique is contraindicated in the setting of thoracoabdominal trauma or a difficult airway (Fig. 30.4).

- The *Bigelow maneuver* is the final method of closed reduction. As in the Allis maneuver, an assistant applies pressure to the anterior spines of the patient's pelvis for stability. One hand is used to apply traction on the affected leg by pulling on the ankle, while the other forearm is placed under the knee. The knee and hip are flexed on the injured leg, and abduction, external rotation, and extension of the hip are performed until the femoral head is in the acetabulum.

- Another novel technique for the reduction of a hip dislocation realized high success rates with no reported neurovascular complications or injuries to the knee. The "Captain Morgan" technique involves placing the physician's knee behind the supine patient's flexed knee and lifting with anterior force, with rotation as needed.

Surgical intervention should be performed, if closed reduction is unsuccessful, bony fragments or soft tissue remains in the joint space, or the joint remains unstable. Open reduction is typically performed using a posterior approach, owing to the decreased rate of avascular necrosis relative to the anterior approach.

COMPLICATIONS

Serious complications include sciatic nerve damage, inability to perform closed reduction, avascular necrosis of femoral head (AVN), secondary osteoarthritis of hip and recurring dislocation.

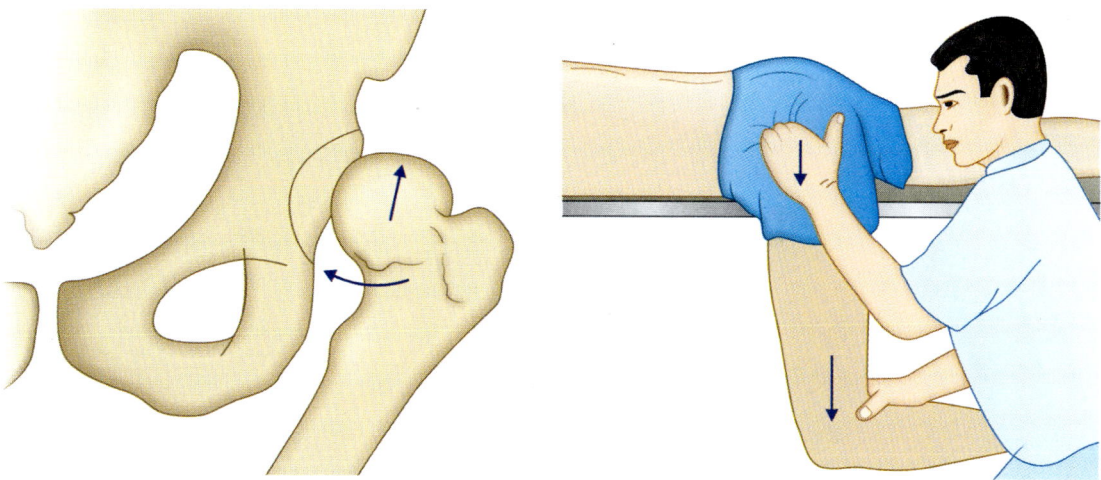

Fig. 30.4: Stimson's method

The sciatic nerve sits just inferoposterior to the hip joint and is injured in approximately 20% of all hip dislocations. These injuries range from nerve contusion to full laceration.

Incidence of AVN of femoral head depends on the time interval for closed reduction in fresh injuries:

- <6 hours: 10%
- If >24 hours: 20–50%

Secondary O-A of hip:

- Incidence: 15–20%

Causes

- AVN
- Instability
- Incongruous reduction
- Cartilage damage at time of dislocation

Other complications include: Myositis ossificans and instability.

ANTERIOR HIP DISLOCATIONS

With an anterior dislocation, the lower limb is lengthened, the hip abducted and the foot is in external rotation.

As the femur head is either anterior in the groin or in the obturator fossa, it can obstruct the femoral vein causing thrombosis and possible pulmonary embolism.

X-ray signs of an anterior hip dislocation are the lesser trochanter being more visible (due to external rotation). The hip is abducted and the femur head is usually inferior to the acetabulum. Shenton's line is also broken.

BIBLIOGRAPHY

- http://emedicine.medscape.com/article/86930-overview
- https://www.youtube.com/watch?v=mAL-Szu7qAc
- https://www.youtube.com/watch?v=WXN9RMjyn4M

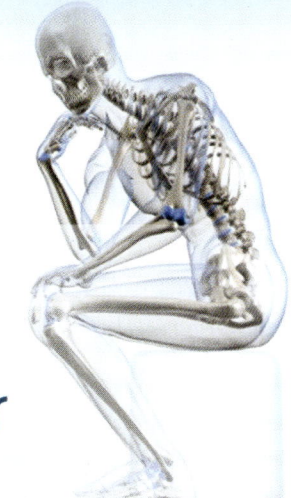

Fracture Neck of Femur

"We come into the world under the brim of the pelvis and go out through the neck of the femur".

- Hip fractures (proximal femoral fractures) occur between the edge of the femoral head and 5 cm below the lesser trochanter. Intracapsular fractures (femoral neck fractures): Between the edge of the femoral head and insertion of the capsule of the hip joint. These can follow relatively minor trauma in the elderly. Fractures in younger patients are usually caused by a high-energy impact. Increased risk in the elderly because of osteoporosis, osteomalacia and falls.
- In the UK, the mortality following a fractured neck of femur is between 20% and 35% within one year in people aged 82, ±7 years, of whom 80% were women.
- Worldwide, the total number of hip fractures is expected to surpass 6 million by the year 2050.

Neck of femur fractures (Fig. 31.1) are considered intracapsular fractures (also called proximal femoral fractures). Intracapsular fractures include:
- Subcapital: Femoral head/neck junction
- Transcervical: Midportion of femoral neck
- Basicervical: Base of femoral neck

Further, severity of a subcapital fracture is graded by Garden classification of hip fractures.

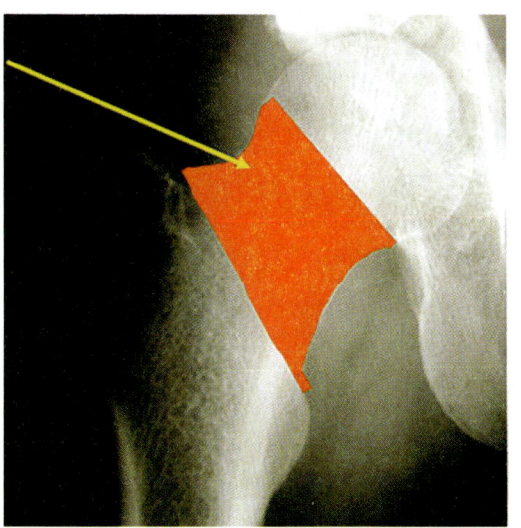

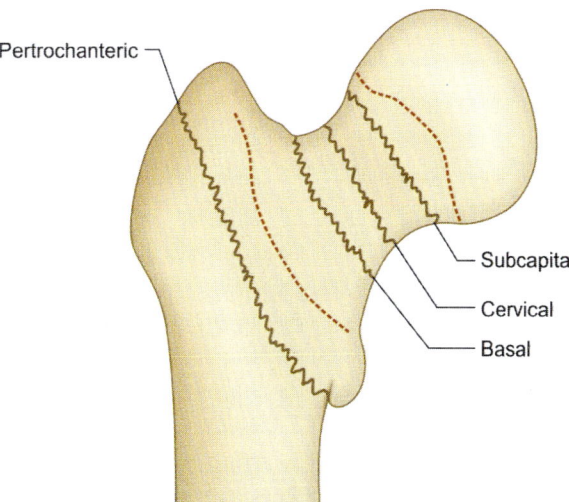

Pertrochanteric

Subcapital

Cervical

Basal

Fig. 31.1: Femoral neck (marked red)

Intracapsular neck of femur fractures are graded by various classifications, including Garden's classification (Fig. 31.2):

- *Garden I:* Trabeculae angulated, inferior cortex intact. No significant displacement.
- *Garden II:* Trabeculae in line but a fracture line is visible from superior to inferior cortex. No significant displacement.
- *Garden III:* Obvious complete fracture line with slight displacement and/or rotation of the femoral head.
- *Garden IV:* Gross, often complete, displacement of the femoral head.
- X-rays of the affected hip usually make the diagnosis obvious; AP (anteroposterior) and lateral views should be obtained.
- The grades correlate with prognosis and the rates of AVN or non-union, with Garden I and II fractures non-displaced and Garden III and IV having a low likelihood of healing and a high risk of osteonecrosis.

RADIOGRAPHIC FEATURES

Plain Film

- Shenton's line disruption: Loss of contour between normally continuous line from medial edge of femoral neck and inferior edge of the superior pubic ramus.
- Lesser trochanter is more prominent due to external rotation of femur.
- Femur often positioned in flexion and external rotation (due to unopposed iliopsoas)
- Asymmetry of lateral femoral neck/head
- Sclerosis in fracture plane
- Smudgy sclerosis from impaction
- Bone trabeculae angulated
- Nondisplaced fractures may be subtle on X-ray.
- In situations where a hip fracture is suspected but not obvious on X-ray, an MRI is the next test of choice. If an MRI is not

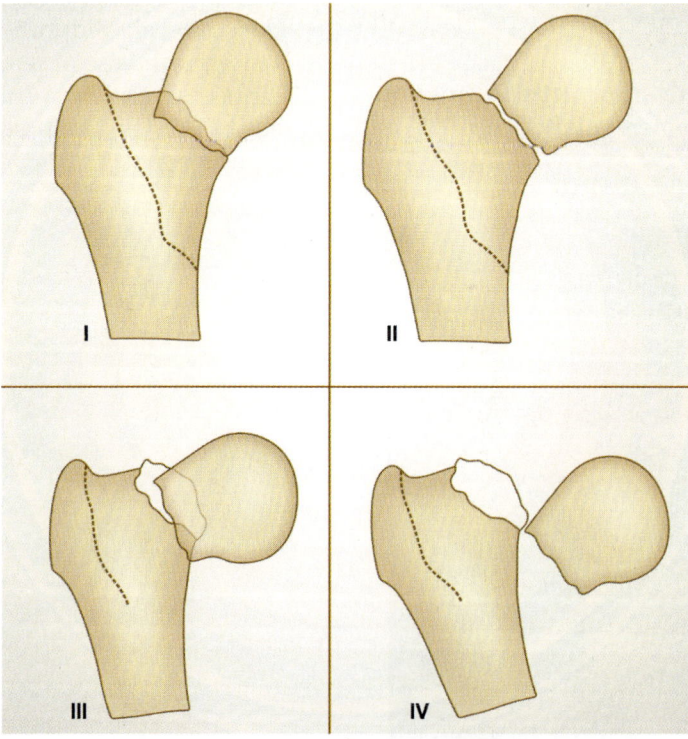

Fig. 31.2: Garden's classification

available or the patient cannot be placed into the scanner, a CT may be used as a substitute. MRI sensitivity for radiographically occult fracture is greater than CT. Bone scan is another useful alternative however, substantial drawbacks include decreased sensitivity, early false negative results, and decreased conspicuity of findings due to age related metabolic changes in the elderly.

MANAGEMENT

The treatment of femoral neck fracture depends primarily on the activity of the patient, the severity of fracture displacement, the age of the fracture, and the degree of osteoporosis present.

Displaced intracapsular fractures may be treated either by reduction and internal fixation in younger fit patients, or by replacement of the femoral head with an arthroplasty in older less fit patients. Patients with pre-existing joint disease, medium or high activity levels and a reasonable life expectancy should have a total hip replacement rather than hemiarthroplasty as primary treatment (Fig. 31.3).

For low-grade fractures (Garden types I and II), standard treatment is fixation of the fracture *in situ* with screws or a sliding screw/plate device. Femoral neck fractures reduced anatomically are best fixed with 3 pins or screws. This treatment can also be offered for displaced fractures after the fracture has been reduced. The incidence of AVN and non-union is decreased by fixation within 12 hours after injury.

The risk of dying from the stress of the surgery and the injury in the first 30 days is about 10%. The prognosis of untreated hip fractures is very poor. The death rate within one year of fractured neck of femur is typically reported as between 20 and 35%.

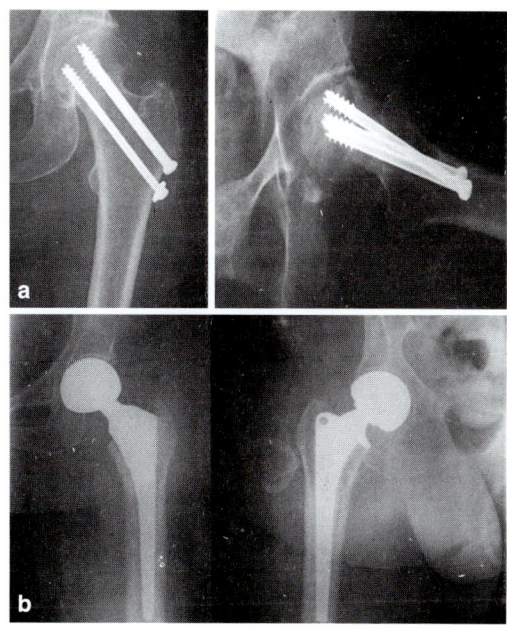

Fig. 31.3: (a) Osteosynthesis and (b) hemiarthroplasty

COMPLICATIONS (Figs 31.4 to 31.6)

- Complications include infection, hemorrhage, non-union, malunion and avascular necrosis.

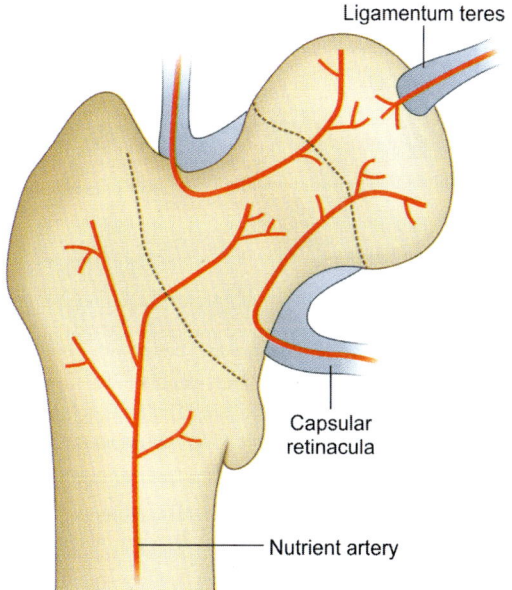

Fig. 31.4: Normal blood supply

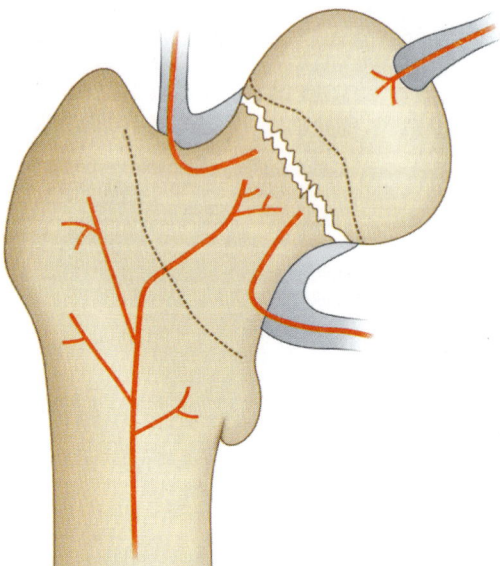

Fig. 31.5: Loss of blood supply to femoral head

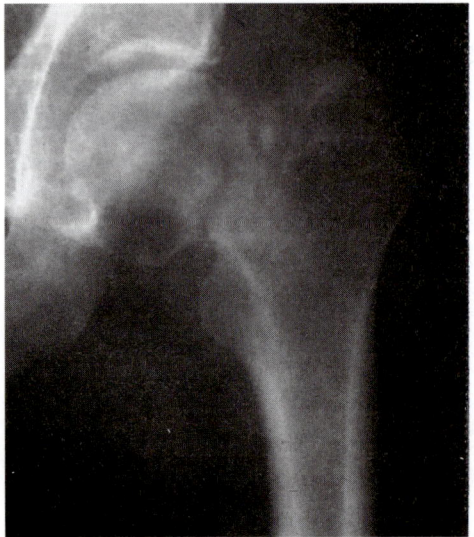

Fig. 31.6: Non-union

- There is a high risk of postoperative complications in the elderly, including pneumonia, myocardial infraction, stroke, deep vein thrombosis, pulmonary embolus and pressure ulcers.
- Reported non-union rates range from 0 to 4% to over 30%. Options for treatment of non-union include repeat internal fixation, bone or muscle-pedicle grafting, valgus osteotomy, and hip arthroplasty.

Avascular Necrosis (AVN) (Fig. 31.7)

The main therapeutic options are femoral head-preserving procedures and joint reconstruction. Among the procedures that preserve the femoral head are joint unloading, femoral head core decompression, electric stimulation, osteotomy, and bone grafting. Joint reconstruction procedures include: Cup arthroplasty, hemi-resurfacing, total hip resurfacing, femoral head replacement and femoral head endoprosthesis.

Patients with hip fractures are at high risk for future fractures including hip, wrist, shoulder, and spine. Currently, only 1 in 4 patients after a hip fracture receives treatment and work up for osteoporosis, the underlying cause of most of the fractures. Current treatment standards include the starting of a bisphosphonate to reduce future fracture risk by up to 50%.

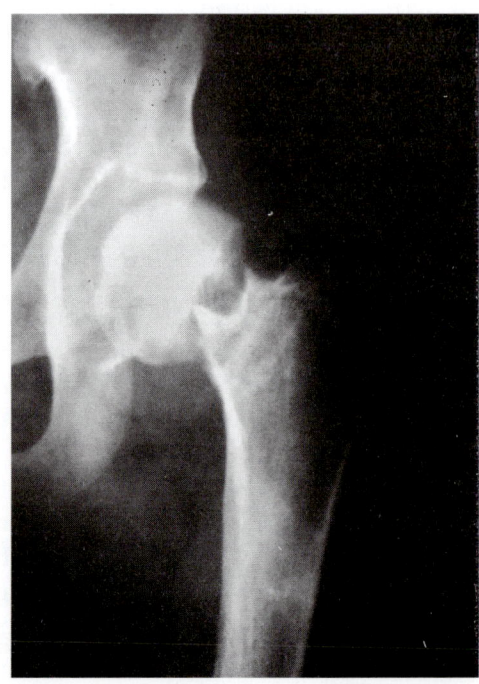

Fig. 31.7: Avascular necrosis

Patients who suffer a fractured neck of femur have a high mortality and morbidity rate with up to 20% needing long-term care post-fracture and a further 30% not returning to their pre-fracture functioning. Hip fracture accounts for 87% of total fragility fractures.

BIBLIOGRAPHY

- http://en.wikipedia.org/wiki/Hip_fracture
- http://radiologymasterclass.co.uk/tutorials/musculoskeletal
- https://www.youtube.com/watch?v=8ZOvoYYxGu0
- http://www.gla.ac.uk/t4/~fbls

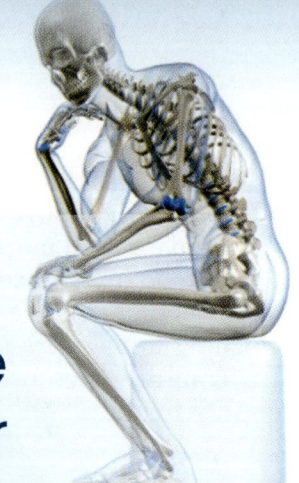

Nonunion Fracture
Neck of Femur

Nonunion and avascular necrosis of the femoral head or a combination of both is the main complication following fractures of the femoral neck. In spite of improved operative techniques, nonunion is still reported in 10–20% of cases. The reason is a combination of unfavorable bio-mechanical and vascular conditions caused by the fracture itself, ignoring general contraindications, poor reduction and inadequate internal fixation.

Usually nonunions are apparent within one year of femoral neck fracture;
- Incidence ranges from 10 to 30%

Three-fourths of patients with nonunion will require reoperation:
- Nonunion is initially suspected when there is pain in groin or buttock, especially on extension of the hip or with weight-bearing.
- These symptoms occur earlier and are more severe than those from AVN.

DEFINITION OF NONUNION
- Fracture where reparative process has halted (Cave 1958)
- A particular fracture not united in the time it normally unites—cannot be uniformly applied to all bones.
- FDA panel definition (1986)
  - Minimum 9 months have elapsed after injury and no progressive sign of healing for 3 months.
  - Cannot be applied universally.

Fractures of shaft of long bone should not be considered nonunion until at least 6 months post injury but in contrast, a central fracture of the femoral neck can sometimes be defined as a nonunion after only 3 months.

WHY IS NONUNION COMMON AFTER FRACTURE NOF?
- Absence of cambium layer of periosteum of femoral neck leads to decrease in the healing potential (Phemister, 1939)
- Continuous synovial bathing
- Avascularity as healing callus comes from the neck shaft side the fracture because of avascularity of the head (Hulth 1961)
- High velocity trauma in young adults

FACTORS CONTRIBUTING TO NONUNION OF FEMORAL NECK
- Inaccurate reduction
- Unsound or loss of fixation
- Vascular insufficiency
- Posterior comminution
- No treatment

Nonunion or loss of reduction can present with groin, hip, or thigh pain that never fully resolves following surgery, or increases after a period of improvement.

Clinical Signs
- Trendelenburg test/sign (Figs 32.1 to 32.5)
- Trendelenburg gait

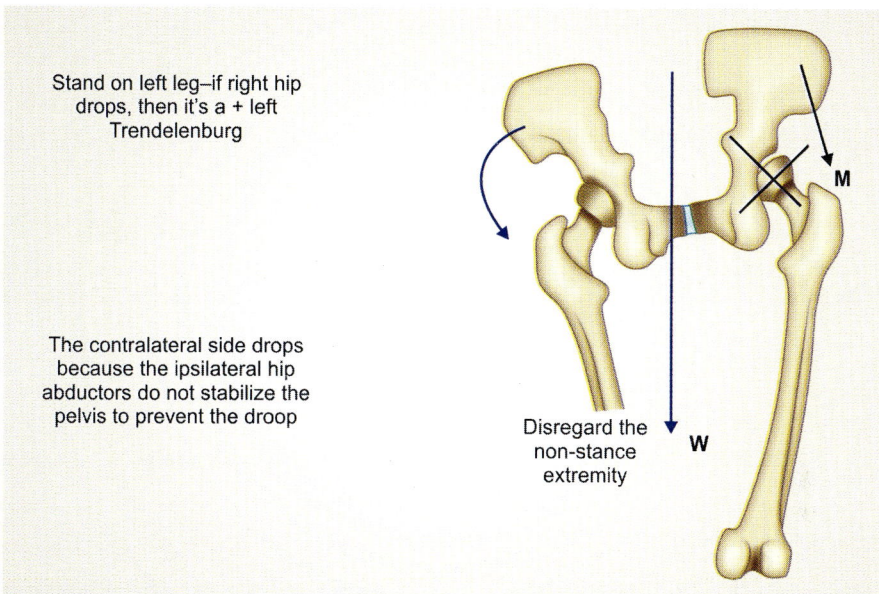

Fig. 32.1: Trendelenburg sign

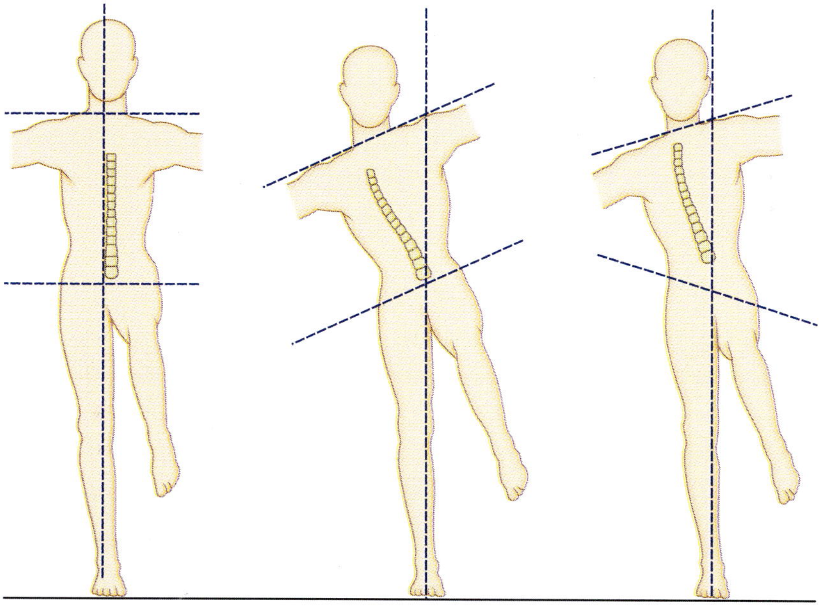

Stand on left leg–if right hip drops, then it's a + left Trendelenburg

The contralateral side drops because the ipsilateral hip abductors do not stabilize the pelvis to prevent the droop

Disregard the non-stance extremity

M

W

Fig. 32.2: Special tests—Trendelenburg test

- Telescopy test (Fig. 32.6)
- True shortening of the limb

- Tomography or high resolution CT scan
- MRI

Investigations

- Plain X-rays
- Bone scanning

TREATMENT

Although prosthetic replacement frequently is considered for the treatment of displaced

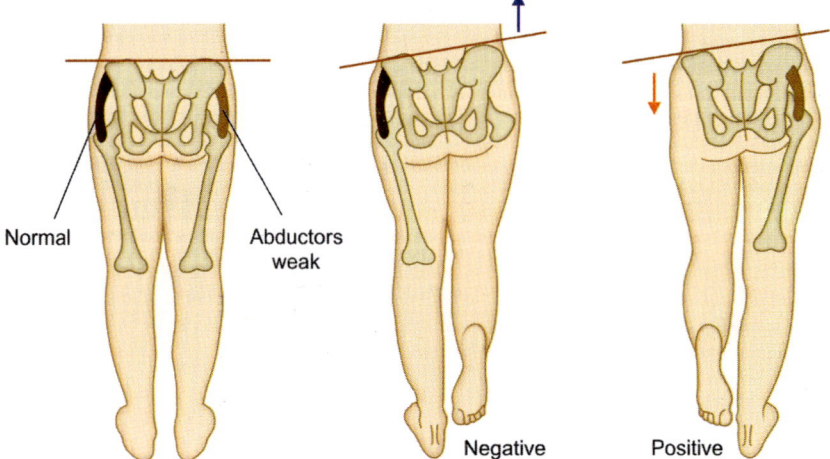

Fig. 32.3: Trendelenburg test

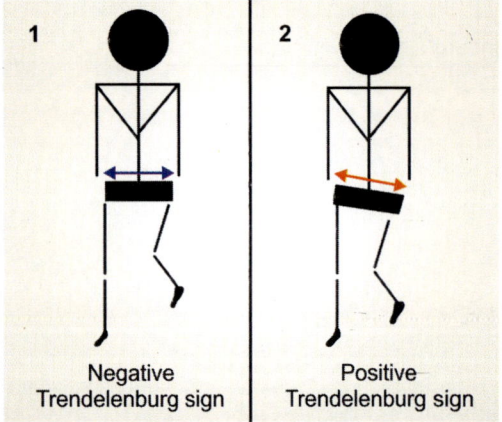

Fig. 32.4: Trendelenburg sign

fractures in elderly patients, efforts are focused on preserving the femoral head in physiologically younger patients. Surgical options are mainly divided into head salvage procedures and sacrificing procedures.

Salvage Procedures

If femoral head is viable and adequate neck is remaining, nonunions can be treated by:

- Fixation alone
- Osteotomy ±fixation
- Muscle pedicle bone grafting ±fixation
- Cortical bone grafting ±fixation
- Cancellous bone grafting ±fixation
- Combination of osteotomy and bone grafting

Fixation Alone

- Could be tried within 3 weeks of injury (late presenters or untreated fractures) which are undisplaced or are reducible.
- In established cases of nonunion, just fixing the head will not suffice (Rocked and Green 1990)

Osteotomy ±Fixation

- Pauwels' osteotomy
- Dickson's geometric osteotomy
- McMurray's osteotomy
- Schanz angulation osteotomy

Pauwels' Osteotomy (1935)

- Mechanical problem rather than a biological one
- Abduction osteotomy at intertrochanteric level
- Converts shearing force into compressive force
- Based on Pauwels' classification
- AVN without segmental collapse is NOT a contraindication.
- 86% union in 50 nonunions, Marti et al (1993).

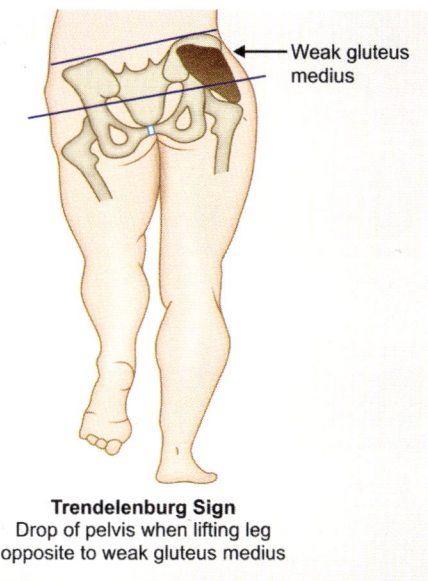

Trendelenburg Sign
Drop of pelvis when lifting leg
opposite to weak gluteus medius

Fig. 32.5: Trendelenburg sign

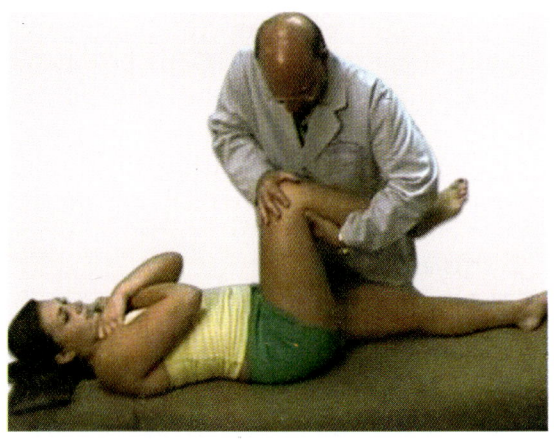

Fig. 32.6: Telescopy test

Dickson's Geometric Osteotomy (1947)

- *Indications:* Nonunion with viable femoral neck and varus displacement
- *Advantages:*
  - Easy to perform
  - Immediate stability can be provided
  - Converts sheer force into compressive force

McMurray's Osteotomy (1936)

- Displacement type of osteotomy
- Puts the shaft beneath the head
- Line of weight-bearing shifted medially
- Makes the fracture line horizontal
- Shortens the lever arm between the trochanter and the hip and leads to early OA changes
- Makes future arthroplasty difficult
- Not practiced and no longer popular

Schanz Angulation Osteotomy

- Made distal to lesser trochanter
- Angulated so as to gain length
- Line of weight-bearing shifted medially
- Not popular

Muscle Pedicle Bone Grafting ±Fixation

- Useful in delayed presenters as well as nonunion
- Insertion quadratus femoris muscle to the femur is mobilised with femoral cortex and is fixed across the fracture site posteriorly.

- Meyer et al (1974)
  - 11% segmental collapse at 2 years
  - 90% union

Muscle Pedicle Bone Grafting ±Bone Grafting

- Bakshi (1983,86,92)
  - Used gluteus minimus with attached bone block
  - Fixed anteriorly
  - Used in proven nonunions with absorbed necks
  - 75% good results
- Pati et al (1998)
  - Used screw fixation + MPBG
  - 11% segmental collapse as compared to 32% with fixation alone in delayed presenters

Cortical Bone Grafting ±Fixation
(Nagi, et al 1998)

- Fibula is used successfully.
- 80% good results in late presenters.
- All bad results were in nonunions.
- Uses single screw + BG.
- Puts the patient in hip spica.
- Patients presenting as late as 10 months were included in the study.

Cancellous Grafting ±Fixation
(Deyerly 1980 & Dickson 1953)

- Promising results
- Window created anteriorly in the head and neck

Sacrifice

- Unipolar arthroplasty
- Bipolar arthroplasty
- Total hip arthroplasty
- Girdlestone arthroplasty

Confirmed Nonunions

Young Adults (20–40) *(Neck is not absorbed and the head is viable)*

- Fixation alone will not work
- Augment it with bone grafting or osteotomy or muscle pedicle bone grafting
- Preserve the head as far as possible

If neck is absorbed and the head is not viable:

- Arthrodesis
- Girdlestone arthroplasty
- Bipolar after proper explanation to the patient, if acetabular cartilage good.
- THR, if articular cartilage is of poor quality.

Middle Age Group (40–60)

- If head is viable and neck is not resorbed:
  - Fixation+ BG
  - Osteotomy, if leg is short.
- If there is segmental collapse: Bipolar or THR
- If no segmental collapse but evidence of:
  - AVN
  - Pauwels' osteotomy
  - Muscle pedicle bone grafting

MANAGEMENT: YOUNG PATIENTS

- In younger patients, refixation with cancellous graft and valgus osteotomy (Figs 32.7 and 32.8) may be indicated.
- In most nonunions, there is a vertical fracture line (causing shear stress rather than compression across the fracture site) and most nonunions have drifted into some varus angulation.
- Valgus intertrochanteric osteotomy

Pauwels classified the femoral neck fractures based on their mechanical behavior. As a logical consequence of his theories, he designed the abduction osteotomy at the intertrochanteric level for the treatment of nonunions which converts shearing forces into compression.

- Makes fracture line more horizontal and converts shear forces at nonunion site to compressive forces, which then promote fracture healing.

The valgization osteotomy, designed by Pauwels, represents a masterly mechanical concept, with which not only healing of the nonunion and osteotomy can be achieved

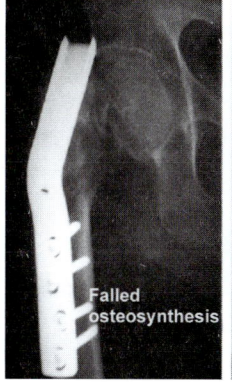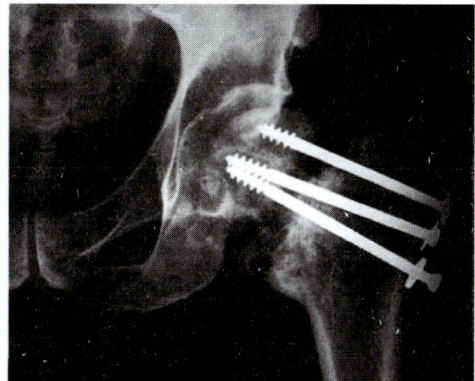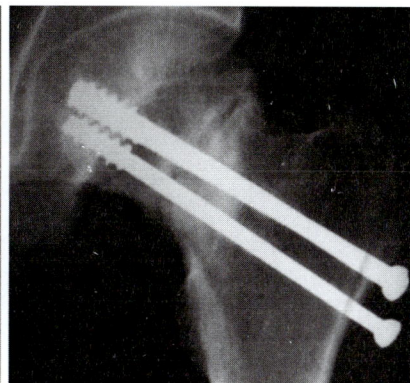

Fig. 32.7: Failed osteosynthesis

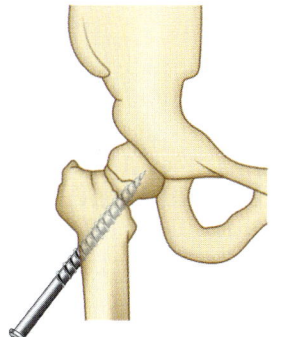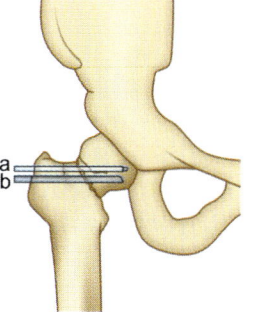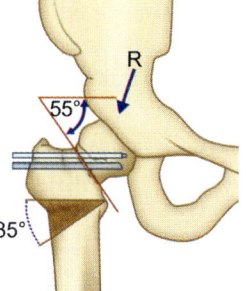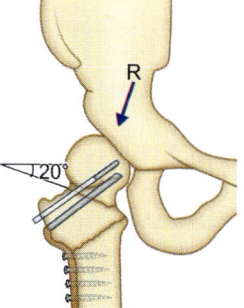

Fig. 32.8: Valgus osteotomy

but also leg length discrepancy, rotational and angular deformity can be corrected at the same time.

• The ideal implant for the valgization osteotomy is the AO 120° fixed angled blade plate. An alternative is the 95° condylar plate which can be bended to any desired angle, creating a shape similar to the 120° plate.

Usually nonunions of the femoral neck are grossly displaced by shortening and rotation. If not, a simple (re)fixation of the initial fracture without complementary osteotomy can be successful, as long as the original fracture line corresponds to the Pauwels' types 1 and 2.

BIBLIOGRAPHY

• http://www.wheelessonline.com/ortho/femoral_neck_non_union
• http://www.ncbi.nlm.nih.gov/pmc/articles/PMC2759582/
• http://www.natboard.edu.in/notice_for_dnb_candidates/Femora_neck.htm

Chapter 33

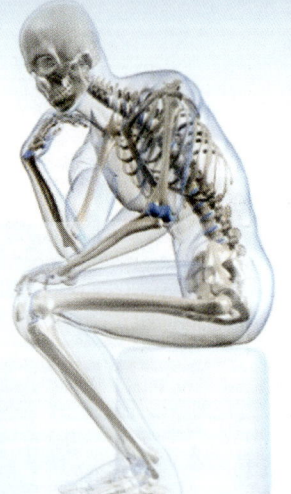

Intertrochanteric Fractures

Worldwide, the total number of hip fractures is expected to surpass 6 million by the year 2050.

Intertrochanteric fractures are breaks of the femur between the greater and the lesser trochanters. They are extracapsular fractures, i.e. outside the hip joint's fibrous capsule. The epidemiology of intertrochanteric fractures is similar to that of femoral neck fractures. Intertrochanteric fractures account for approximately 38 to 50% of all hip fractures.

In-hospital mortality of 6.3% and 30.8% in one year have been reported, with men's mortality rate double that of women's. One in 15 elderly patients admitted with hip fractures will die in hospital; out of those who survive, one-third will die within the first year. Three or more comorbidities are the strongest risk factors for mortality with chest infections and heart failure leading.

Intertrochanteric (IT) femur fractures comprise approximately ½ of all hip fractures caused by a low-energy mechanism such as a fall from standing height. These fragility hip fractures occur in a characteristic population with risk factors including increasing age, female gender, osteoporosis, a history of falls, and gait abnormalities.

Intertrochanteric fractures can be divided into two categories: Stable and unstable. Stable fractures are those in which the femur is broken into two or three parts. Unstable fractures are those in which the femur is broken into four parts or the fracture is of the reverse oblique pattern. Reverse oblique fractures are unstable because of the femur's tendency to displace medially (Figs 33.1 and 33.2).

The most often used classification system for intertrochanteric fractures is based on the stability of the fracture pattern and the ease in achieving a stable reduction. This classification was introduced by Evans in 1949 and accurately differentiates stable fractures (standard oblique fracture pattern) from unstable fractures (reverse oblique fracture pattern). The stability of intertrochanteric fractures depends on the integrity of the posteromedial cortex, and instability increases with comminution of the fracture, extension of the fracture into the subtrochanteric region, and the presence of a reverse oblique fracture pattern.

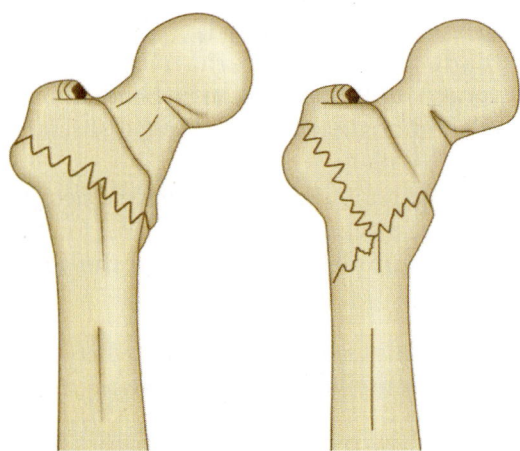

Fig. 33.1: Standard oblique fracture

Fig. 33.2: Reverse oblique fracture

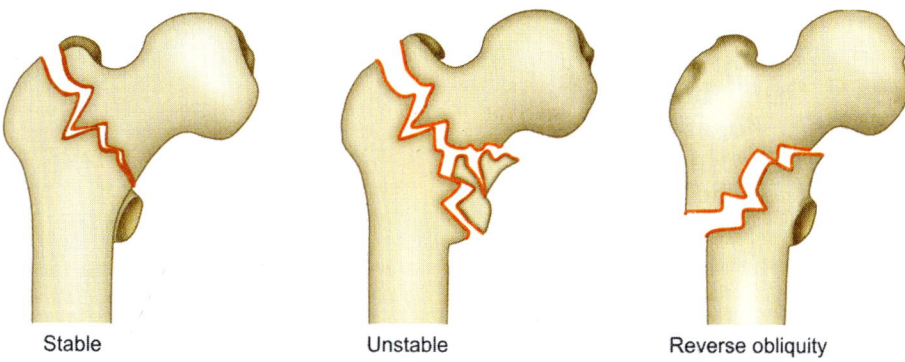

| Stable | Unstable | Reverse obliquity |

Fig. 33.3: Stable and unstable fractures

CLASSIFICATION

Intertrochanteric fractures can be classified (Evans, 1949) as the following types (Fig. 33.3):

i. Non-displaced with no comminution
ii. Displaced with no comminution;
iii. Displaced with greater trochanteric (posterolateral) comminution;
iv. Displaced with lesser trochanteric (posteromedial); and
v. Reverse obliquity

Modified Boyd Classification

- Type I—21%
  - Nondisplaced and stable
- Type II—36%
  - Stable, but displaced fractures
  - Stable construct with pin and plate
- Type III—28%
  - Unstable with pin and plate (Fig. 33.4)
  - Large posteromedial comminution
- Type IV—15%

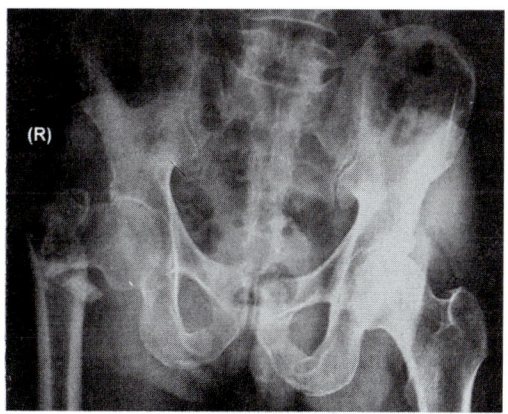

Fig. 33.4: Unstable fracture

  - Intertrochanteric with subtrochanteric component

Differences between Fracture Neck of Femur and Intertrochanteric Fracture

Add 'extra' for intertrochanteric fracture, e.g. extra-force, extra-decade, extra-external deformity (Table 33.1).

Tabe 33.1: Differences between fracture neck of femur and intertrochanteric fracture

Feature	Fracture neck of femur		Intertrochanteric fracture
Mechanism of injury	Trivial fall	E	Major fall
Age of the patient	6th decade	X	7th decade
External rotation deformity	Mild to moderate	T	Severe
Swelling	Minimal	R	More marked
Haemorrhage	Minimal	A	Significant
Shortening	Minimal	More	
Treatment	DHS/Hemi A'plasty	DHS/Nailing	
Complications	AVN and nonunion	Malunion and shortening	

MANAGEMENT

Surgery is almost always the recommended treatment as the morbidity and mortality associated with nonoperative treatment historically have been high. The fixation method is guided by the fracture pattern; standard options include the sliding hip screw, intramedullary nail, or fixed angle plate.

Treatment of Stable Fractures

If the fracture is stable, treatment is with a sliding hip screw (Fig. 33.5) coupled to a side plate that is screwed onto the femoral shaft. The screw provides proximal fragment fixation. It is set inside a telescoping barrel that allows impaction of the bone, which promotes fracture union. The lateral buttress must be intact so that the screw will not stop sliding.

Treatment of Unstable Fractures

Approximately 5% of fractures are extremely unstable, and the direction of the fracture is

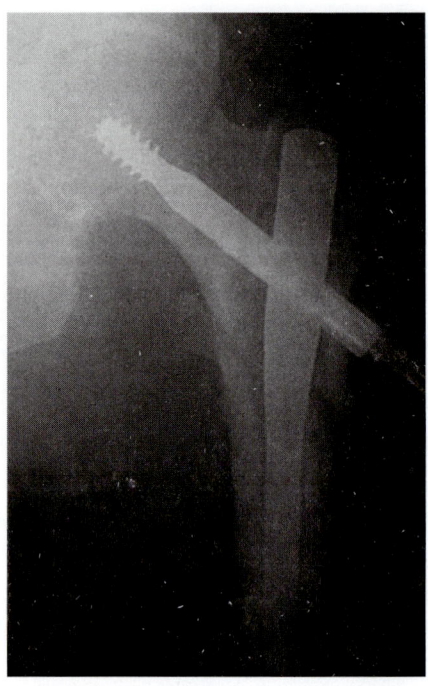

Fig. 33.6: Intramedullary hip screw

parallel to the femoral neck. This fracture type is called the reverse oblique pattern. A high rate of failure occurs, if the fracture is treated with a sliding hip screw and a side plate. Because of the angle of the fracture, there is no bone laterally to stop the screw from sliding. In such cases, an intramedullary hip screw is indicated (Fig. 33.6).

Postoperatively, patients should receive thromboembolic prophylaxis and should be mobilized. The amount of weight-bearing allowed is proportional to fracture stability; although mentally alert patients seem to auto-regulate their weight-bearing correctly.

Calcar Replacing Prosthesis

Indications
- Salvage of failure of fixation
- Severe comminution
- Rheumatoid arthritis

Problems
- High cost

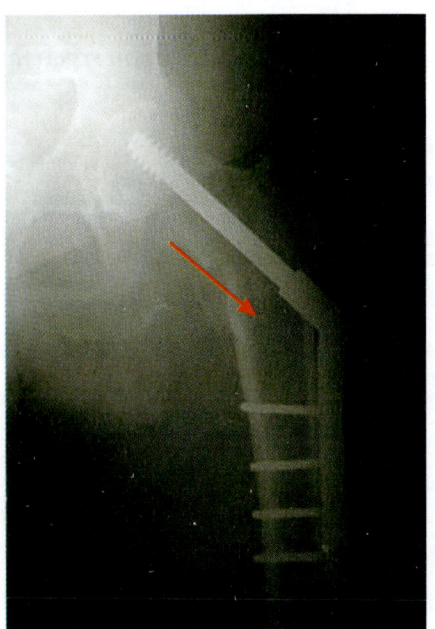

Fig. 33.5: Sliding hip screw

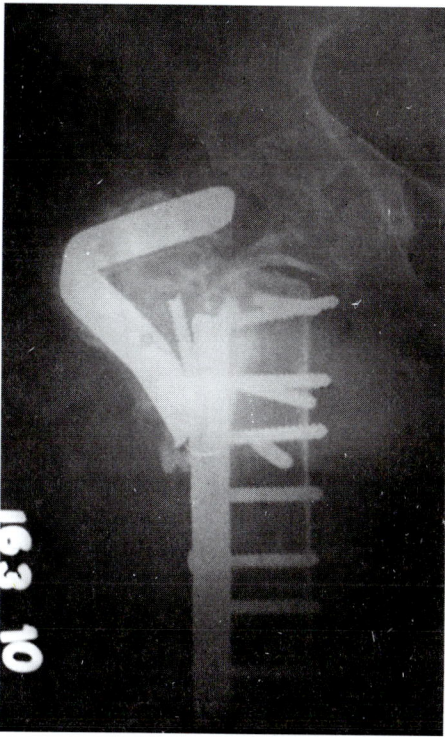

Fig. 33.7: Implant failure

- Higher morbidity/mortality
- High risk of dislocation

COMPLICATIONS

Complications for intertrochanteric fractures are similar to those for femoral neck fractures and include infection, thromboembolism, pressure sores, and malunion (varus). Other complications include:

1. Implant failure (Fig. 33.7) and screw cut out—6% of cases
2. Nonunion is rare—1% of cases
3. Infection—2–5%
4. Malrotation
5. Periprosthetic fracture

BIBLIOGRAPHY

- http://www.boneschool.com/hip/hip-fractures/intertrochanteric-fractures
- https://www.youtube.com/watch?v=zaEBxJBD_EM
- https://www.youtube.com/watch?v=2_2a-bBOyno

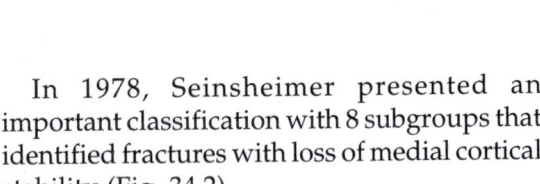

Chapter 34

Subtrochanteric Fracture

The subtrochanteric region of the femur, arbitrarily designated as the region between the lesser trochanter and a point 5 cm distal, consists predominantly of cortical bone. Healing in this region is predominantly through a primary cortical healing. Thus, the fracture is quite slow to consolidate.

Subtrochanteric fractures (Fig. 34.1) account for approximately 10–30% of all hip fractures, and they affect persons of all ages. Most frequently, these fractures are seen in two age groups, namely older osteopenic patients after a low-energy fall and younger patients involved in high-energy trauma. Axial loading forces through the hip joint create a large moment arm, with significant lateral tensile stresses and medial compressive loads. In addition to the bending forces, muscle forces at the hip also create torsional effects that lead to significant rotational shear forces.

In 1978, Seinsheimer presented an important classification with 8 subgroups that identified fractures with loss of medial cortical stability (Fig. 34.2).

AO CLASSIFICATION (Fig. 34.3)

Type A: Simple fracture (two part fracture)

A1	Spiral
A2	Oblique
A3	Transverse

Type B: Wedge fracture (fracture with butterfly fragment)

B1	Spiral wedge
B2	Bending wedge
B3	Communited wedge (fragmented wedge)

Type C: Complex comminuted fractures

C1	Complex spiral
C2	Complex segmental
C3	Complex irregular

FIELDING'S CLASSIFICATION OF SUBTROCHANTERIC FRACTURES

Type	Description
I	Fracture is at the level of the lesser trochanter
II	Fracture is 2.5 to 5 cm below the lesser trochanter
III	Fracture is 5 to 7.5 cm below the lesser trochanter

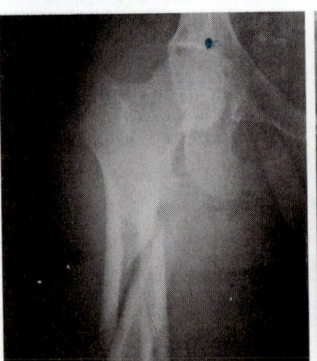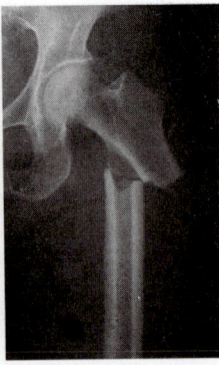

Fig. 34.1: Subtrochanteric fracture

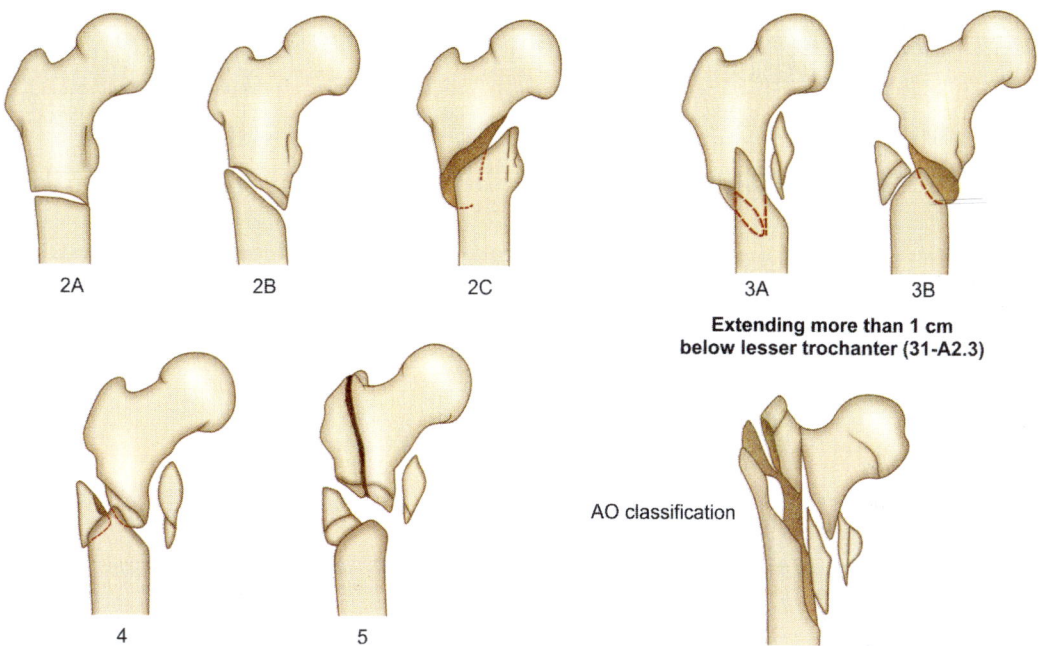

2A   2B   2C   3A   3B

**Extending more than 1 cm
below lesser trochanter (31-A2.3)**

4   5

AO classification

Fig. 34.2: Seinsheimer classification

RUSSELL-TAYLOR CLASSIFICATION OF SUBTROCHANTERIC FRACTURE OF FEMUR

The Russell-Taylor system is based on the lesser trochanter continuity and whether the fracture extends posteriorly into the greater trochanter and involves the piriformis fossa (Table 34.1 and Fig. 34.4).

Table 34.1: Russell-Taylor classification

Type	Description
I	Fracture does not extend into piriformis fossa
Ia	Comminution and fracture lines extend from below lesser trochanter to femoral isthmus
Ib	Fracture lines and comminution involve area of lesser trochanter to isthmus
II	Fracture extends proximally into greater trochanter and involves piriformis fossa
IIa	No significant comminution or fracture of lesser trochanter
IIb	Significant comminution of medial femoral cortex and loss of continuity of lesser trochanter

TREATMENT

The goals of treatment are important to recognize and include anatomic alignment, early mobilization, and effective rehabilitation. Current indications for surgical treatment include displaced and nondisplaced fractures in adults, fractures in patients with multiple traumatic injuries, open fractures, severe ipsilateral extremity injuries, and pathologic fractures.

Surgical treatment can be divided into three main techniques: Open reduction with plates and screws, intramedullary fixation and external fixation (Figs 34.5 to 34.7). Fixed angle plates may be used to fix these fractures. Anatomically contoured locking plates are now available for subtrochanteric fractures. Intramedullary nails are emerging as the treatment of choice for subtrochanteric fractures. The most widely used nails are either centromedullary (contained within the medullary canal) or cephalomedullary (including those that affix to the femoral neck and head).

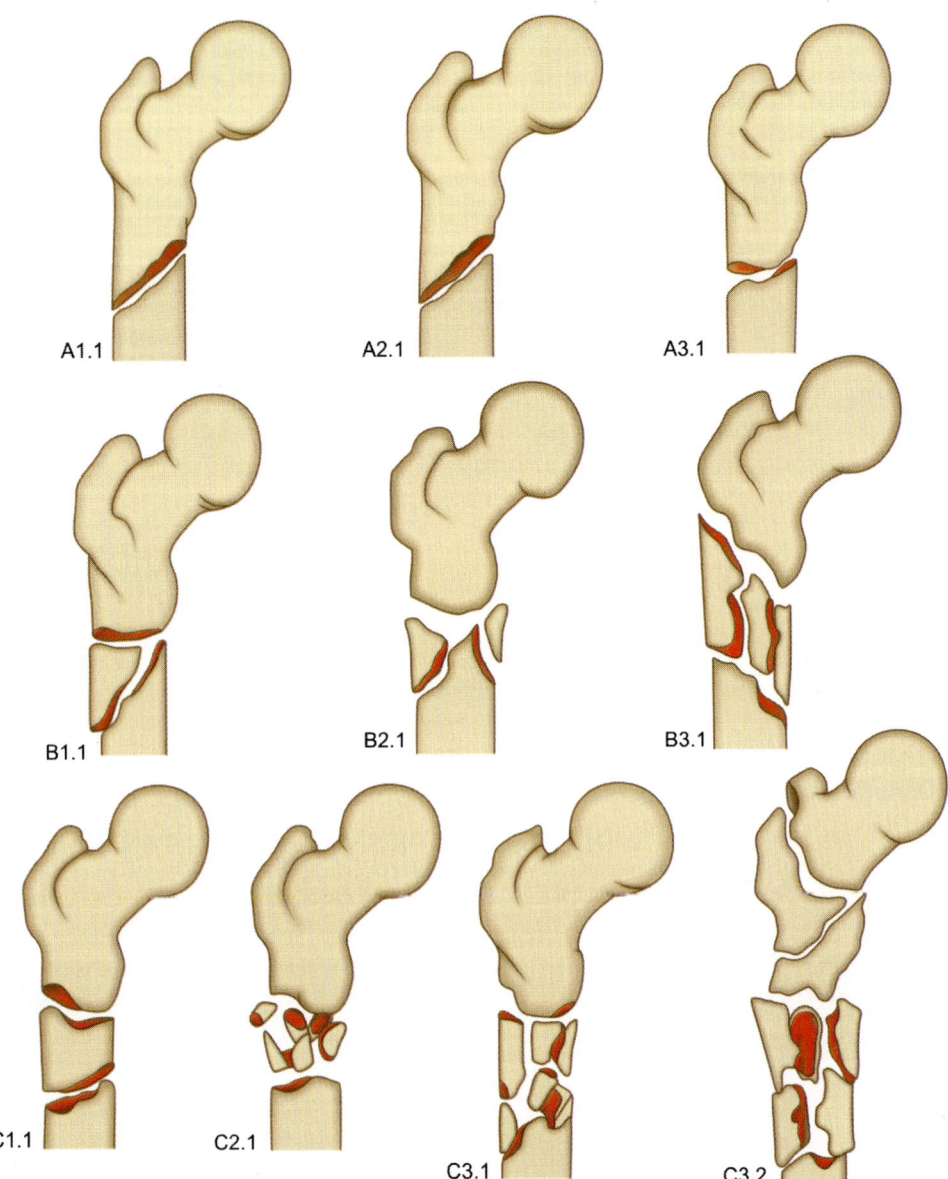

Fig. 34.3: AO classification

Table 34.2: Treatment recommendations based on Russell-Taylor classification of subtrochanteric fractures

Type	Fracture description	Treatment
Ia	Piriformis fossa and lesser trochanter intact	Standard interlocking IM nail
Ib	Piriformis fossa intact, lesser trochanter fractured	Reconstruction IM nail
IIa	Piriformis fossa fractured, lesser trochanter intact	Hip screw or reconstruction IM nail
IIb	Piriformis fossa and lesser trochanter fractured	Hip screw with bone graft or reconstruction IM nail

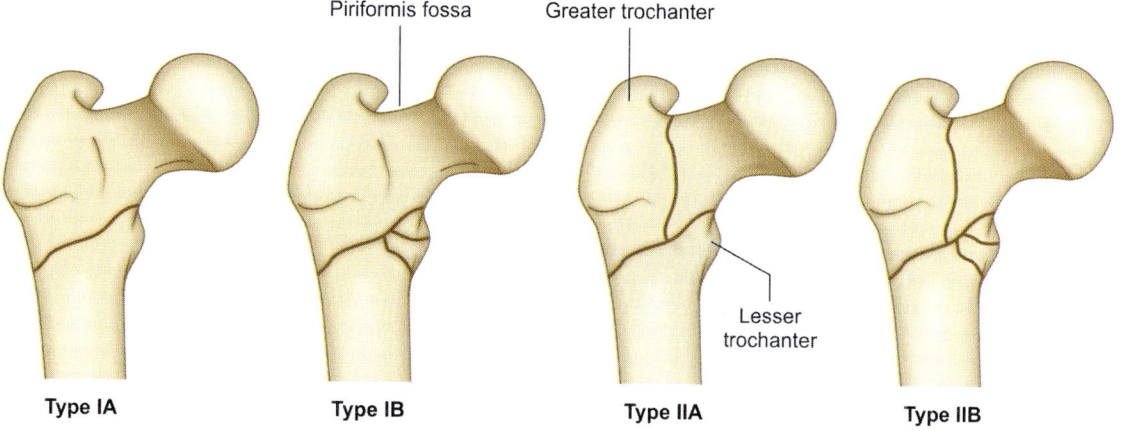

Fig. 34.4: Russell-Taylor classification

Type IA Type IB Type IIA Type IIB

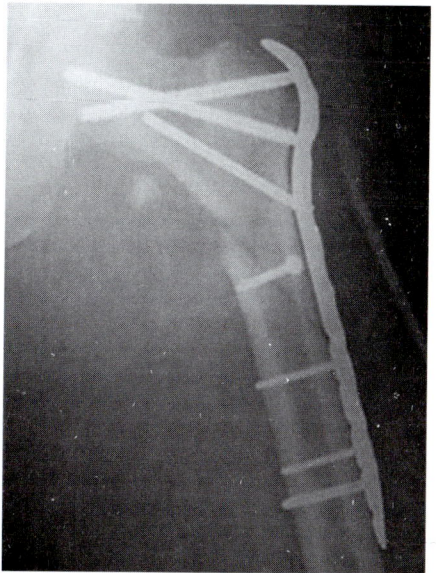

Fig. 34.5: Locking plate

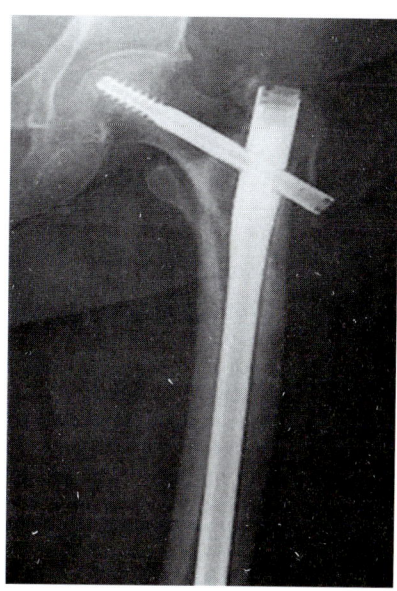

Fig. 34.6: Intramedullary nail

COMPLICATIONS

Common complications include: Nonunion, varus malunion, failure of fixation, deep vein thrombosis and wound infection.

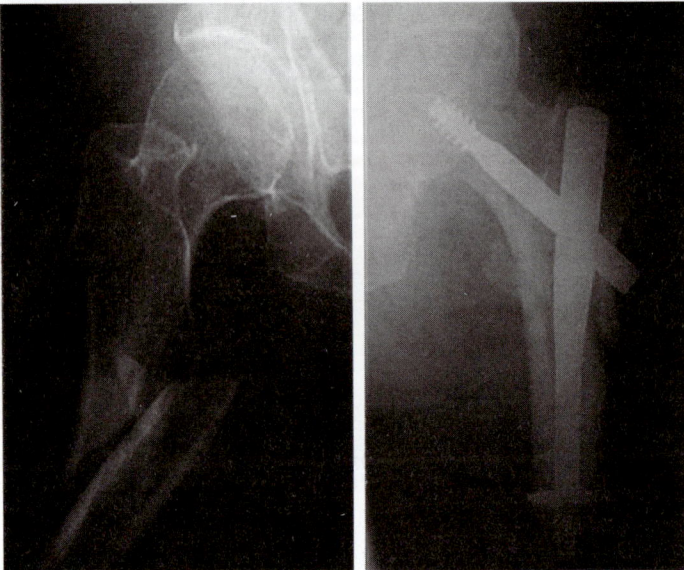

Fig. 34.7: Intramedullary nail

BIBLIOGRAPHY

- https://www.youtube.com/watch?v=cHd7afhOOqU
- https://emedicine.medscape.com/article/1247329
- www.orthobullets.com/trauma/1039

Fracture Shaft of Femur

- High energy injuries, frequently associated with life-threatening conditions.
- The annual incidence of midshaft femur fractures is approximately 10 per 100,000 person-years
- The incidence peaks among the young, decreasing after age 20, and then again in the elderly
- *Initial evaluation:* Advanced Trauma Life Support (ATLS) should be initiated.
- *Neurovascular:* Must record and document distal neurovascular status.

CLASSIFICATION

Classification of fracture shaft of femur is given in Table 35.1.

TREATMENT

Surgical stabilization within 24 hours is associated with:

- Decreased pulmonary complications (ARDS)
- Decreased thromboembolic events
- Improved rehabilitation

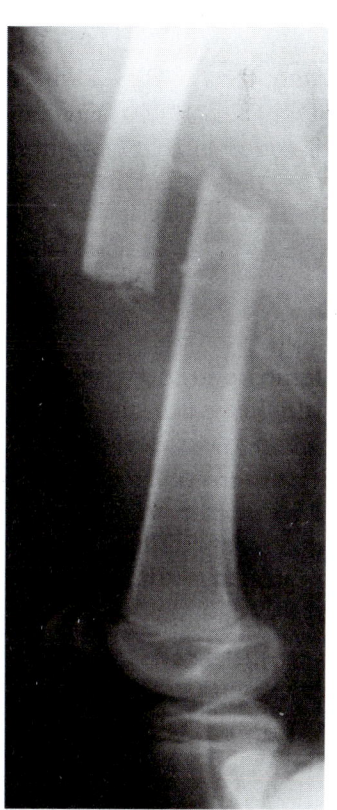

Fig. 35.1: Fracture of femoral shaft

Table 35.1: Winquist and Hansen classification

Type 0	No comminution
Type I	Insignificant amount of comminution
Type II	Greater than 50% cortical contact
Type III	Less than 50% cortical contact
Type IV	Segmental fracture with no contact between proximal and distal fragment

The current favoured treatment of femoral shaft fractures is with statically locked reamed intramedullary nailing. Alternatives include: Traction with or without cast bracing, plate osteosynthesis and external fixation.

COMPLICATIONS

- Heterotopic ossification
  - Incidence: 25%
- Pudendal nerve injury
  - Incidence: 10% when using fracture table with traction
- Femoral artery or nerve injury
  - Incidence: Rare
- Malunion
  - Incidence:
    - o Proximal fractures: 30%
    - o Distal fractures: 10%

- Delayed union
  - Treatment—dynamization of nail with or without bone grafting
- Nonunion
  - Incidence: <10%
  - Treatment—reamed exchange nailing
- Infection
  - Incidence: < 1%
  - Treatment:
    - o Removal of nail and reaming of canal
    - o External fixation used if fracture not healed

BIBLIOGRAPHY

- http://www.orthobullets.com/trauma/1040/femoral-shaft-fractures
- http://emedicine.medscape.com/article/824856-overview
- https://www.youtube.com/watch?v= MI2Jvgt9Z8c
- https://www.youtube.com/watch?v= lk9U3vxGE4A

Fractures of Distal Femur

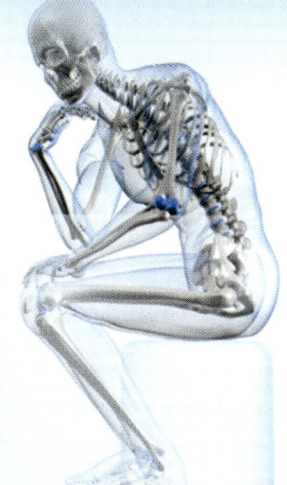

- Defined as fractures from articular surface to 5 cm above metaphyseal flare.
- The estimated frequency is 0.4% with an epidemiology that varies: There is a classic bimodal distribution, with a frequency peak for men in their 30s and a peak for elderly women; however, at present it is found predominantly in women and in the elderly with more than 50% of patients who are over 65.
- Distal femur fractures represents about 7% of all femur fractures in adults, and are notoriously difficult to treat.

Fractures of the distal femur may be extra-articular or have an intra-articular component. Mismanagement of any of these fractures can result in abnormalities of alignment of the load-bearing axis of the lower limb and/or rotational deformities. These can have profound biomechanical consequences.

AO CLASSIFICATION

- Type A = extra-articular
  Treatment = retrograde IM nail or ORIF usually via minimal lateral approach
- Type B = unicondylar fractures
  Treatment = percutaneous lag screw fixation +/- plating
- Type C = intra-articular fractures
  Treatment = ORIF via modified lateral para patellar arthrotomy
- Periprosthetic distal femur fracture
  Treatment = Lateral locked plating with indirect reduction

- Elderly osteoporotic patients with severe comminution—consider primary total knee arthroplasty.

TREATMENT
Nonoperative

Hinged knee brace with immediate ROM, NWB for 6 weeks

Indications (rare):
- Nondisplaced fractures
- Nonambulatory patient
- Patient with significant comorbidities

Operative

For an extra-articular fracture, all therapeutic options are possible and mini-invasive surgery can be performed. In case of an intra-articular fracture, open reduction and internal plate fixation should be performed with the patient on a standard operating table.

Open Reduction Internal Fixation
Indications
- Displaced fracture
- Intra-articular fracture
- Nonunion

Goals
- Need anatomic reduction of joint
- Stable fixation of articular component to shaft
- Preserve vascularity

Techniques: Simple screw fixation is proposed in the presence of a frontal or sagittal unicondylar fracture. Blade plate or dynamic compression/locking plate fixation is indicated in extra-articular fractures, sagittal unicondylar fractures or supracondylar and intercondylar fractures. Total knee arthroplasty is reserved for complex fractures in the elderly.

Postoperative

- Early ROM of knee important
- Non-weight bearing or touch toe weight-bearing for 6–8 weeks
- Quadriceps and hamstring strength exercises.

Retrograde IM Nail

Indications

- Good for supracondylar fracture without significant comminution.
- Preferred implant in osteoporotic bone

External Fixation

External fixation should bridge the knee when there is intra-articular involvement.

COMPLICATIONS

- Symptomatic hardware
  - Lateral plate
    - Pain with knee flexion/extension due to IT band contact with plate
  - Medial screw irritation
    - Excessively long screws can irritate medial soft tissues.
    - Determine appropriate intercondylar screw length by obtaining an AP radiograph of the knee with the leg internally rotated 30°.
- Malunions
  - Most commonly associated with plating
  - Functional results satisfactory, if malalignment is within 5° in any plane.

- Nonunions
  - Treatment with revision ORIF and autograft indicated.
  - Consider changing fixation technique to improve biomechanics.

SUPRACONDYLAR FRACTURE OF FEMUR (Fig. 36.1)

Supracondylar region is the area which is 9 cm from the articular surface of the knee joint. Of all femoral fractures, approximately 4–7% are distal femur fractures. The incidence of supracondylar fracture after total knee arthroplasty is approximately 1%.

Bimodal demographic presentation:
- Low energy osteoporotic fractures in elderly patients
- High energy in young patients

AO Classification (Fig. 36.2)

1. Type 33A: Extra-articular fracture
   - A1: Simple
   - A2: Metaphyseal wedge and/or fragmented wedge
   - A3: Metaphyseal complex
2. Type 33B: Partial articular fracture
   - B1: Lateral condyle, sagittal
   - B2: Medial condyle, sagittal
   - B3: Frontal

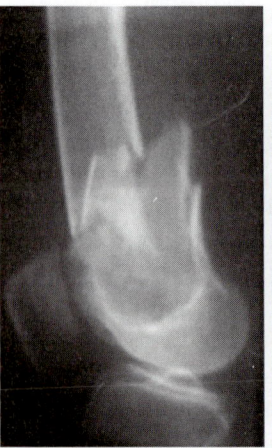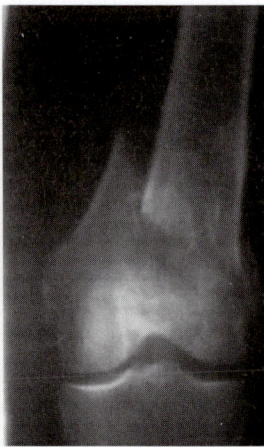

Fig. 36.1: Supracondylar fracture of femur

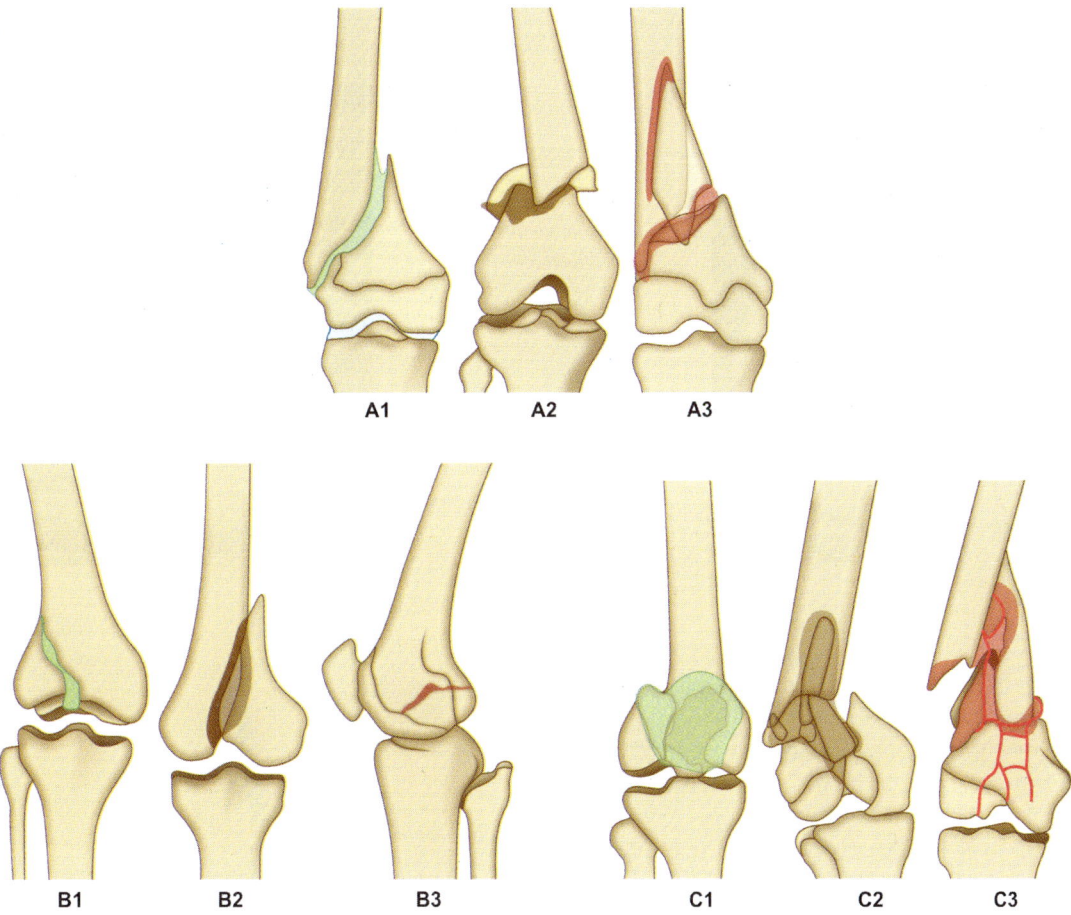

Fig. 36.2: AO classification

3. Type 33C: Complete articular fracture
  • C1: Articular simple, metaphyseal simple
  • C2: Articular simple, metaphyseal multi-fragmentary
  • C3: Articular multifragmentary

Hoffa fracture is a type of supracondylar distal femoral fracture, it is intra-articular and is characterized by a fracture in the coronal plane. Hoffa fragments are more commonly unicondylar and usually originate from the lateral femoral condyle. They can be occasionally bicondylar.

Management

Successful management of the distal femoral fracture is possible with adherence to the basic principles of anatomic reduction, stable fixation, and early motion.

Except in extreme circumstances, operative treatment for supracondylar femoral fractures is the standard, while nonsurgical treatment has largely fallen out of favor as the result of further advances in technique and implants. Fractures of the distal femur shaft are more difficult to treat conservatively. The gastrocnemius muscle crosses the knee and pulls the distal fragment into flexion thus causing a posterior angulation.

Implant selection is determined on the basis of the characteristics of the fracture, the bone quality, the needs of the patient, and the experience of the surgeon.

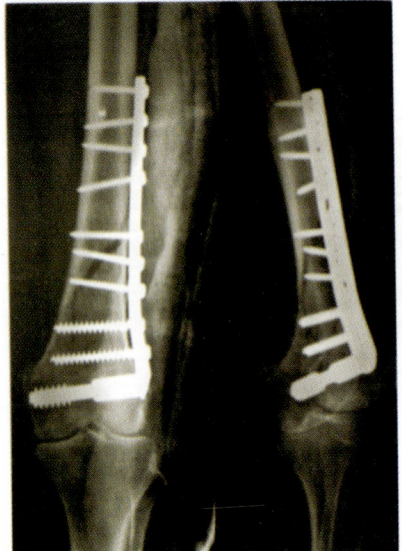
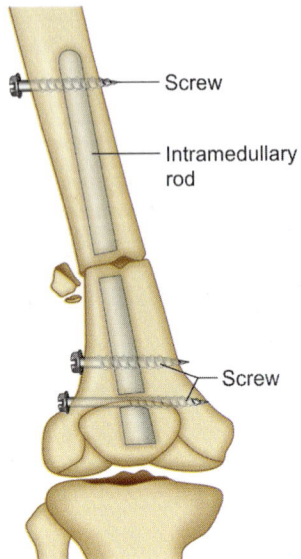
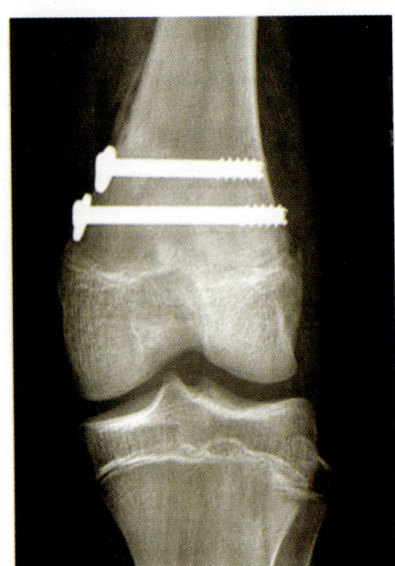

Fig. 36.3: Internal fixation

For an extra-articular fracture, all therapeutic options are possible and mini-invasive surgery can be performed. Best known internal fixator system for distal femur is LISS (less invasive stabilization system—Synthes), which has the option to be introduced percutaneously, by minimally invasive techniques (Fig. 36.3). Submuscular plate insertion reduces the nonunion rate.

Antegrade/retrograde nailing is the other option.

Simple screw fixation is proposed in the presence of a frontal or sagittal unicondylar fracture.

Blade plates/DCP/LCP are other implants used to treat these fractures. The goal of locking plate is to provide better stability in fragile bone. Primary stability of the plate is independent of the friction effect as the screw presses the plate, and is obtained by locking the screw into the plate. Plate design is usually anatomical which allows it to be used as a "reduction mold", molding the bone to the plate.

All types of fractures can be treated with locking plates and a classic or mini-invasive surgical approach is possible.

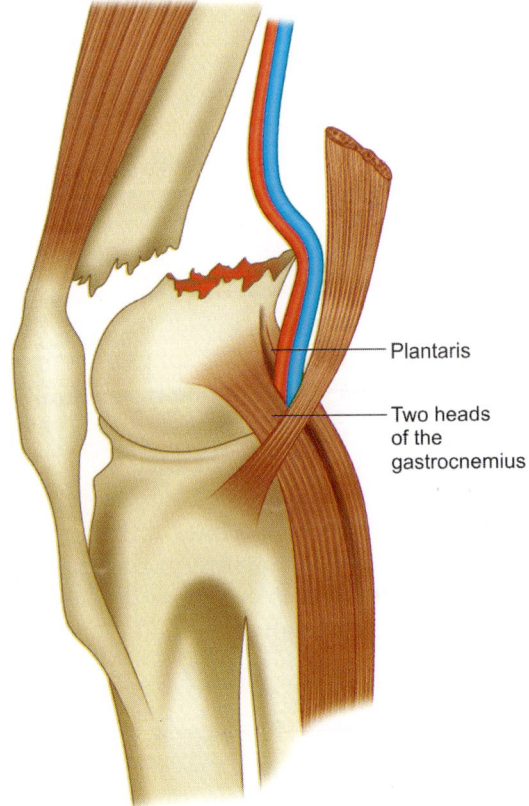

Fig. 36.4: Damage to popliteal artery

Complications

Damage to popliteal artery is rare, but is a serious complication (Fig. 36.4).

- Nonunion
- Malunion
- Infection
- Failure of fixation
- Painful hardware
- Compartment syndrome
- DVT/PE
- Heterotopic ossification
- Extension contracture

BIBLIOGRAPHY

- http://www.sciencedirect.com/science/article/pii/S1877056813000200
- https://www.youtube.com/watch?v=ZlyPYEdtjHM
- https://www2.aofoundation.org/
- www.rcsed.ac.uk/.../femur

Fractures of Patella

Patella fractures account for approximately 1% of all skeletal injuries. Patella fractures become problematic, if the extensor mechanism of the knee is nonfunctional, articular congruity is lost, or stiffness of the knee joint ensues.

Disruption of the extensor mechanism renders the patient unable to extend the knee against gravity and usually implies that a tear is present in the medial and lateral quadriceps expansion (Fig. 37.1).

Most patella fractures can be adequately visualized and classified by using standard anteroposterior (AP), lateral, and axial (Merchant or sunrise) radiographs of the knee (Figs 37.2 and 37.3).

Can be described based on fracture pattern (Fig. 37.4):

- Nondisplaced
- Transverse
- Pole or sleeve (upper or lower)

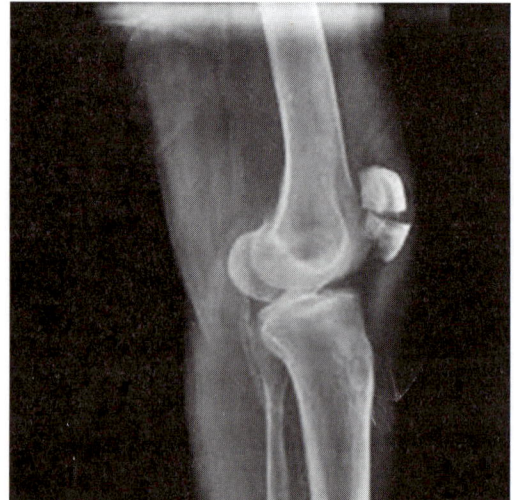

Fig. 37.2: AP view

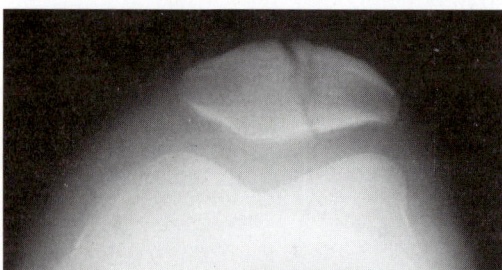

Fig. 37.3: Axial view

- Vertical
- Marginal
- Osteochondral
- Comminuted (stellate)

If the fracture is not displaced and the extensor mechanism is intact, the fracture may

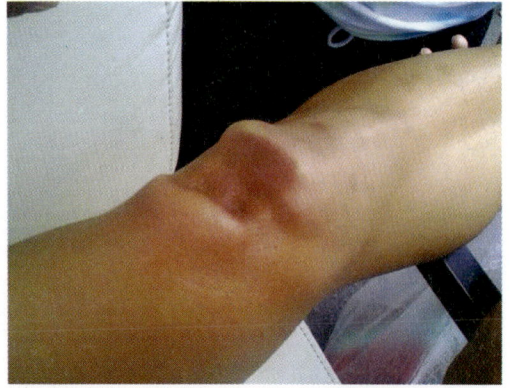

Fig. 37.1: Visible gap in fracture patella

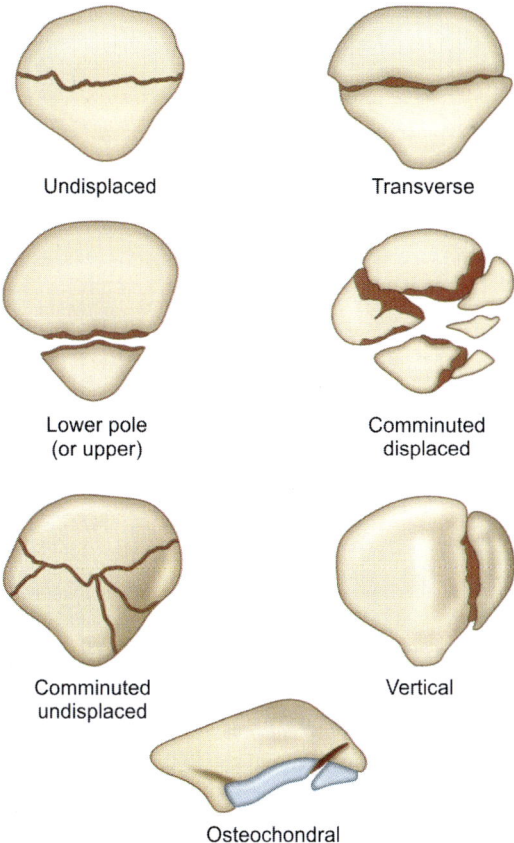

Undisplaced

Transverse

Lower pole
(or upper)

Comminuted
displaced

Comminuted
undisplaced

Vertical

Osteochondral

Fig. 37.4: Patellar fracture patterns

be treated by means of immobilization. This usually involves placing the affected extremity in a cylinder cast for 4–6 weeks. The patient is allowed to bear weight in the cast.

Indications for operative treatment of a patella fracture include:

- Disruption of the extensor mechanism
- Articular incongruity with more than 2 mm of step off
- More than 3 mm of separation between primary fracture fragments

The biomechanical principle of tension band fixation is to convert a tensile force into a compressive force while the knee is flexed. By placing a tension band at the anterior surface, this tensile force is converted into a compressive force, thereby aiding in fracture healing.

Modifications of the tension band technique include the use of cannulated screws instead of K-wires (Figs 37.5 to 37.7).

After fixation of a patella fracture, closing the arthrotomy and repairing the retinacula are vital. These measures add to the healing of the extensor mechanism and help prevent patellar subluxation.

Postoperative rehabilitation is dependent on the fracture pattern, the stability of fixation, and the status of the soft tissue.

Circumferential cerclage wires are helpful for stellate fractures. If the fracture is at the most proximal or distal pole, adequate fixation may not be achievable with hardware. In such cases, nonabsorbable heavy suture material can be used for the repair. This involves placing several sets of suture in the patellar or quadriceps tendon, using a locking and running stitch.

In rare instances (e.g. cases of severe and irreparable comminution), a partial or a total patellectomy must be performed. Because the long-term outcomes with these techniques are poor, they should be used only as a last resort. With a partial patellectomy involving at least one-third of the patella, a loss of motion of approximately 18° can be expected. With a total patellectomy, loss of motion, loss of strength, and knee instability with stair climbing occur. Therefore, it is essential to try to salvage as much patella as possible in all fractures.

COMPLICATIONS

- Infection
- Stiffness of knee joint
- Hardware prominence
- Loss of fixation or reduction

PROGNOSIS

The prognosis depends primarily on the quality of articular restoration. Any intra-articular incongruities lead to post-traumatic arthritis.

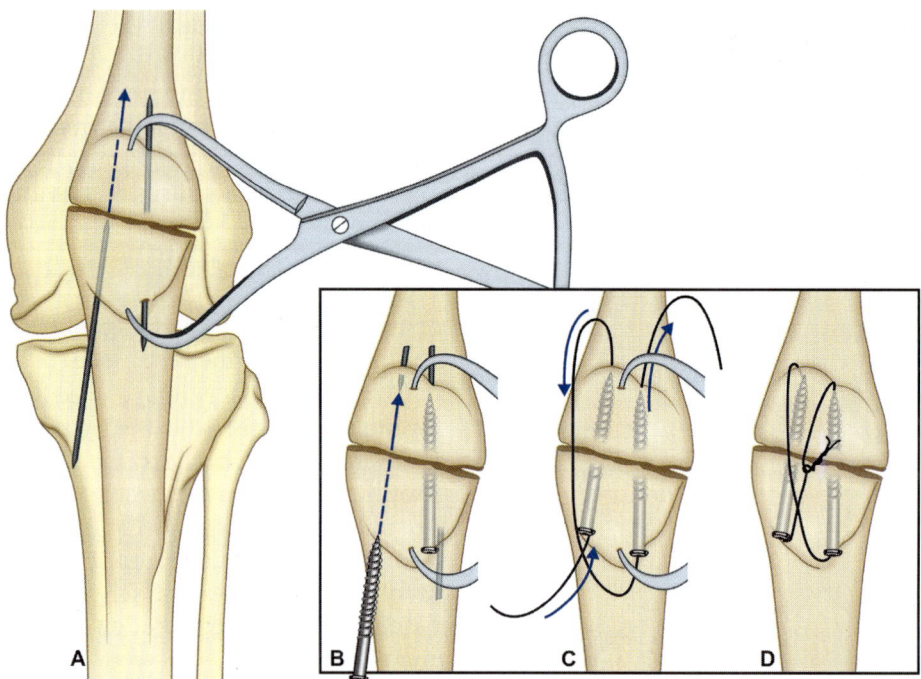

Fig. 37.5: Tension band wiring: Transverse patellar fracture fixation technique using tension band cable and cannulated screws: (A) After reducing the fracture with a clamp, two parallel K-wires are drilled from inferior to superior. (B) K-wires replaced with guidewires. Cannulated screws inserted along guidewires. (C) Titanium cable threaded through screws, starting with head of medial screw. (D) Cable tightened anteriorly and excess cable cut away

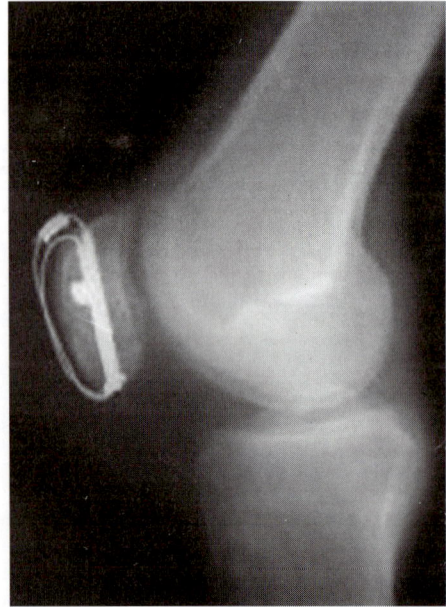

Fig. 37.6: Postoperative X-ray knee

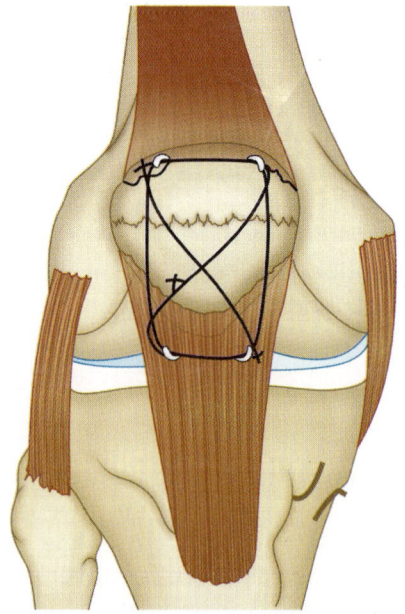

Fig. 37.7: Technique of tension bnad wiring

If arthrofibrosis develops, it may require manipulation with the patient under anesthesia or arthroscopic release of adhesions.

Bioabsorbable fixation methods may reduce the frequency of hardware-related symptoms.

BIBLIOGRAPHY

- http://emedicine.medscape.com/article/1249384-treatment#a1133
- https://www.youtube.com/watch?v=Qe6VNxxOJaw
- https://www.youtube.com/watch?v=ZhdU9EnfNNA

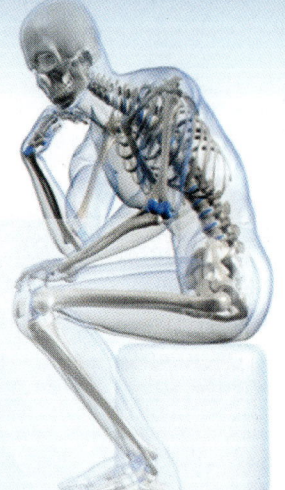

Chapter 38

Tibial Plateau Fractures

Sir Astley Cooper first described fractures of the proximal tibia in 1825. Sarmiento popularized functional cast bracing of most tibial condylar fractures. The increased frequency of tibial plateau fractures in older females is due to the increased prevalence of osteoporosis in these individuals. Tibial plateau fractures in younger patients are commonly the result of high-energy injuries. The most common mechanism resulting in a tibial plateau fracture is a valgus force with axial loading. Of these fractures, 80% are motor vehicle-related injuries, and the remainder are sports-related injuries. A bumper- or fender-related injury from a vehicle-pedestrian collision constitutes more than 25% of tibial plateau fractures.

CLASSIFICATION

Schatzker et al proposed a classification system of condyle fractures based on the fracture pattern and fragment anatomy. This classification system, which is widely accepted and used today, divides these fractures into the six types (Figs 38.1 and 38.2):

- *Type I:* This is a wedge or split fracture of the lateral aspect of the plateau, usually as a result of valgus and axial forces; the wedge fragment is not compressed (depressed), because the underlying cancellous bone is strong; this pattern is usually seen in younger patients.
- *Type II:* This is a lateral wedge or split fracture associated with compression; the mechanism of injury is similar to that of a type I fracture, but the underlying bone may be osteoporotic and unable to resist depression, or the force may have been greater.
- *Type III:* This is a pure compression fracture of the lateral plateau; as a result of an axial force, the depression is usually located laterally or centrally, but it may involve any portion of the articular surface.
- *Type IV:* This is a fracture that involves the medial plateau; as a result of either varus or axial compression forces, the pattern may be either split alone or split with compression; because this fracture involves the larger and stronger medial plateau.
- *Type V:* This fracture includes split elements of both the medial and the lateral condyles and may include medial or lateral articular compression, usually as a result of a pure axial force occurring while the knee is in extension.
- *Type VI:* This is a complex, bicondylar fracture in which the condylar components separate from the diaphysis; depression and impaction of fracture fragments are the rule.

Approximately 50% of the knees with closed tibial plateau fractures have injuries of the menisci and cruciate ligaments that usually require surgical repair.

Most tibial plateau fractures are easy to identify on standard anteroposterior (AP) and lateral projections of the knee. Lipo-

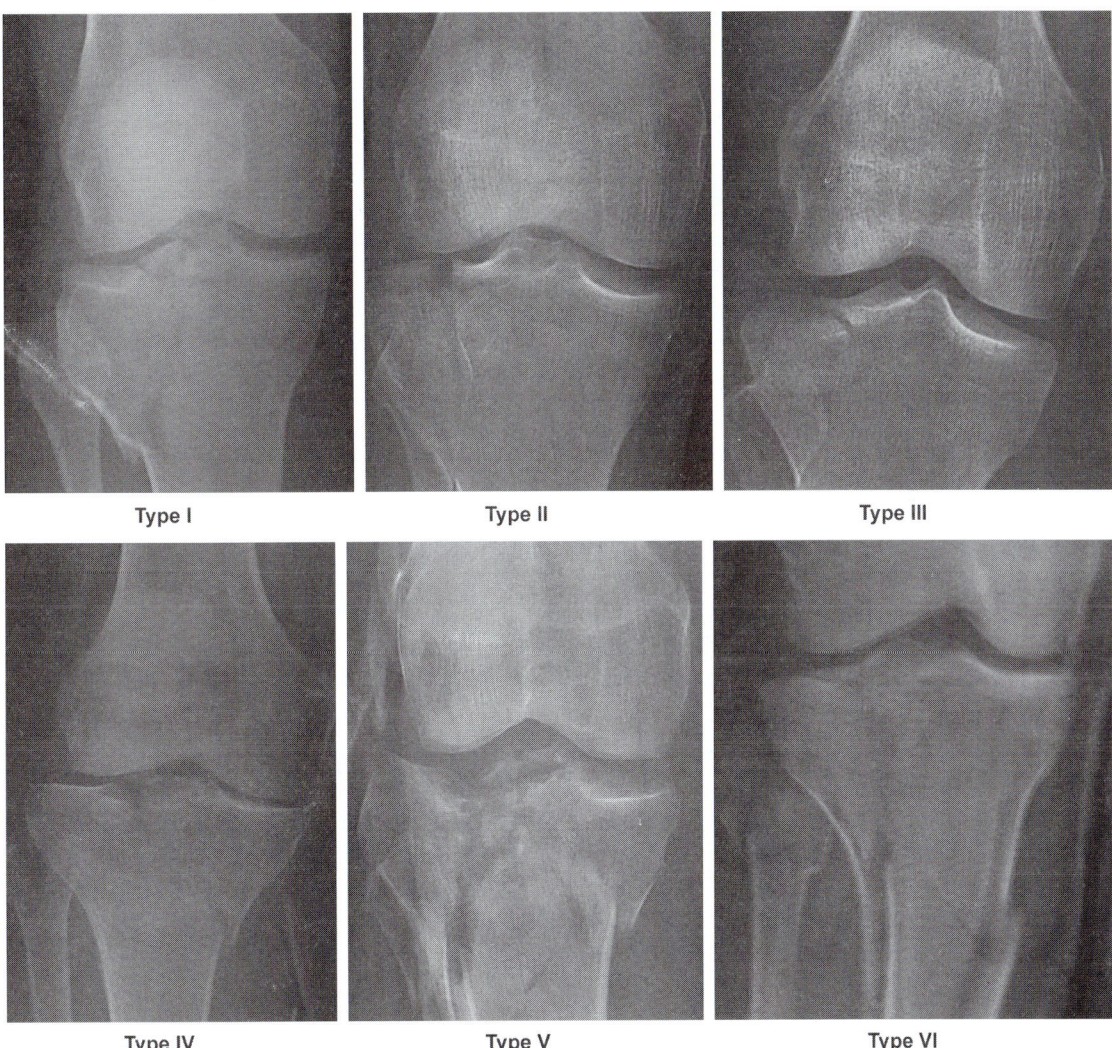

Type I   Type II   Type III

Type IV   Type V   Type VI

Fig. 38.1: Schatzker types

haemarthrosis results from an intra-articular fracture with escape of fat and blood from the bone marrow into the joint, and is most frequently seen in the knee, associated with a tibial plateau fracture or distal femoral fracture.

By acquiring thin axial slices through the knee and reconstructing the image data in the sagittal and coronal planes, computed tomography (CT) provides more detailed information. The information obtained from a CT scan can help determine the best surgical approach based on the fracture planes seen on the computer images.

Magnetic resonance imaging (MRI) is acknowledged as a reliable and accurate tool for assessing meniscal, collateral, and cruciate ligamentous injury, as well as for identifying occult fractures of the tibial plateau.

MANAGEMENT

The ultimate goals of tibial plateau fracture treatment are to re-establish joint stability, alignment, and articular congruity while

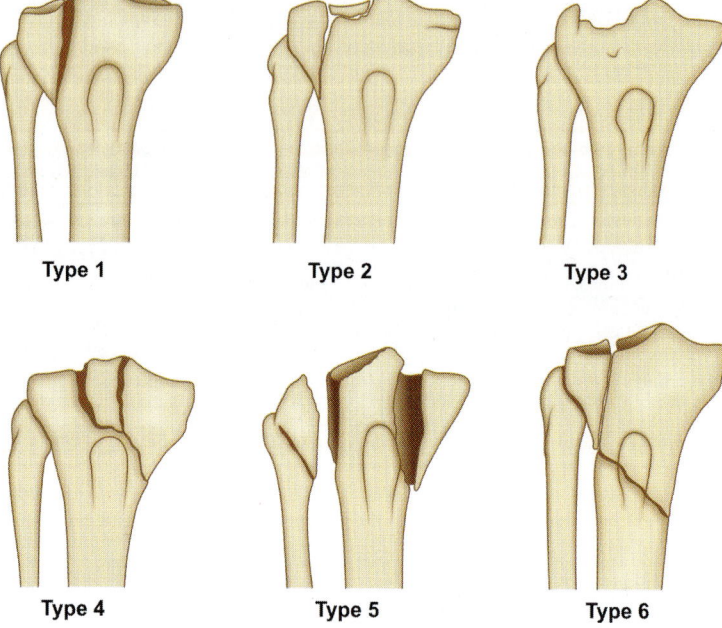

Type 1   Type 2   Type 3

Type 4   Type 5   Type 6

Fig. 38.2: Types of tibial plateau fractures

preserving full range of motion. Fracture displacement ranging from 4–10 mm can be treated nonoperatively; however, a depressed fragment greater than 5 mm should be elevated and grafted.

Open or arthroscopic-assisted techniques are considered for fractures with displacement, depression of the condylar surfaces, or both.

Internal fixation can be accomplished by means of the following:
- Biologic fixation—screw fixation, minimally invasive plate osteosynthesis, least invasive stabilization system
- Arthroscopic-assisted fixation
- Conventional double plating

External fixation can be accomplished with the following:
- Ilizarov fixator
- Hybrid fixator

Follow-up

Non-weight-bearing precautions generally continue for 12 weeks. Active flexion and passive extension are encouraged for 6 weeks, after which active knee extension is started. Active knee extension is delayed, if open reduction and internal fixation of a tibial tubercle avulsion was required.

COMPLICATIONS

Early
- Compartment syndrome
- Vascular injuries
- Swelling and wound-healing problems
- Infections
- Deep vein thrombosis
- Nerve injuries

Late
- Knee stiffness
- Knee instability
- Angular deformities
- Late collapse
- Malunion
- Secondary osteoarthrosis of knee joint

Summary

The goal of tibial plateau fracture management is a stable, well-aligned, congruent joint, with a painless range of motion and function. Minimally displaced stable fractures should be treated with protected mobilization. The treatment of displaced tibial plateau fractures, however, remains controversial. Surgical reduction and stabilization of displaced tibial plateau fractures, when indicated, requires careful evaluation of both the "personality" of the fracture and the soft tissue envelope. The timing of surgery and the handling of the soft tissue in this region are critical to treatment success. After restoration of a congruent joint surface, bone grafting and buttress plating are usually needed to allow early range of motion and optimize treatment outcome.

BIBLIOGRAPHY

- htthttp://emedicine.medscape.com/article/1249872-overviewp://emedicine.medscape.com/article/1249872-treatment#d13
- https://en.wikipedia.org/wiki/Tibial_plateau_fracture
- https://www.youtube.com/watch?v=0sOfB-FET34
- https://www.youtube.com/watch?v=Vji4F9v7uo4

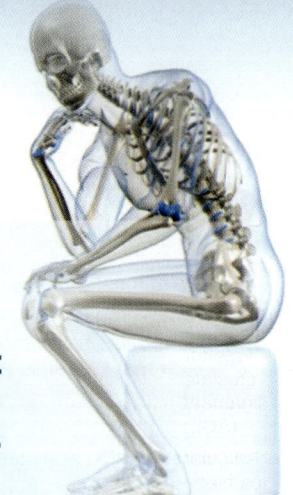

Ligamentous Injuries of the Knee Joint

LIGAMENTOUS ANATOMY

Anterior cruciate ligament is the most common ligament to be injured. The ACL is often stretched and/or torn during a sudden twisting motion (when the feet stay planted one way, but the knees turn the other way). Skiing, basketball, and football are sports that have a higher risk of ACL injuries. However, the PCL injury usually occurs with sudden, direct impact, such as in a car accident or during a football tackle. Medial collateral ligament (MCL) is injured more often than the lateral collateral ligament (LCL) (Figs 39.1 to 39.7).

Ligamentous Anatomy

- Anterior cruciate ligament (ACL)—prevents anterior tibial translation
- Posterior cruciate ligament (PCL)—prevents posterior tibial translation
- Medial collateral ligament (MCL)—protects against valgus stress
- Lateral collateral ligament (LCL)—protects against varus stress

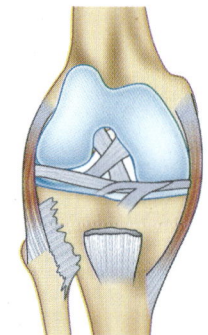

Fig. 39.1: Anatomy of knee

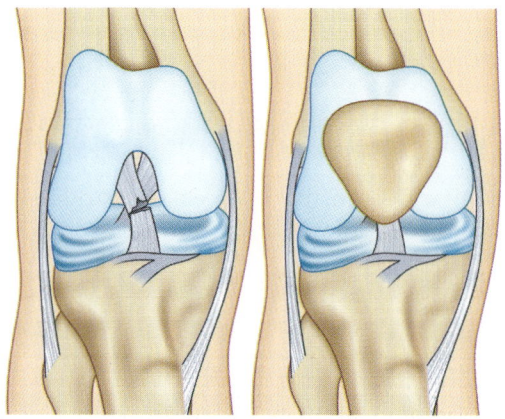

Fig. 39.2: Knee joint ligaments

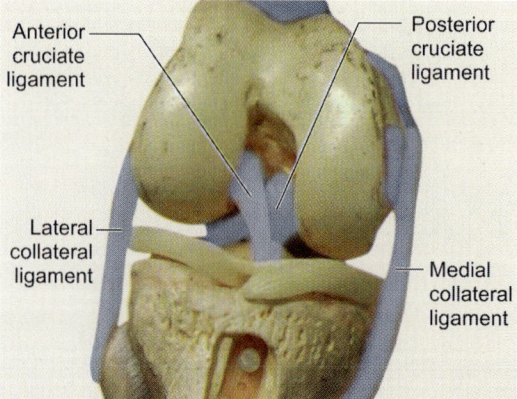

Fig. 39.3: Knee ligaments

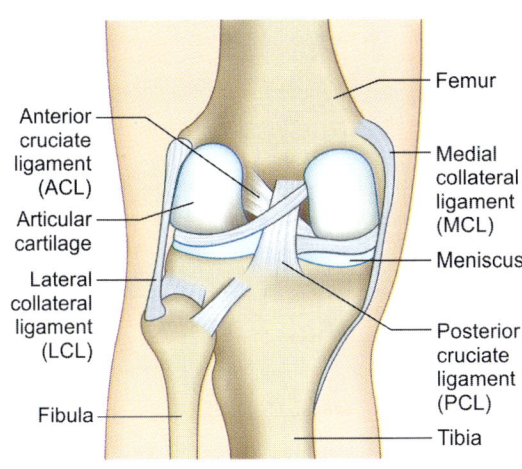

Fig. 39.4: Left knee from behind

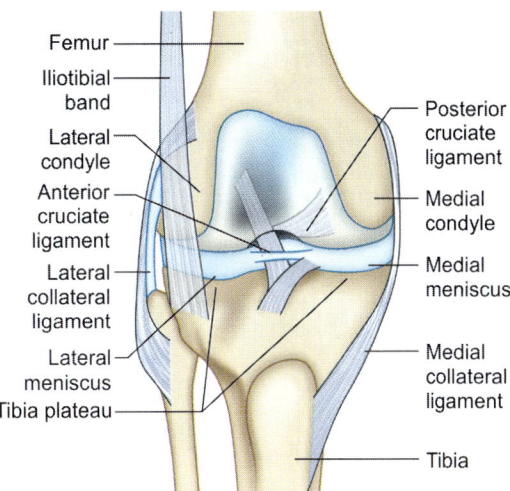

Fig. 39.5: View inside of the knee (knee cap removed)

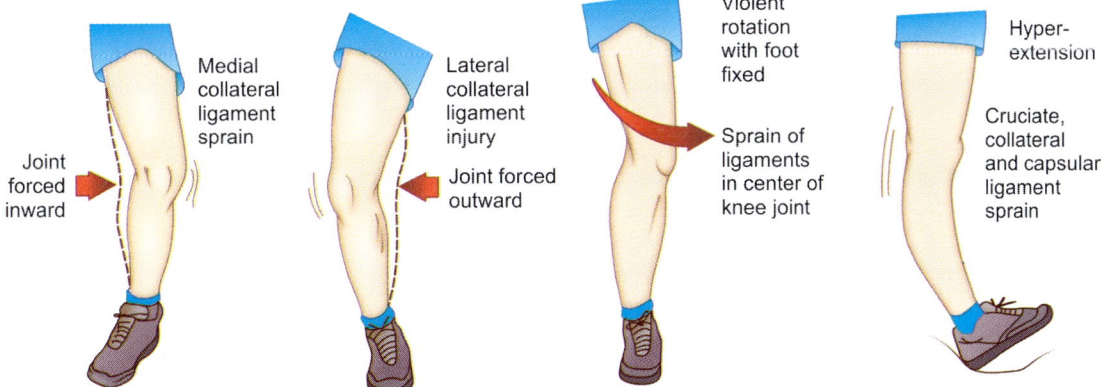

Fig. 39.6: Mechanism of injury

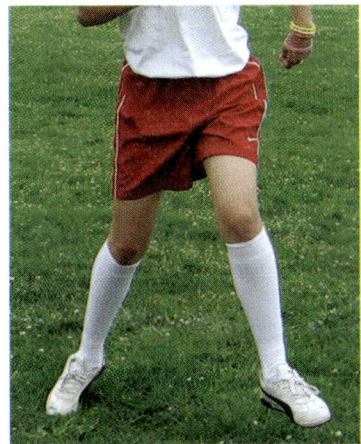

Fig. 39.7: Twisting injury of knee while playing

Early medical treatment for knee ligament injury may include, but is not limited to, the following:

- Rest
- Ice pack application (to reduce swelling that occurs within hours of the injury)
- Compression (from an elastic bandage or brace)
- Elevation
- Pain relievers

ANTERIOR CRUCIATE LIGAMENT INJURY

ACL injuries occur when an individual stops suddenly or plants his/her foot hard into the

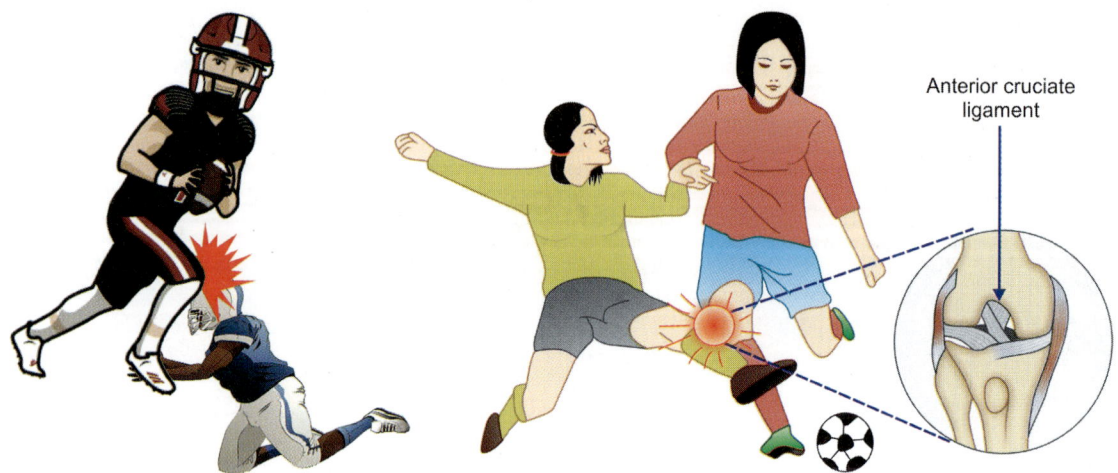

Anterior cruciate ligament

Fig. 39.8: Sports-related injury

ground (cutting). ACL failure has also been linked to heavy or stiff-legged landing; the knee rotating while landing, especially when the knee is in an unnatural position. ACL tears occur for two reasons: The failure load of the ligament and the mechanical load applied to it. Women in sports such as association football, basketball, and tennis are significantly more prone to ACL injuries than men (Fig. 39.8).

The combination of "pop" during a twisting movement or rapid deceleration, together with inability to continue participation, and followed by early swelling, is said to indicate a 90% probability of rupture of the anterior cruciate ligament. An ACL tear can present with a popping sound heard after impact, swelling after a couple of hours, severe pain when bending the knee, and buckling or locking of the knee during movement.

Clinical Diagnosis

In an athlete with an acute traumatic knee effusion, the Lachman test, anterior drawer test, and pivot shift test are clinical examinations that aid in making the diagnosis of an ACL tear.

Anterior Drawer Test

The anterior drawer test is performed with the patient supine with the knee flexed to 90°. The

examiner grasps the tibia just below the knee joint, with the examiner's thumbs placed on either side of the patellar tendon. The tibia is pulled forward. An increased amount of anterior tibial translation compared with the opposite leg or a lack of a firm end point suggests a torn ACL (Fig. 39.9).

Lachman Test

The Lachman test is performed with the patient supine. The injured knee is flexed to 30°. The examiner places 1 hand behind the tibia with the examiner's thumb on the tibial tubercle and the other hand on the patient's lower thigh. The tibia is pulled anteriorly. Examinations of both knees are compared. Increased anterior movement of the tibia relative to the femur without a firm end-point compared with the examination of the uninjured knee suggests a torn ACL (Fig. 39.10).

Both the Lachman and anterior drawer tests require a relaxed patient without hamstring guarding.

Pivot Shift Test

The pivot shift test is performed with the patient supine and the knee extended. The examiner stresses the lateral side of the knee while gradually flexing the patient's knee. A

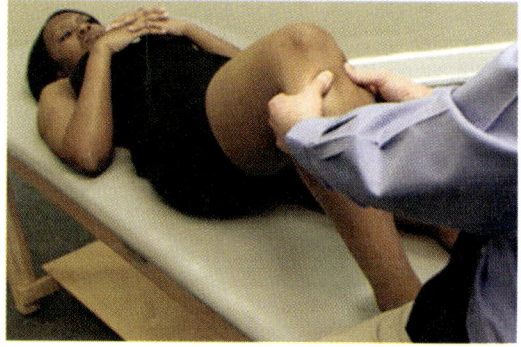

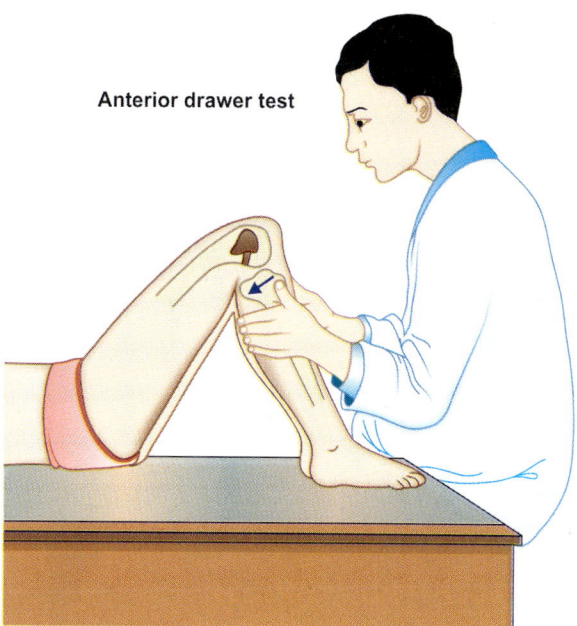

Anterior drawer test

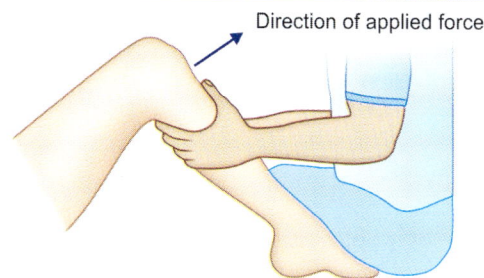

Direction of applied force

Fig. 39.9: Anterior drawer's test

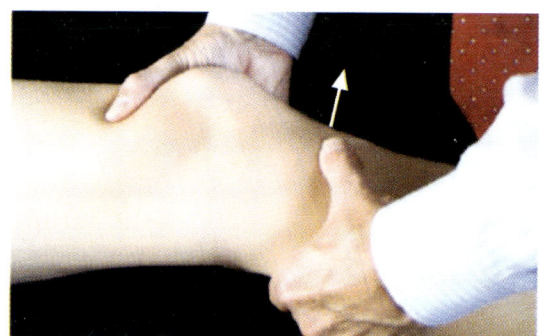

Fig. 39.10: Lachman's test

"clunk" sensation occurs when the partly subluxated tibia relocates in relation to the femur, indicating that the ACL is torn (Fig. 39.11).

The Lachman test is considered the most accurate of the three commonly performed clinical tests for an acute ACL tear, showing a pooled sensitivity of 85% and a pooled specificity of 94%.

O' Donoghue's Triad

1. Medial collateral ligament

2. Medial meniscus

3. Anterior cruciate ligament rupture.

Non-Surgical Treatment

Non-surgical management is indicated in patients with:

- Partial tears and no instability symptoms
- Complete tears and no symptoms of knee instability
- Who do light manual work or live sedentary lifestyles
- Whose growth plates are still open (children)

Patients who have suffered an ACL injury should be evaluated for other injuries that often occur in combination with an ACL tear (Fig. 39.12) and include cartilage/meniscus injuries, bone bruises, PCL tears, posterolateral injuries and collateral ligament injuries.

The pivot-shift test, anterior drawer test and Lachman test are used during the clinical examination of suspected ACL injury.

The term for non-surgical treatment for ACL rupture is "conservative management",

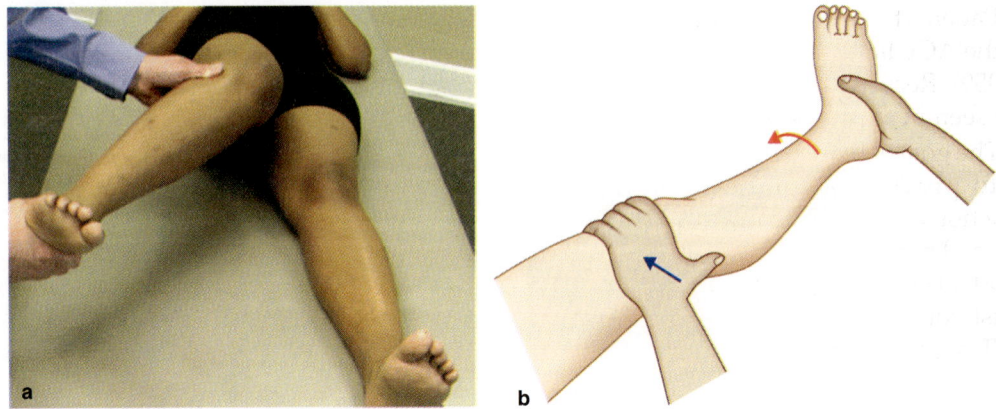

Fig. 39.11a and b: Pivot shift test

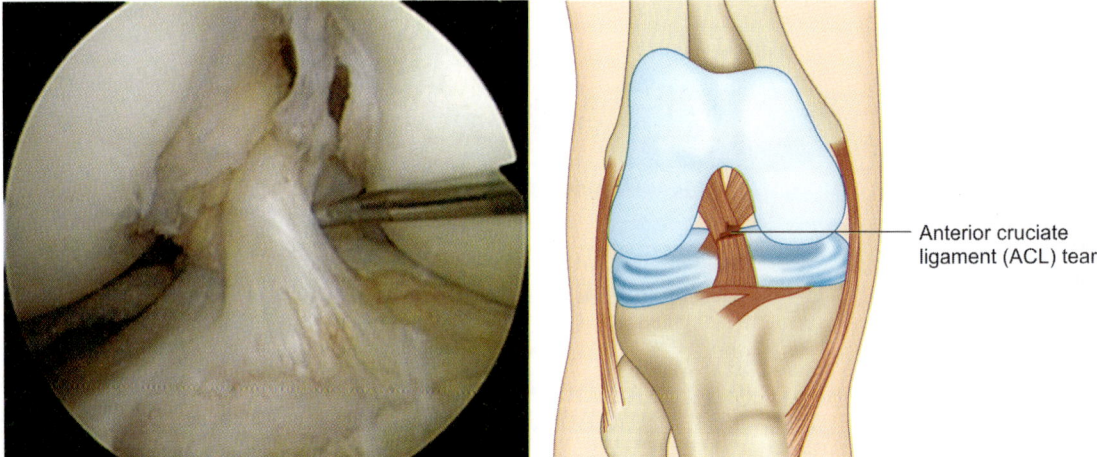

Anterior cruciate
ligament (ACL) tear

Fig. 39.12: Anterior cruciate ligament (ACL) tear

and it often includes physical therapy and using a knee brace. Instability associated with ACL deficiency increases the risk of other knee injuries such as a torn meniscus, so sports with cutting and twisting motions are problematic and surgery is often recommended in those circumstances.

If surgery is decided upon, either because obvious instability interferes with activities of daily living, or because the knee is subject to repeated, severe, provocative maneuvers, such as the case of the competitive athlete involved in cutting and rapid deceleration, etc., then several issues need to be decided upon.

- *Timing:* Immediate repair is usually avoided and initial swelling and inflammatory reaction allowed to subside.
- *Choice of graft material:* Autograft or allograft.
- *Choice of anterior cruciate ligament augmentation:* Patellar tendon or hamstring tendon.

The grafts commonly used to replace the ACL include:

- Patellar tendon autograft (autograft comes from the patient)
- Hamstring tendon autograft
- Quadriceps tendon autograft
- Allograft (taken from a cadaver) patellar tendon, Achilles tendon, semitendinosus, gracilis, or posterior tibialis tendon

Patients treated with surgical reconstruction of the ACL have long-term success rates of 82 to 95%. Recurrent instability and graft failure are seen in approximately 8% of patients.

The goal of the ACL reconstruction surgery is to prevent instability and restore the function of the torn ligament, creating a stable knee. This allows the patient to return to sports. There are certain factors that the patient must consider when deciding for or against ACL surgery (Figs 39.13 to 39.15).

In the most common ACL reconstruction technique, bone tunnels are drilled into the tibia and the femur to place the ACL graft in almost the same position as the torn ACL. Variations on this surgical technique include the "two-incision," "over-the-top," and "double-bundle" types of ACL reconstructions, which may be used because of the preference of the surgeon or special circumstances (revision ACL reconstruction, open growth plates) (Figs 39.16 to 39.18).

The pitfalls of the patellar tendon autograft are:
- Postoperative pain behind the kneecap
- Pain with kneeling
- Slightly increased risk of postoperative stiffness
- Low risk of patella fracture

Hamstring Tendon Autograft

The semitendinosus hamstring tendon on the inner side of the knee is used in creating the hamstring tendon autograft for ACL reconstruction. Some surgeons use an additional tendon, the gracilis, which is attached below the knee in the same area. This creates a two- or four-strand tendon graft (Fig. 39.19).

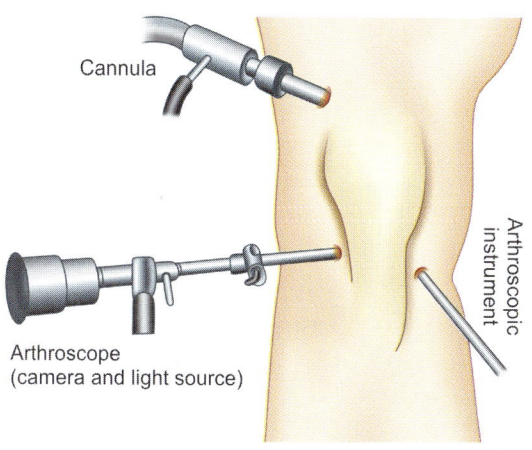

Fig. 39.13: Knee arthroscopy

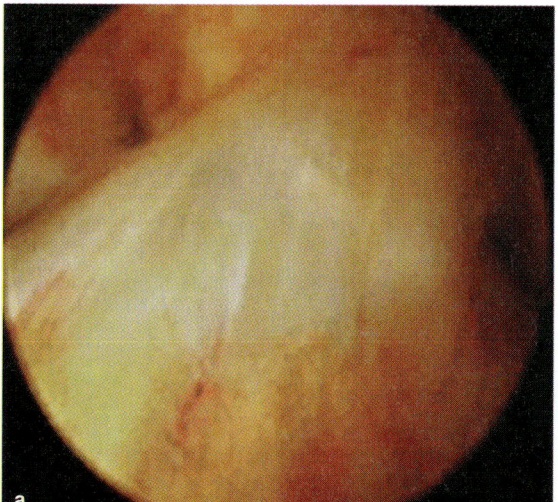

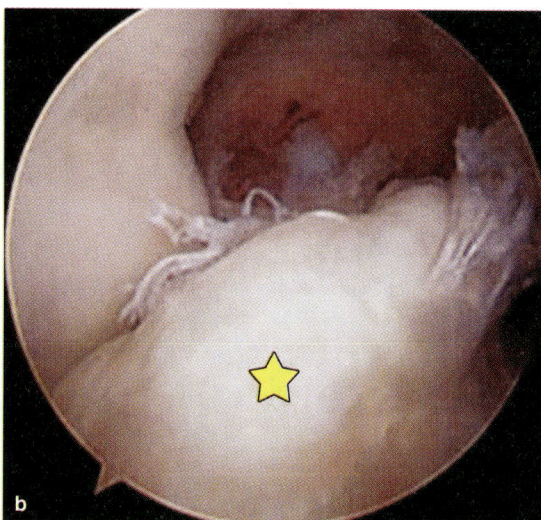

Fig. 39.14: (a) Arthroscopic picture of the normal ACL. (b) Arthroscopic picture of torn ACL (yellow star)

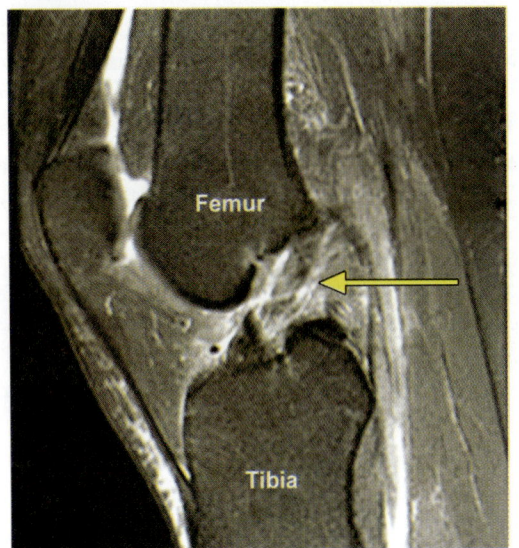

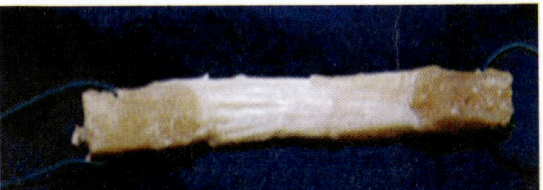

Fig. 39.16: Patellar tendon autograft prepared for ACL reconstruction

Fig. 39.15: MRI of complete ACL tear. The ACL fibers have been disrupted and the ACL appears wavy in appearance (yellow arrow)

common mechanism of injury in motor vehicle accidents is a dashboard injury or direct force to the proximal anterior tibia. Sports related injuries result from hyperflexion of the knee with the foot typically plantar flexed. The latter mechanism is the most common cause of isolated PCL injuries, while in the trauma population as many as 95% of patients with knee injuries have combined ligamentous damage.

POSTERIOR CRUCIATE LIGAMENT INJURY

Posterior cruciate ligament (PCL) injuries have a reported incidence of between 3 and 37%, depending on the clinical setting. The most

Clinical Tests

Posterior Tibial Sag Sign

To observe posterior tibial sag (Fig. 39.20), place patient supine and put 90° of flexion at the

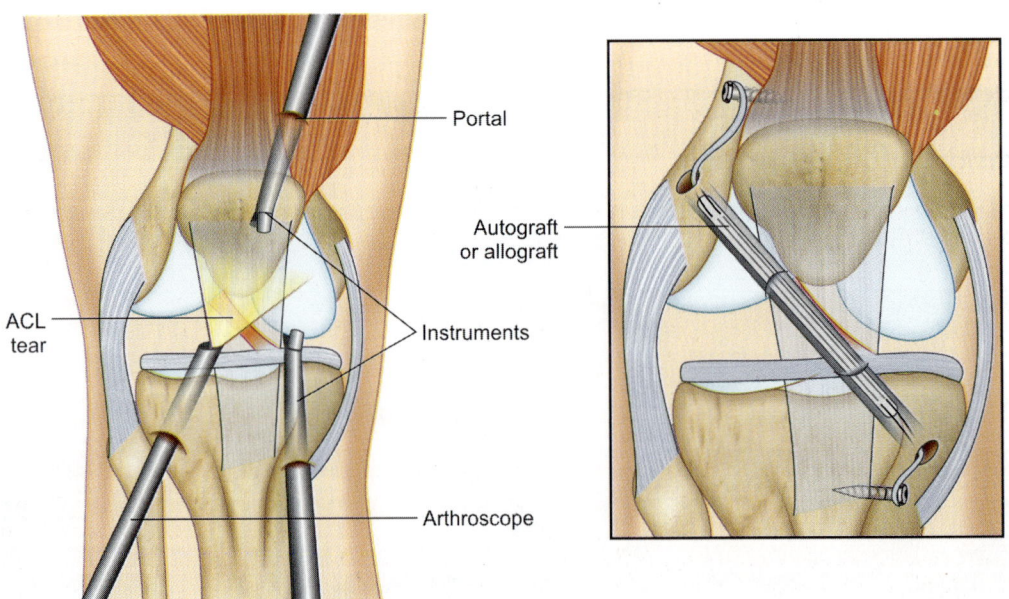

Fig. 39.17: ACL repair

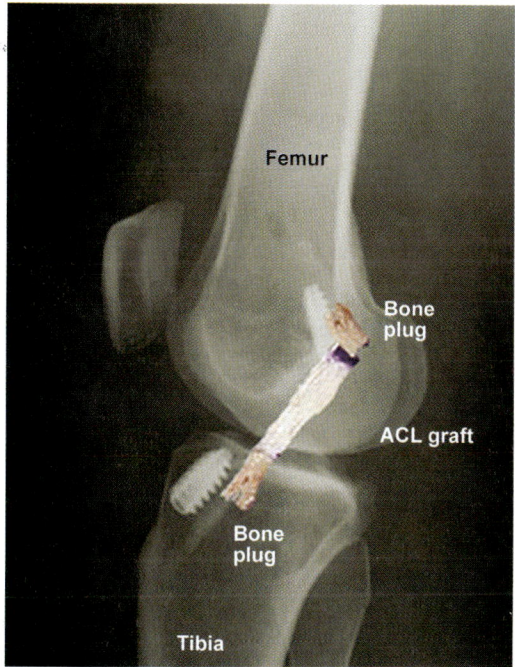

Fig. 39.18: Postoperative X-ray after ACL patellar tendon reconstruction (with picture of graft superimposed) shows graft position and bone plugs fixation with metal interference screws

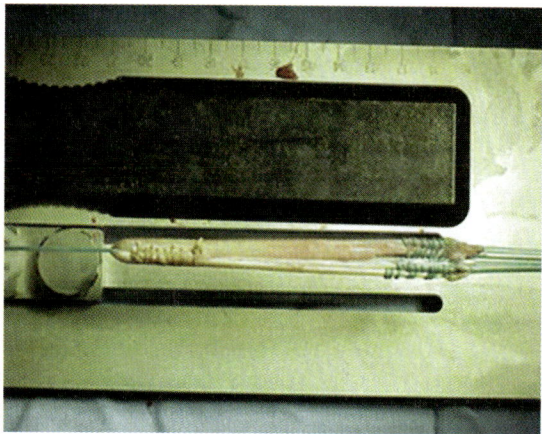

Fig. 39.19: Hamstring tendon autograft prepared for ACL reconstruction

placed flat on the table. The examiner imparts a posterior force to the proximal tibia, and if the tibia can be displaced 0–5 mm or if there is side-to-side asymmetry, a grade I injury is indicated. If the tibia can be displaced 5–10 mm or the tibial plateau can move posteriorly even with femoral condyles, a grade II injury is indicated. If the tibia can be moved more than 10 mm posteriorly or the tibial plateau moves behind the femoral condyles, a grade III injury is indicated.

The internal and external rotation of the foot during the posterior drawer test can assess different structures. If the foot is placed in internal rotation, the PCL and tibial collateral ligaments are tested. If the foot is placed in external rotation, the PCL, LCL, and postero-lateral corner are tested.

knee and hip. In such a position, gravity pulls posteriorly on the tibia, and in the case of PCL disruption, the tibia falls even or behind the femoral condyles. Comparison should be made to the opposite knee (Fig. 39.21).

Posterior Drawer Test (Fig. 39.22)

The patient is placed supine with both knees flexed to 90° and the feet in neutral rotation

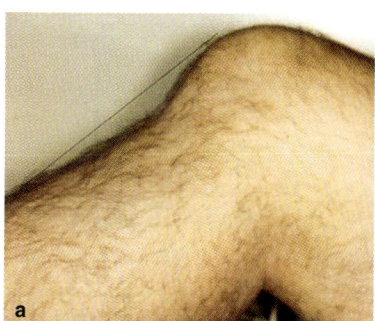
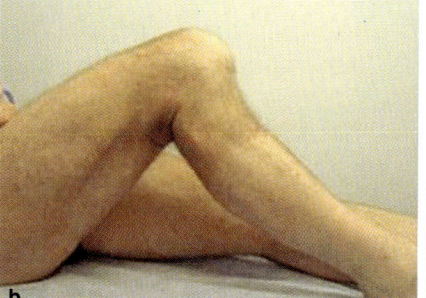
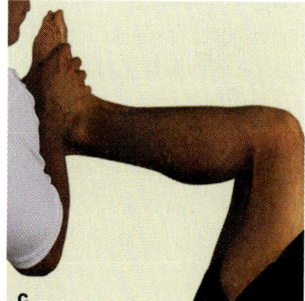

Fig. 39.20: Posterior tibial sag sign

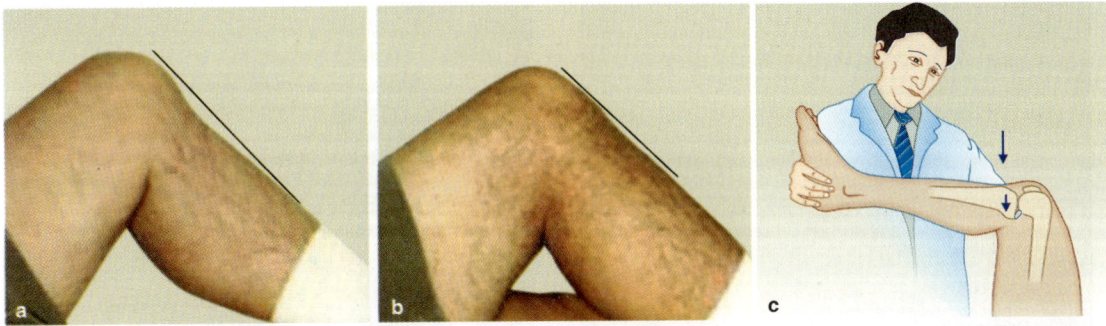

Fig. 39.21: Posterior tibial sag sign: (a and b) Demonstrates the clinical finding of the posterior tibial sag sign. A line drawn parallel to the patella accentuates the posterior tibial sag. (c) Demonstrates the quadriceps active drawer test described by Daniels. With the knee in 70–90° of flexion, the extensor mechanism is contracted, pulling the tibia anteriorly into a reduced position

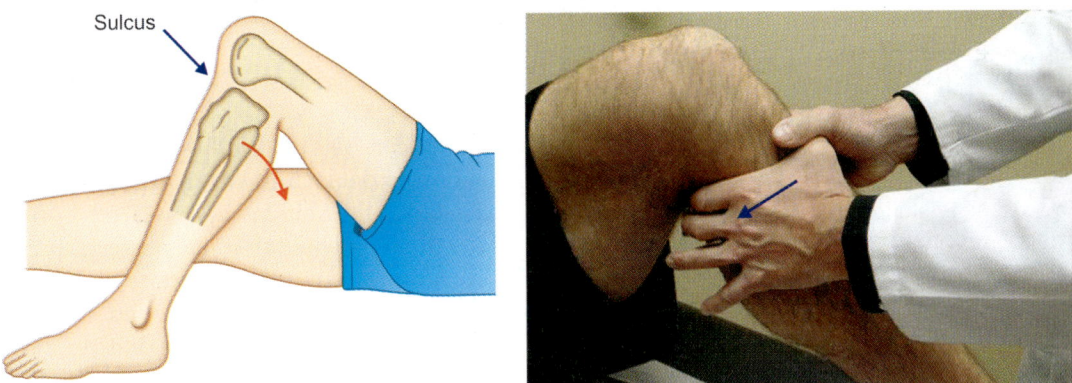

Fig. 39.22: Posterior drawer test

False-positive Lachman Test

The Lachman test is performed to assess the integrity of the ACL. In a knee with a deficient PCL, the starting position of the tibial plateau is posterior to normal. Since the starting point is posterior, there seems to be increased anterior laxity. This results in a false-positive Lachman test. The endpoint of the Lachman test is still firm with PCL disruption (Fig. 39.23).

Isolated PCL injuries have a very good prognosis. However, a PCL injury combined with posterolateral corner injury has a less favorable prognosis.

Treatment

The course of rehabilitation for a PCL injury is dependent on the degree of injury and type of treatment rendered (i.e. operative vs nonoperative).

Isolated, partial PCL injuries (grades I and II) can best be treated nonoperatively while complete injuries (grade III) may require operative treatment based on clinical symptoms. All combined ligamentous injuries usually respond best with surgical management.

Overall, rehabilitation for a PCL injury should take longer than for an ACL injury.

Historically, controversy in treatment modalities exists because of the lack of knowledge of the natural history of this injury; in addition, reported surgical results are variable. When surgical reconstruction is considered, graft recommendations include the following:

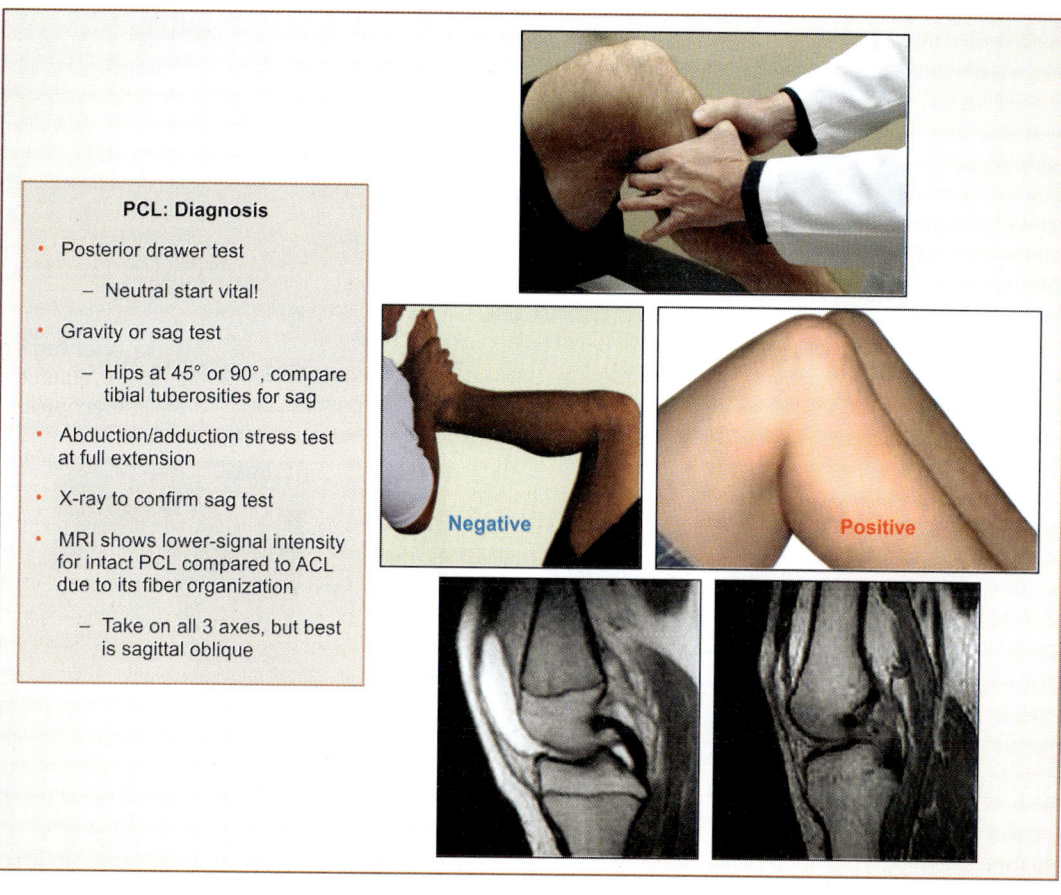

PCL: Diagnosis

- Posterior drawer test
  - Neutral start vital!
- Gravity or sag test
  - Hips at 45° or 90°, compare tibial tuberosities for sag
- Abduction/adduction stress test at full extension
- X-ray to confirm sag test
- MRI shows lower-signal intensity for intact PCL compared to ACL due to its fiber organization
  - Take on all 3 axes, but best is sagittal oblique

Negative   Positive

Fig. 39.23: Diagnosis of PCL tear

- *Autograft*
  - Patellar tendon
  - Quadriceps tendon
  - Hamstring tendons
  - Medial head of gastrocnemius
- *Allograft*
  - Achilles tendon
  - Patellar tendon
  - Quadriceps tendon
  - Hamstring tendons

Complications

Possible complications associated with PCL injury include:

- Initial stiffness
- Instability
- Progressive arthritis
- Postoperative complications

MEDIAL COLLATERAL LIGAMENT INJURY

Medial collateral ligament injury of the knee is the most common ligament injury and occurs in all age groups. It is more common in sports persons especially in sports like football, hockey, wrestling and other contact sports (Fig. 39.24).

O'Donoghue Classification

- *Isolated grade I MCL injury (mild):* MCL has few torn fibres but no loss of ligamentous integrity.
- *Isolated grade II MCL injury (moderate):* MCL is partially torn. However, the fibres are still

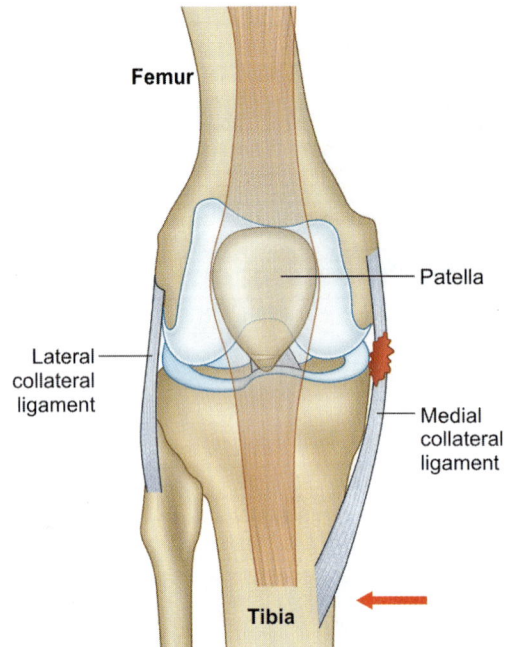

Fig. 39.24: Force outwards—a "valgus" force (red arrow) may stretch or tear the MCL

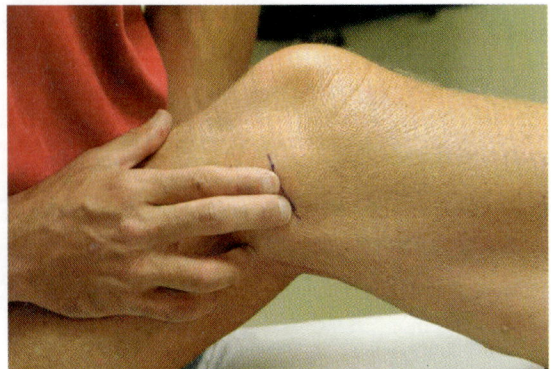

Fig. 39.25: Tenderness over lateral side of knee joint

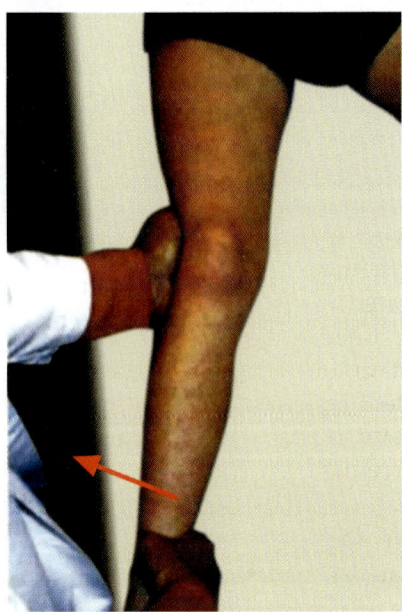

Fig. 39.26: Valgus stress test

opposed. There might be mild pathological laxity, which may or may not be symptomatic.

- *Isolated grade III MCL injury (severe):* Integrity of the MCL is completely disrupted. There is significant pathological laxity of the knee with valgus stress.

AMA Committee Classification

MCL injuries are classified based on the amount of medial joint opening when a valgus load is applied at 20° to 30° of knee flexion:

- Grade I: 0 to 5 mm of opening
- Grade II: 5 to 10 mm of opening
- Grade III: >10 mm of opening

Clinical Diagnosis (Fig. 39.25)

Valgus Stress Test

This test is done to check the integrity of medial collateral ligament and is done in full knee extension and 30° of flexion. The examiner supports the thigh with one hand applies lateral force on the leg with other hand. Comparison with the opposite knee is always done (Fig. 39.26).

Treatment

In acute setting, the standard treatment for sprains is followed which includes rest, ice, compression, and elevation. The severity of the injury dictates further treatment.

Grade I and II injuries are treated nonoperatively. An appropriate knee orthosis is applied and protective weight-bearing is

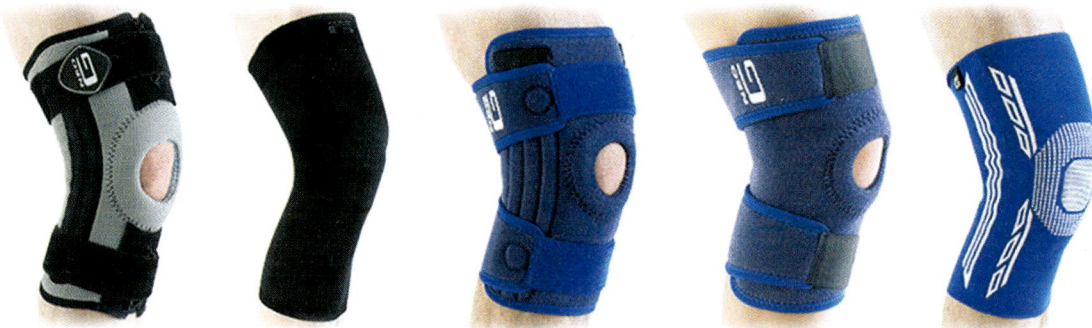

Fig. 39.27: Various types of knee braces used for MCL injury of knee

instituted with crutches (Fig. 39.27). This is continued until a normal gait is obtained. Most of the grade III injuries are also treated nonoperatively either in long leg cast or hinged knee orthosis and protective weight-bearing for 1–2 weeks. After that, range of motion exercises are started which are followed in due course with quadriceps strengthening.

Isolated medial collateral ligament injury rarely needs operative repair. Another indication for surgical intervention would be persistent instability, with surgery consisting of tissue repair and imbrication. Often, reinforcement with an allograft is necessary.

LATERAL COLLATERAL LIGAMENT INJURY

The patient commonly reports a history of varus force applied to the knee (Fig. 39.28).

Clinical Diagnosis

Varus Stress Test (Fig. 39.29)

- The patient is in the supine position with the knee flexed 20–25°. The examiner places one hand on the medial knee and grasps the lateral ankle with other hand. The knee is adducted. Pain and excessive laxity indicate injury to the LCL.
- Then perform the same technique as above with the knee extended. If pain and laxity are still present, injury to the posterior capsule may be present.

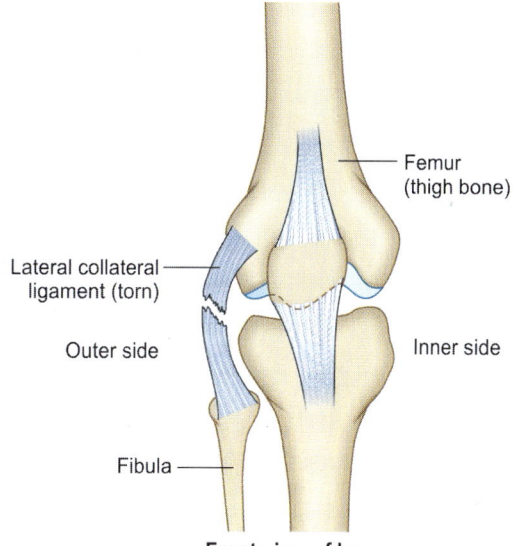

Front view of knee

Fig. 39.28: Lateral collateral ligament tear

Injury severity:
- Grade I: Less than 5 cm laxity (partial tear)
- Grade II: 5–10 cm laxity
- Grade III: More than 10 cm laxity (complete tear)

Indications for plain knee radiographs in suspected knee ligamentous injuries (Pittsburgh decision rules) are blunt trauma or a fall with one of the following criteria:

- The patient is unable to walk 4 weight-bearing steps.
- The patient is older than 50 years or younger than 12 years.

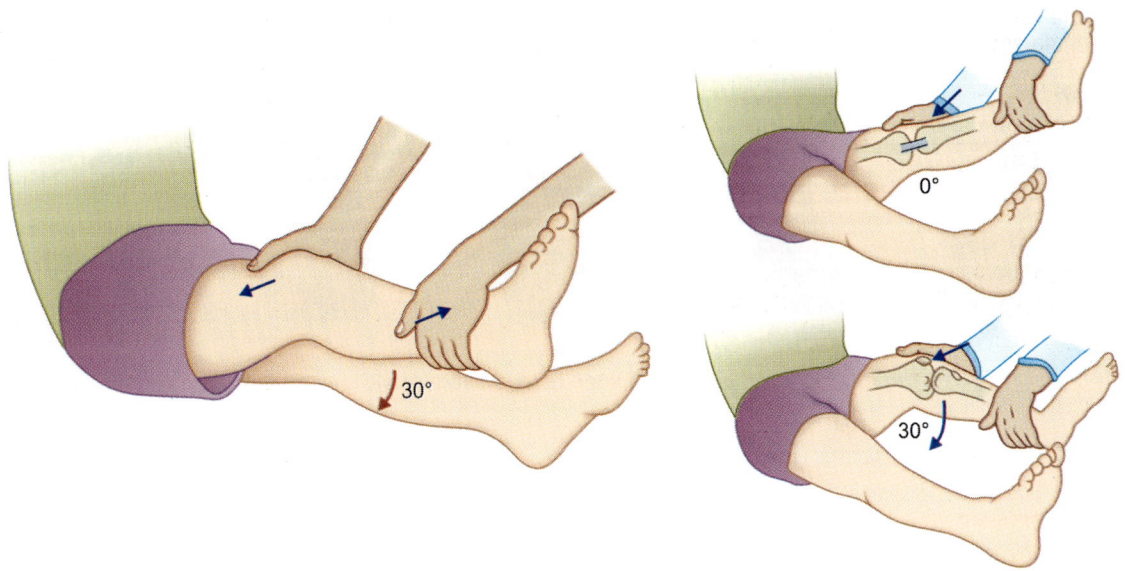

Fig. 39.29: Varus stress test

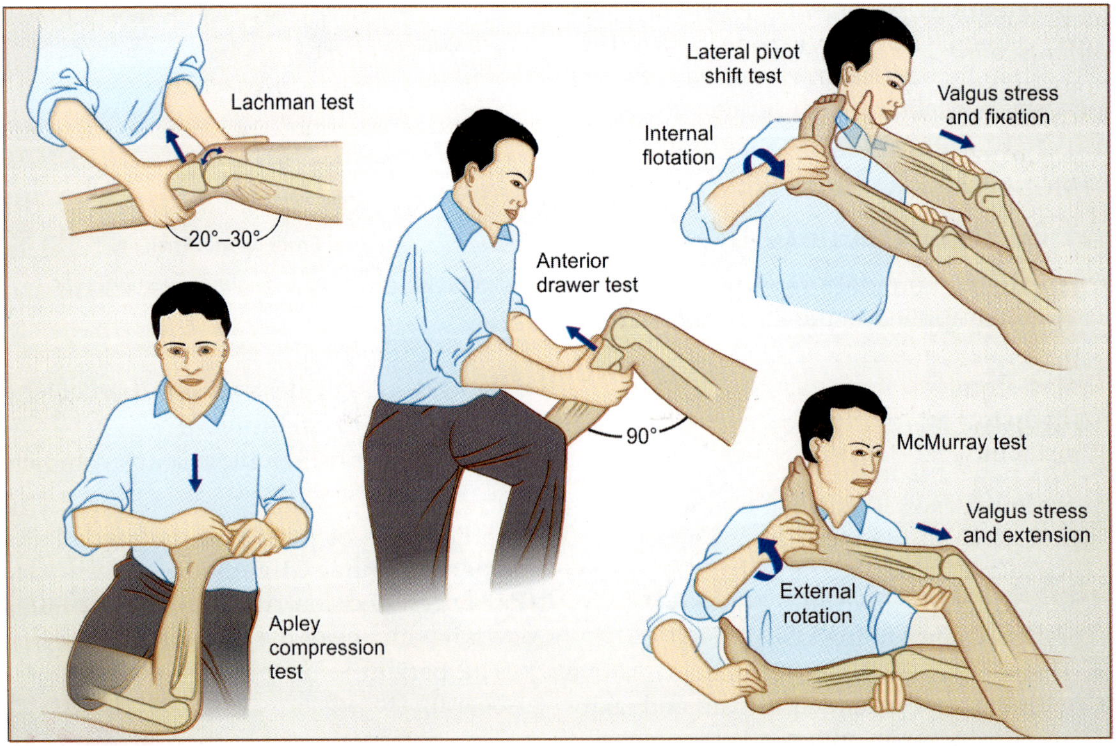

Fig. 39.30: Special clinical tests for knee joint

Table 39.1: Diagnostic tests for ligament injuries (Fig. 30.30)

Tests that evaluate collateral ligaments
- Valgus stress test
- Varus stress test

Tests that evaluate the anterior cruciate ligament
- Anterior drawer test
- Lachman test
- Nirschl modified Lachman test
- Pivot shift test
- Flexion rotation drawer test
- Crossover test

Tests that evaluate the posterior cruciate ligament
- Posterior drawer test
- Posterior sag test
- Quadriceps contraction test
- External rotation test
- Reverse pivot shift test

Treatment

Lateral collateral ligament (LCL) injuries heal more slowly than do MCL injuries, due to the difference in collagen density. Recommendations for the treatment of LCL injuries include:

- *Grades I and II:* These injuries are treated according to a regimen similar to that for MCL injuries of the same severity. A hinged brace is used for 4–6 weeks.

- *Grade III:* Severe LCL injuries typically are treated surgically due to rotational instability, because they usually involve the posterolateral corner of the knee. Patients may require bracing and physical therapy for up to 3 months in order to prevent later instability.

Historical Clues to Knee Injury Diagnoses

Noncontact injury with "pop"	ACL tear
Contact injury with "pop"	MCL or LCL tear, meniscus tear, fracture
Acute swelling	ACL tear, PCL tear, fracture, knee dislocation, patellar dislocation
Lateral blow to the knee	MCL tear
Medial blow to the knee	LCL tear
Knee "gave out" or "buckled"	ACL tear, patellar dislocation
Fall onto a flexed knee	PCL tear

Complications

- Chronic pain in the region
- Weakness of the knee
- Instability of the knee
- Peroneal nerve injury

BIBLIOGRAPHY

- http://www.consultant360.com
- http://orthoinfo.aaos.org/topic.cfm?
- http://radiopaedia.org
- https://youtube/DcDi_6YvJa4
- https://youtube/uSu02FvA8pc
- https://www.youtube.com/watch?v=xEhj3OLOFXY
- http://www0.sun.ac.za/ortho/audio
- https://www.youtube.com/watch?v=P3eXIhubscQ
- https://www.youtube.com/watch?v=uDbhg_bZ0fk
- https://www.youtube.com/watch?v=vEQw-G1Vr18
- https://www.youtube.com/watch?v=3mKZ8iwF1WI

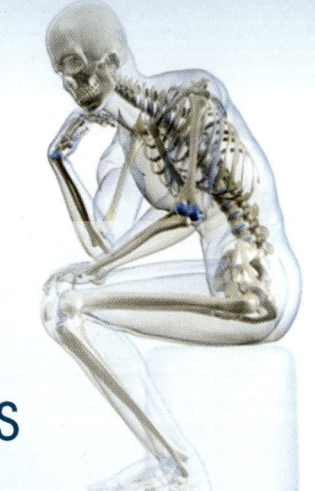

Meniscal Injuries

Meniscal injuries may be the most common knee injury. Meniscus tears are sometimes related to trauma, but significant trauma is not necessary. A sudden twist or repeated squatting can tear the meniscus. Meniscal injuries may be the most common knee injury. A meniscal tear tends to be more frequent in sports that have rough contact or pivoting sports such as soccer. The prevalence of acute meniscal tears is 61 cases per 100,000 persons.

The overall male-to-female incidence is approximately 2.5:1. The peak incidence of meniscal injury for males is in those aged 31–40 years. For females, the peak incidence is in those aged 11–20 years.

Meniscal tears can occur in isolation or in combination with a ligamentous injury. The meniscus in the knee is usually damaged by a twist occurring on a slightly flexed knee. A partial or total tear of a meniscus may occur when a person quickly twists or rotates the upper leg while the foot stays planted. Repeated or prolonged squatting can also tear the meniscus.

In patients older than 65 years, the rate of degenerative meniscal tears is 60%.

Because the posterior horn of the medial meniscus has the least movement, it is at greatest risk for disruption.

The most abundant component of the menisci is collagen (75%)—mainly type I collagen (>90%) but it also contains types II, III, V, and VI. Most meniscal tissue is avascular and depends on passive diffusion and

mechanical pumping to provide nutrition to the fibrocytes within the meniscal substance. The limited peripheral blood supply originates from the medial and lateral inferior and superior geniculate arteries.

The neuroanatomy of the meniscus is not well described. However, the distribution of neural elements has been demonstrated in essentially the same anatomic distribution as the vascular supply. The anterior and posterior horns are the most richly innervated, and the body innervation follows the pattern along the periphery.

The medial meniscus is more commonly injured because it is firmly attached to the medial collateral ligament and joint capsule. The lateral meniscus, on the outside of the knee, is more circular in shape. The lateral meniscus is more mobile than the medial meniscus as there is no attachment to the lateral collateral ligament or joint capsule (Fig. 40.1).

SIGNS AND SYMPTOMS

Most meniscal injuries can be diagnosed by obtaining a detailed history. Important points to address include:

- Mechanism of injury (e.g. twisting, squatting, changes in position)
- Pain (commonly intermittent and usually localized to the joint line)
- Mechanical complaints (e.g. clicking, catching, locking, pinching, or a sensation of giving way)

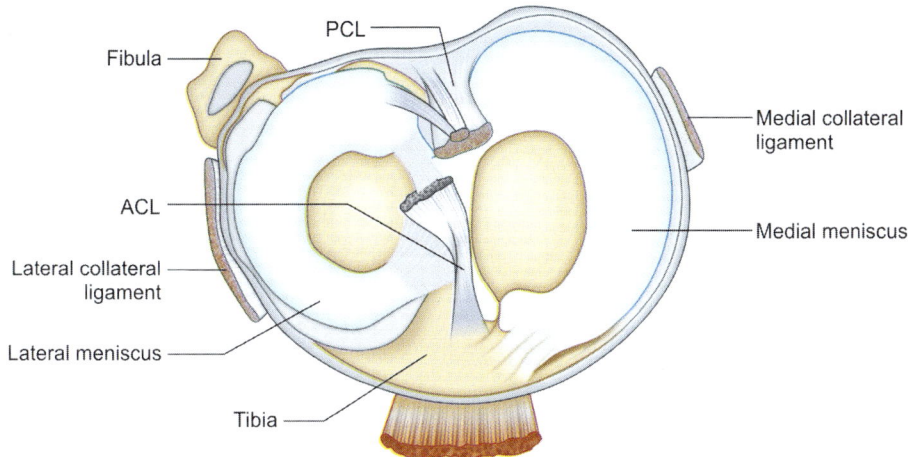

Fig. 40.1: Knee joint anatomy

- Swelling (usually delayed, sometimes absent; degenerative tears often manifest with recurrent effusions)

Physical findings that are significant in the examination of a patient with a possible meniscus injury include the following:

- Joint line tenderness (77–86% of patients with a meniscal tear) (Fig. 40.2)
- Effusion (~50% of patients presenting with a meniscal tear) (Fig. 40.3)
- Impaired range of motion: A mechanical block to motion or frank locking can occur with displaced tears; restricted motion commonly results from pain or swelling.

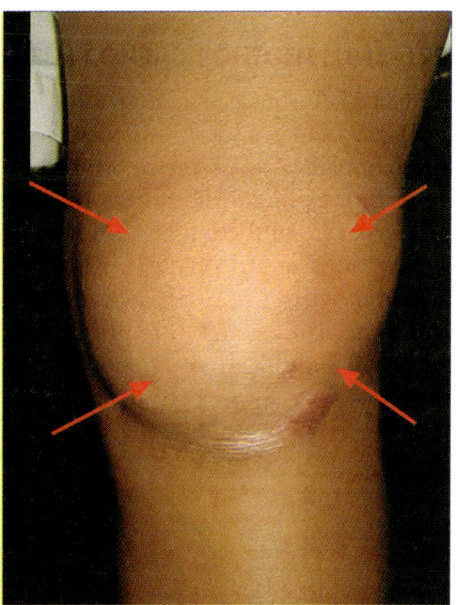

Fig. 40.3: Knee effusion

PROVOCATIVE MANEUVERS

These techniques cause impingement by creating compression and/or shearing forces on the torn meniscus between the femoral and tibial surfaces.

The McMurray Test

This maneuver usually elicits pain or a reproducible click in the presence of a meniscal

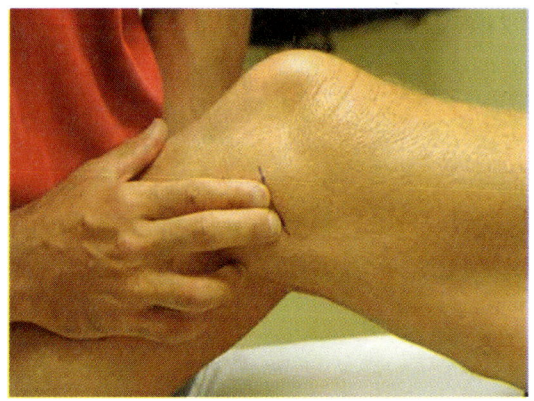

Fig. 40.2: Joint line tenderness

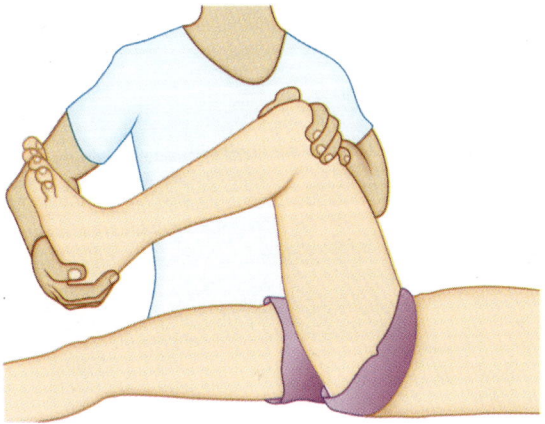

Fig. 40.4: McMurray test

tear. The medial meniscus is evaluated by extending the fully flexed knee with the foot/tibia externally rotated while a valgus stress is applied. The lateral meniscus is evaluated by extending the knee from the fully flexed position, with the foot/tibia internally rotated while a varus stress is applied to the knee. One of the examiner's hands should be palpating the joint line during the maneuver (Fig. 40.4).

The Steinmann Test

Tibial rotation is performed with the patient seated and the knee flexed 90°. Asymmetric pain is created with external (medial meniscus) or internal (lateral meniscus) rotation (Fig. 40.5).

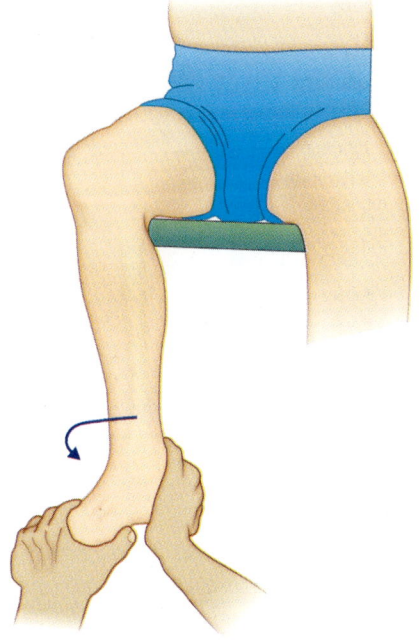

Fig. 40.5: Steinmann test

The Apley Test (Fig. 40.6)

This maneuver is performed with the patient prone and the knee flexed 90°. An axial load is applied through the heel as the lower leg is internally and externally rotated. This grinding maneuver is suggestive of meniscal pathology, if pain is elicited at the medial or lateral joint.

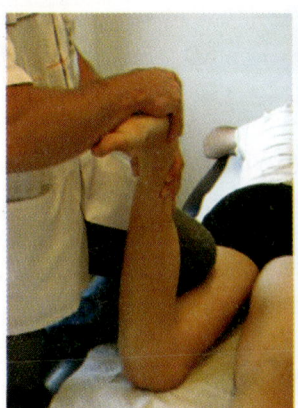
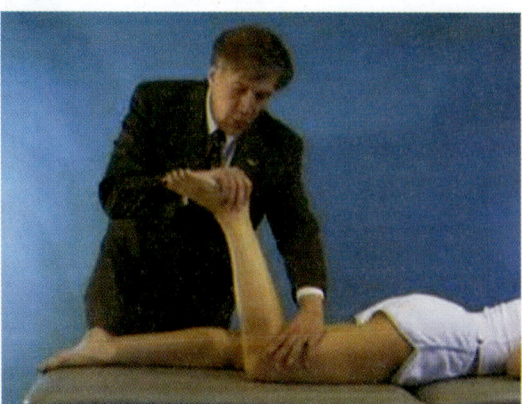

Fig. 40.6: Apley's grinding test

The Thessaly Test (Fig. 40.7)

This maneuver is performed with the patient standing on one leg and the knee flexed to 5° and 20° while holding the examiner's hand for balance. From this position, the patient is asked to internally and externally rotate the knee. Pain or a locking or catching sensation at the medial or lateral joint line is suggestive of meniscal tears.

The Cooper's Sign

This is present in over 92% of tears. It is a subjective symptom of pain in the affected knee when turning over in bed at night.

TYPES OF MENISCAL TEARS

The classification of meniscal tears provides a description of pathoanatomy. The types of meniscus tears include (Fig. 40.8):

- Longitudinal tears that may take the shape of a bucket handle, if displaced
- Radial tears
- Parrot-beak or oblique flap tears
- Horizontal tears

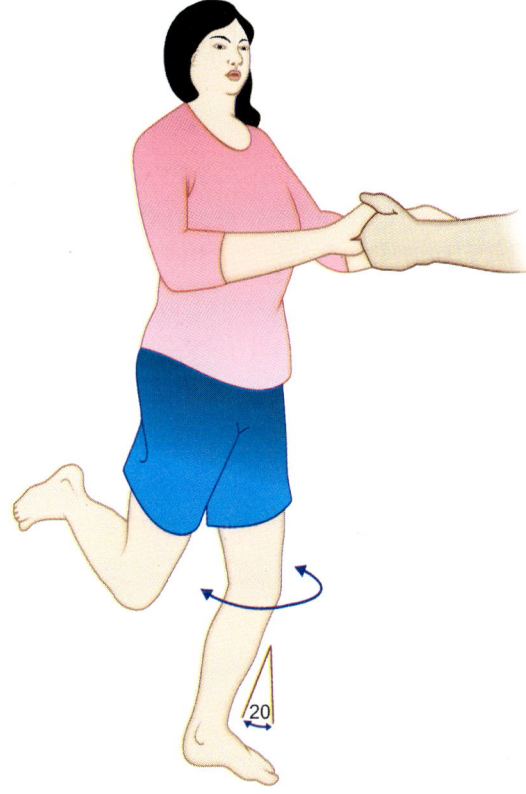

Fig. 40.7: Thessaly test

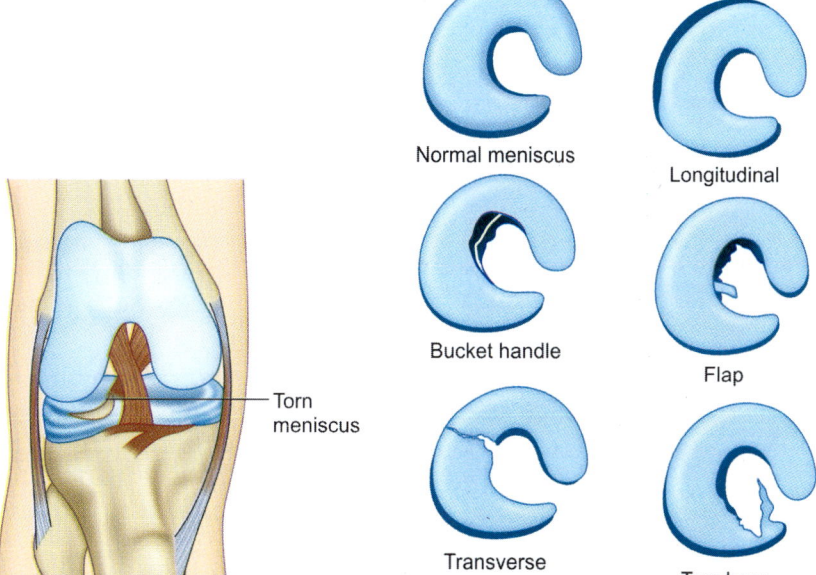

Normal meniscus

Bucket handle

Transverse

Longitudinal

Flap

Torn horn

Torn meniscus

Fig. 40.8: Types of meniscal tear

- Root tears
- Complex tears that combine variants of the above

MRI Scan (Fig. 40.9)

Abnormal meniscal signals on MRI are classified into the following groups:
- Grade I—small area of increased signal within the meniscus
- Grade II—linear area of increased signal that does not extend to an articulating surface
- Grade III—abnormal increased signal that reaches the surface or edge of the meniscus (indicative of meniscal tearing)
- Root tears—meniscal extrusion of at least 3 mm in the mid-coronal plane

We, as physicians, need to treat the patient, and not the MRI scan.

Arthroscopy

- In the hands of a competent arthroscopist, arthroscopy is considered the best tool for meniscal tear diagnosis, with sensitivity, specificity, and accuracy approaching 100%.

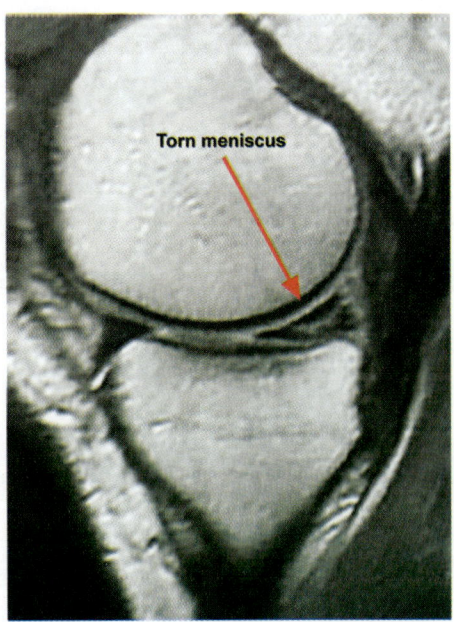

Fig. 40.9: Meniscal tear on MRI scan

- Arthroscopy is therapeutic and diagnostic and thus offers the advantage of immediate treatment of most disorders.

TREATMENT

The following factors have to be considered before deciding the choice of treatment:
- The patient's activity level
- The patient's age
- The location of the tear and the type of tear
- When the injury happened
- Injury symptoms
- Any other associated injuries

Conservative treatment should be attempted in all but the most severe cases. In the acute phase, such treatment may include:
- Home physical therapy program
- Simple rest with activity modification
- Ice
- Nonsteroidal anti-inflammatory drugs (NSAIDs)

Small tears in the meniscus that are not dislodged may heal, or may eventually be symptom-free. Larger tears that displace and tears associated with instability, are less likely to heal. Tears in the outer one-third of the meniscus are more likely to heal than tears toward the inside of the meniscus because the blood supply is better in the outer region.

If conservative treatment does not lead to resolution, surgical treatment is considered.

Surgical options (arthroscopic or open) include (Fig. 40.10):
- *Partial meniscectomy:* The treatment of choice for tears in the avascular portion of the meniscus or complex tears that are not amenable to repair
- *Meniscus repair:* Recommended for tears that occur in the vascular region (red zone or red-white zone), are longer than 1 cm, root tears, involve greater than 50% of the meniscal thickness, and are unstable to arthroscopic probing
- *In cases of previous total or subtotal meniscectomy, meniscus transplantation:* A

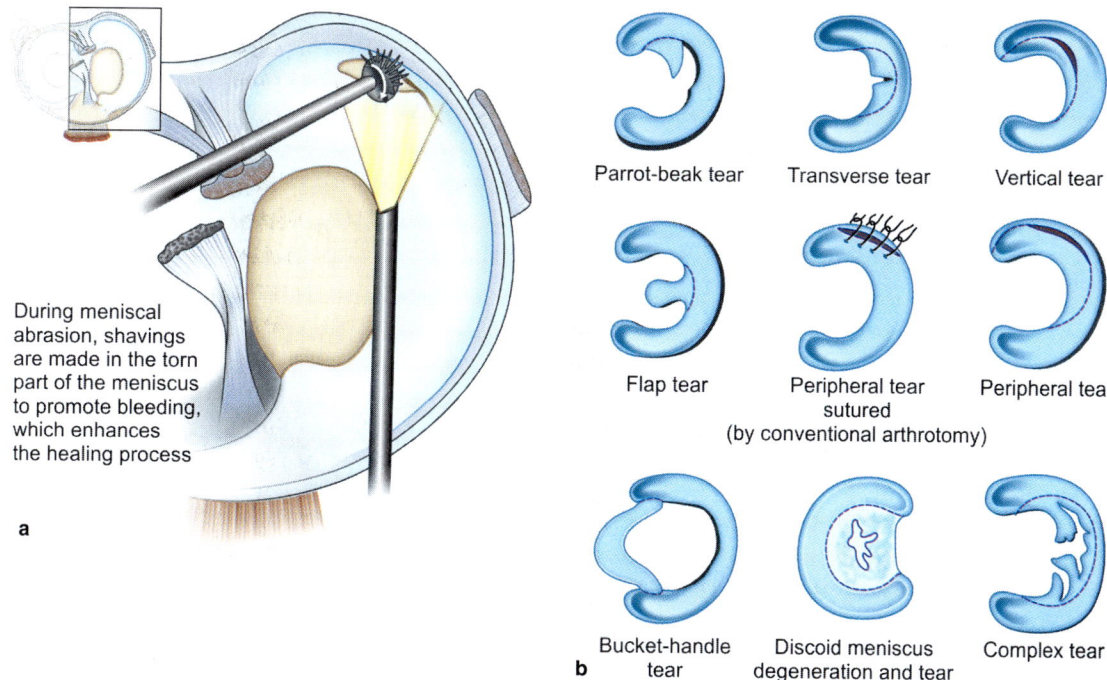

During meniscal abrasion, shavings are made in the torn part of the meniscus to promote bleeding, which enhances the healing process

a

Parrot-beak tear   Transverse tear   Vertical tear

Flap tear   Peripheral tear sutured (by conventional arthrotomy)   Peripheral tear

Bucket-handle tear   Discoid meniscus degeneration and tear   Complex tear

b

Fig. 40.10a and b: Meniscal surgery

relatively new procedure for which specific indications and long-term results have not yet been clearly established.

- *Collagen meniscus implant:* This is a scaffold of collagen inserted into the patient's knee. Over time, a new meniscus may grow within the joint. This procedure is currently in FDA trials in the United States and has just been approved as an accepted surgical procedure in Europe.

- *Meniscal transplant:* This procedure involves transplanting a meniscus from a donor into the injured knee. Only a limited number of surgeons perform this procedure on a routine basis. The long-term outcomes are still being evaluated.

- The basic principle of meniscus surgery is to save the meniscus.

- Most meniscal tears do not heal because they are in an anatomic area that has no blood supply.

- The definitive treatment for meniscal tears is arthroscopic surgery.

Return to play after a meniscus injury is expected. The timing varies and depends on the injury, treatment, and rehabilitation protocol. In many cases, athletes can return to their sport as soon as 2–3 weeks status post arthroscopic partial meniscectomy or 6–8 weeks status post meniscal repair.

In patients with untreated tears, enlargement of the tear and arthrosis are common. In patients who are status post partial meniscectomy, arthrosis is also a concern. However, arthroscopists are hopeful that long-term outcome studies will demonstrate that a partial meniscectomy can delay or prevent the degenerative changes noted by Fairbanks in patients who had open total meniscectomy.

BIBLIOGRAPHY

- emedicine.medscape.com
- http://thesteadmanclinic.com/meniscus/diag.asp
- https://www.youtube.com/watch?v=WuVHWZX91KY
- https://www.youtube.com/watch?v=kB98kPLOcBM

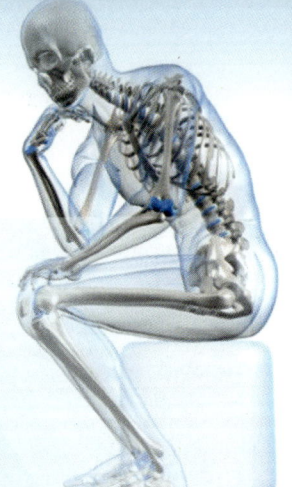

Closed Fractures of Both Bones of Leg

Tibial shaft fractures are the most common long bone fracture and usually involve the fibula as well. Tibial shaft fractures usually present with a history of major trauma.

Maisonneuve fractures involve a fracture of the proximal fibula in association with a fractured medial malleolus (or injured deltoid ligament) and diastasis of the distal tibiofibular syndesmosis. Patients present with proximal fibular pain in addition to medial ankle pain. This is an unstable ankle injury (Fig. 41.1).

Pedestrians struck by motor vehicles with lower extremity fractures have a high incidence of concomitant spine, chest, or intra-abdominal injuries. These patients may need additional radiographic tests to rule out these injuries when clinically indicated.

There are several ways to classify closed tibial shaft fractures, depending on whether the goal is to communicate the bone injury (fracture pattern) or the soft-tissue injury associated with the fracture. Most surgeons classify tibial shaft fractures with simple descriptive terms such as proximal, middle, or distal in addition to transverse, oblique, spiral, segmental, or comminuted.

The two most commonly used classification systems are the AO/OTA (Arbeitsgemein-schaft für Osteosynthesefragen/Orthopaedic Trauma Association) classification of bone injury and the Tscherne and Gotzen

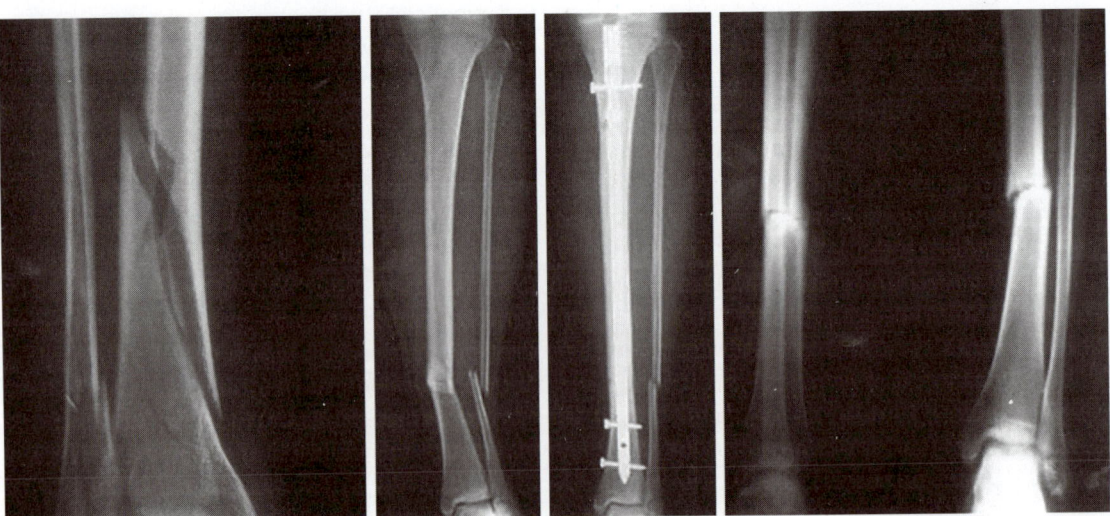

Fig. 41.1: Closed fracture both bones of leg

classification of soft-tissue injury associated with closed tibial shaft fractures.

TREATMENT

Tibial shaft fractures that are closed may be treated with cast immobilization, if alignment is good or with intramedullary nailing.

In summary, the advantages of cast immobilization over intramedullary nail fixation include a negligible risk of infection, few problems with knee pain, and no need for hardware removal. However, the advantages of intramedullary nailing include better control of alignment (including shortening, angulation, and rotation), the ability to institute an early range of motion of the knee and ankle, improved mobility of the patient, the need for less frequent follow-up, and earlier return to work (Fig. 41.2).

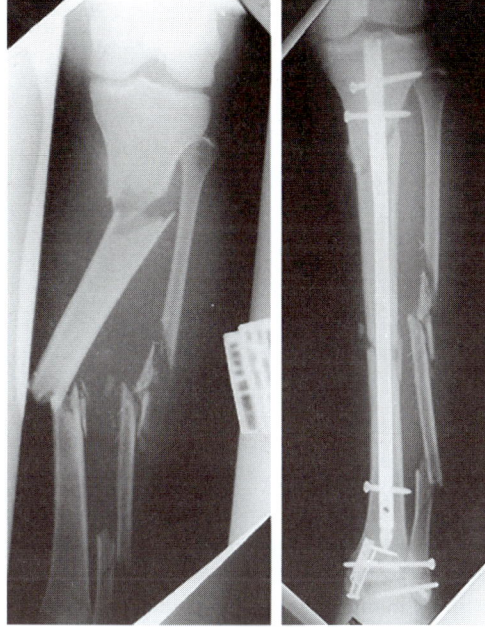

Fig. 41.2: Interlocking nails

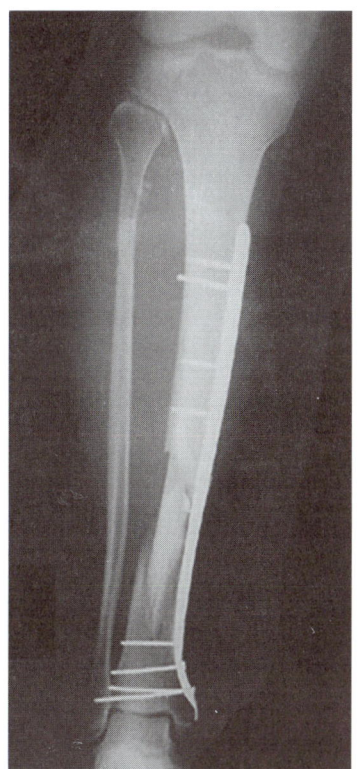

Fig. 41.3: Plate and screws

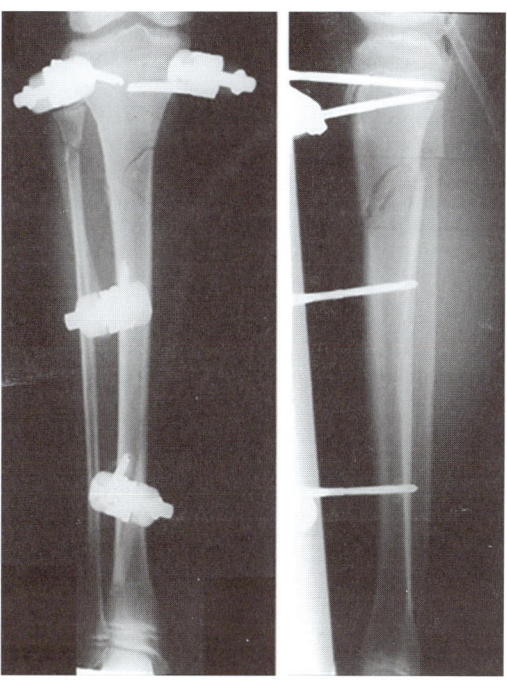

Fig. 41.4: External fixation

Plates are primarily indicated for metaphyseal injuries. Because of the tenuous soft-tissue coverage of the tibia, plate fixation has typically been associated with an unacceptably high prevalence of wound complications, especially when it has been performed for more severe open fractures.

A plate may be applied to the medial (subcutaneous) or lateral (submuscular) border of the tibia. Lateral application is less likely to result in soft-tissue problems, and it may be better biomechanically since the plate functions as a tension band, if the fracture is stable. For percutaneous plate fixation, a prebent plate is applied medially through a small incision. With this technique, a longer plate is used, with screws placed near the fracture and near the ends of the plate (Fig. 41.3).

Provisional external fixation is the initial treatment of choice for high-energy closed or open fractures when the viability of the limb is threatened (Fig. 41.4).

COMPLICATIONS

The following complications may be noted:
- Neurovascular compromise
- Compartment syndrome
- Peroneal nerve injury
- Infection
- Gangrene
- Osteomyelitis
- Delayed union, nonunion, or malunion
- Amputation or skin loss
- Post-traumatic arthritis
- Fat embolism

BIBLIOGRAPHY

- http://emedicine.medscape.com/
- http://www.orthobullets.com/

Chapter
42

Open Fractures of Both Bones of Leg

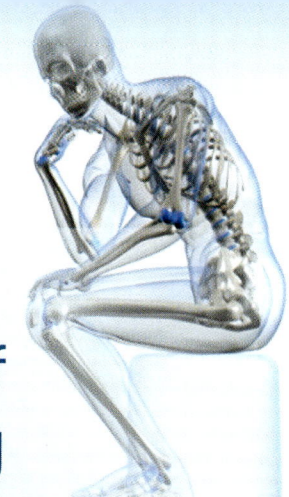

Open fractures of the tibia are the commonest of open long-bone fractures, perhaps because of its thin anteromedial soft-tissue coverage. Due to the subcutaneous position of the tibia, fractures of the tibia more commonly result in an open fracture than any other long bone (Fig. 42.1).

They are caused by various mechanisms, ranging from low-energy twisting forces to high-energy motor vehicle crashes or penetrating injuries (gun shots, blasts).

It has been estimated that between 3.5 and 6 million fractures occur in the United States annually. More than 4.5 million open fractures occur per year in India.

Open tibial fractures can present as isolated injuries or in the context of a multiply injured patient. The patient's clinical status must dictate the primary and ongoing treatment of the open tibial fracture. Thorough evaluation of the entire patient is essential before focusing on the injured leg (Fig. 42.2).

The **Gustilo-Anderson classification** divides soft-tissue wounding of open fractures into three grades—I, II and III (Table 42.1).

The III grade was later further subdivided into types IIIA, IIIB and IIIC (Table 42.2).

The second classification system, the MESS, was originally designed as an objective tool to assist the surgeon in decision-making for amputation vs limb salvage in complex lower extremity trauma. This rating scale takes into consideration the skeletal and soft tissue damage, limb ischemia time, presence of shock, and the patient's age. It has been suggested that a score of greater than or equal to 7 is predictive of amputation with nearly 100% accuracy.

Table 42.1: Gustilo and Anderson classification of open fractures

Type	Description
I	Skin wound less than 1 cm
	Clean
	Simple fracture pattern
II	Skin wound more than 1 cm
	Soft-tissue damage not extensive
	No flaps or avulsions
	Simple fracture pattern
III	High-energy injury involving extensive soft-tissue damage
	Or multifragmentary fracture, segmental fractures, or bone loss irrespective of the size of skin wound
	Or severe crush injuries
	Or vascular injury requiring repair
	Or severe contamination including farmyard injuries

Table 42.2: Gustilo classification of type III open fractures

Type	Description
IIIA	Adequate soft-tissue cover of bone despite extensive soft-tissue damage
IIIB	Extensive soft-tissue injury with periosteal stripping and bone exposure
	Major wound contamination
IIIC	Open fracture with arterial injury requiring repair

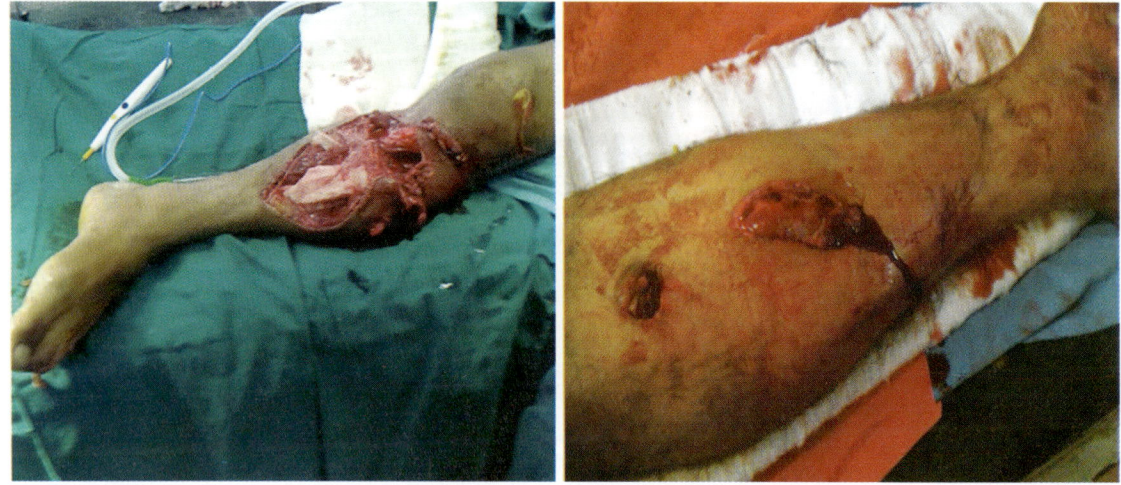

Fig. 42.1: Open fracture tibia

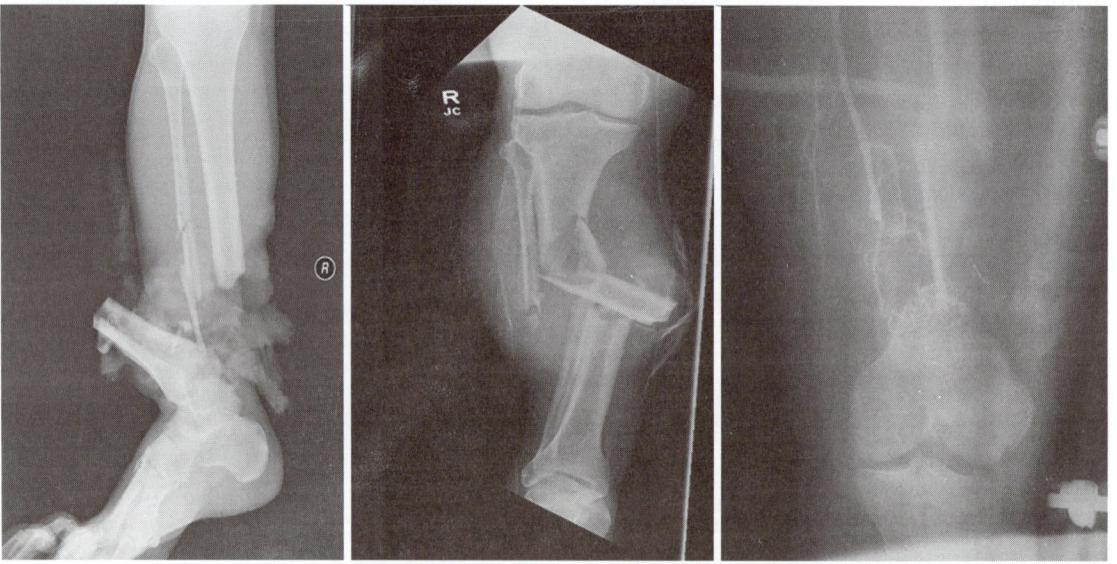

Fig. 42.2: X-rays of open fracture tibia

INITIAL ASSESSMENT

The initial evaluation of a patient with an open fracture of a limb should always follow the principles and guidelines of the Advanced Trauma Life Support System. Other concomitant serious and, possibly, life-threatening injuries should be sought. Any further assessment of the site of the open fracture, apart from control of active bleeding, should be deferred for the secondary survey.

If an open wound is identified, it should immediately be covered with a sterile dressing. It should not be again inspected until the patient is in the OR for debridement. All open fractures are by definition contaminated and must be treated as such. Infection risks also differ by fracture type and have been reported to be ranging from 0 to 2% for Type I fractures, 2 to 10% for Type II fractures, and 10 to 50% for Type III fractures.

NEUROVASCULAR ASSESSMENT

The dorsalis pedis and posterior tibial pulses should be palpated in the foot. Reduced pulses require urgent further assessment.

Motor function in each of the four leg compartments should be evaluated (toe flexion, toe extension, ankle eversion and plantar flexion).

Test sensation of the following nerves:
- Tibial (plantar surface of foot)
- Seep peroneal (dorsal web space between 1st and 2nd toe)
- Superficial peroneal (dorsal lateral foot)
- Saphenous (medial foot)

This may not be possible in all patients (i.e. intubated, multiple injured, comatose), but should be always be attempted and documented.

In severe trauma to the leg, preservation of plantar sensation has been thought to be an important prognostic factor in deciding whether salvage of the limb is worthwhile.

Evaluation for compartment syndrome is critical.

Severe pain and tense swelling are strong suggestions of this problem.

Goals of open fracture management are well known and include the prevention of infection, achievement of bony union, and the restoration of function. The treatment of open fractures requires the simultaneous management of both skeletal and soft-tissue injuries.

As in all open fracture injuries, the patient must receive anti-tetanus prophylaxis and appropriate antibiotic coverage. Any patient presenting with an open fracture who has not completed the tetanus toxoid immunization or has not had their booster in the last 5 years should be given a tetanus toxoid booster. If the wound is prone to contamination with *Clostridium tetani*, the tetanus toxoid should be combined with 250–500 IU of human tetanus immune globulin (HTIG). Furthermore, if more than 10 years has elapsed since the last tetanus booster or the patient's immune system is compromised, both the tetanus toxoid and HTIG should be given. Antibiotics should be given intravenously as soon as possible. The duration of antibiotic therapy in the treatment of open fractures has been suggested to be between 1 and 3 days without any solid agreement on a firm end point. Local antibiotic delivery must be considered when extensive contamination is present. This is commonly done with an "antibiotic bead-pouch" construct formed with antibiotic powder and polymethyl-methacrylate (PMMA) cement.

Generally, all open fractures are treated with coverage for typical skin bacteria, often a 1st generation cephalosporin. Higher grade open fracture wounds will require additional coverage for gram-negative organisms. With soil or barnyard injuries, high-dose penicillin should be added to cover possible clostridial infection (gas gangrene).

For type I fractures, the rate of infection is 0–2%, for type II 2–7%, for type IIIA 7%, for type IIIB 10–50% and for type IIIC 25–50% (with a rate of amputation of 50% or more). The overall infection rate for type III fractures is from 10–25% (Gustilo 1990).

GENERAL PRINCIPLES OF DEBRIDEMENT

Initial surgical intervention should be conducted as soon as possible, but the classic 6-hour rule does not seem to be supported in the literature.

It is important to perform a thorough surgical debridement in an organized manner. Starting with the skin, each layer is debrided systematically. One can imagine a clock face; wound debridement starts at the 12 o'clock position and continues in a clockwise manner around the circumference of the wound. This is repeated for each layer down to the level of the bone. Necrotic tissue is removed and only viable tissue is left behind. The exception is skin, where none is removed unless obviously necrotic.

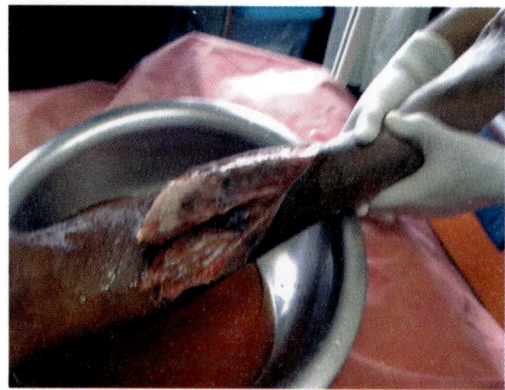

Fig. 42.3: Wound debridement

The quality of the muscle tissue is assessed using the classic 4 Cs (Fig. 42.3):
- Color (red or brown)
- Consistency (how does the muscle feel)
- Capillary Circulation (does it bleed?)
- Contractility (responds to pinch or electro-cautery)

Temporary Fixation

Temporary stabilization of the tibia is chosen in situations where future débridements are felt to be necessary. This is most common in the high-grade open fractures.

Temporary stabilization, usually achieved with an external fixator (Fig. 42.4), minimizes additional soft-tissue injury. This fixation facilitates access to the wound for inspection between débridements.

It also allows simple, rapid disassembly for repeated wound debridement when necessary.

Vacuum-Assisted Closure (VAC)

Negative pressure wound dressings (VACs) can provide helpful temporary coverage of an open wound. They reduce external wound contamination, remove edema fluid, help to shrink wounds, and promote growth of granulation tissue, even over exposed bone. Such dressings may allow definitive closure by the subsequent use of split thickness skin grafts, instead of more complex flaps.

Repeat Debridement

Repeated debridement may be necessary in the higher grade open fracture wounds when there is a concern for additional necrotic tissue or when initial wounds were so badly contaminated that a second look is necessary. This procedure should be repeated, generally every 2–3 days, until only healthy, viable tissue remains and no further necrotic tissue is found on follow-up débridements.

Wound Closure

Options for wound closure in the treatment of open fractures include primary closure of the skin, split-thickness skin-grafting, and the use of either free or local muscle flaps.

The wound is closed, when the surgeon believes no further débridements are necessary. This may be done primarily, but is often done after a secondary procedure.

When skin grafting or soft-tissue flaps are necessary, they should be done as soon as possible. For this reason, an expert in these techniques should be consulted early.

Optimally, coverage should occur within the first two weeks after injury.

There is sufficient evidence to support a more aggressive approach to the open wound. While in less severe grades (I to IIIA), a secondary wound closure seems to yield the best results; in grade-IIIB and grade-IIIC fractures, delayed wound care with repeated debridement and extended exposure of the deep structures results in additional tissue loss through desiccation and infection. In such cases, immediate or very early wound cover through microvascular free-flap transfer minimizes the complications and improves the final outcome provided that appropriate facilities and expertise are available.

Definitive fixation is considered, when:
- The patients clinical status is optimized.
- The wounds are healthy and the soft-tissue envelope will allow for chosen surgical approach.
- A good preoperative plan has been created.

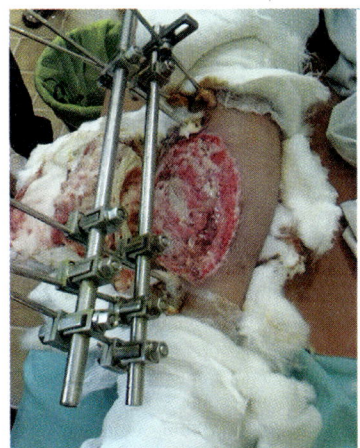
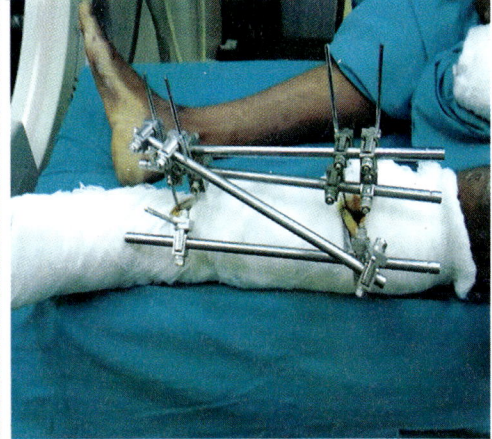
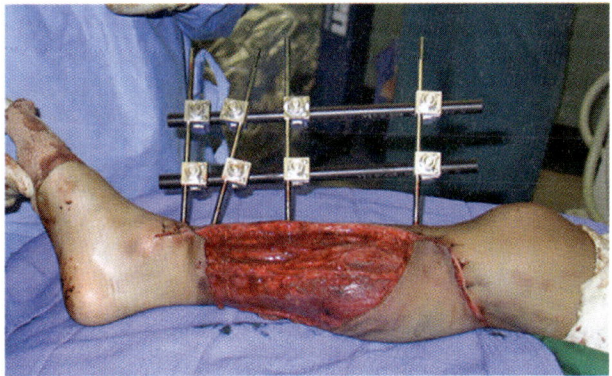

Fig. 42.4: External fixator

COMPLICATIONS

Open tibial fractures have higher rates of non-union, infection, and compartmental syndrome.

Osteomyelitis may occur and can be acute, subacute, or chronic. It may surface many months or years after injury.

Pin-site infections are common with external fixator treatment. Chronic osteo-myelitis in the pin sites is relatively common.

Summary

Open fractures of the tibial shaft are limb threatening and potentially life-threatening emergencies. Compared to closed fractures, they have a significantly higher risk of infection, nonunion, wound healing complications, and often require multiple surgeries for definitive care. Optimal treatment involves appropriate initial evaluation and administration of antibiotics, urgent operative debridement and skeletal stabilization (usually by IM nailing or external fixator). Repeated soft tissue debridement may be required and soft tissue closure or flap coverage.

BIBLIOGRAPHY

- https://www2.aofoundation.org
- https://ispub.com/IJOS
- http://sjs.sagepub.com
- http://www.bjj.boneandjoint.org.uk
- https://www.youtube.com/watch?v=DDYqz8F93kw
- https://www.youtube.com/watch?v=MS4hF9NxJYc

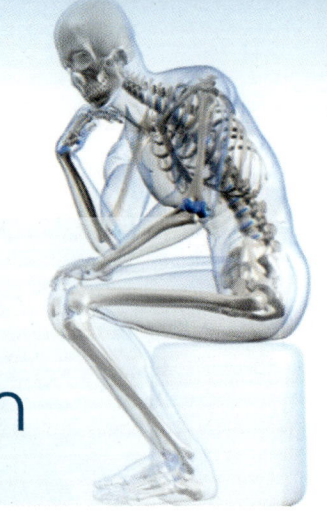

Ankle Sprain

Ankle sprains are very common injuries. Nearly 25,000 people do it everyday. The most common ankle sprain occurs on the lateral side of the ankle. This is an extremely common injury which affects many people during a wide variety of activities (Fig. 43.1).

An ankle sprain is usually that of an inversion-type twist of the foot, followed by pain and swelling. The most commonly injured site is the lateral ankle complex, which is composed of the anterior talofibular, calcaneofibular, and posterior talofibular ligaments (Fig. 43.2).

Ankle sprains are classified into the following three grades (Fig. 43.3):
- *Grade 1 injuries* involve a stretch of the ligament with microscopic tearing but not macroscopic tearing. Generally, little swelling is present, with little or no functional loss and no joint instability. The patient is able to fully or partially bear weight.
- *Grade 2 injuries* stretch the ligament with partial tearing, moderate-to-severe swelling, ecchymosis, moderate functional loss, and mild-to-moderate joint instability.

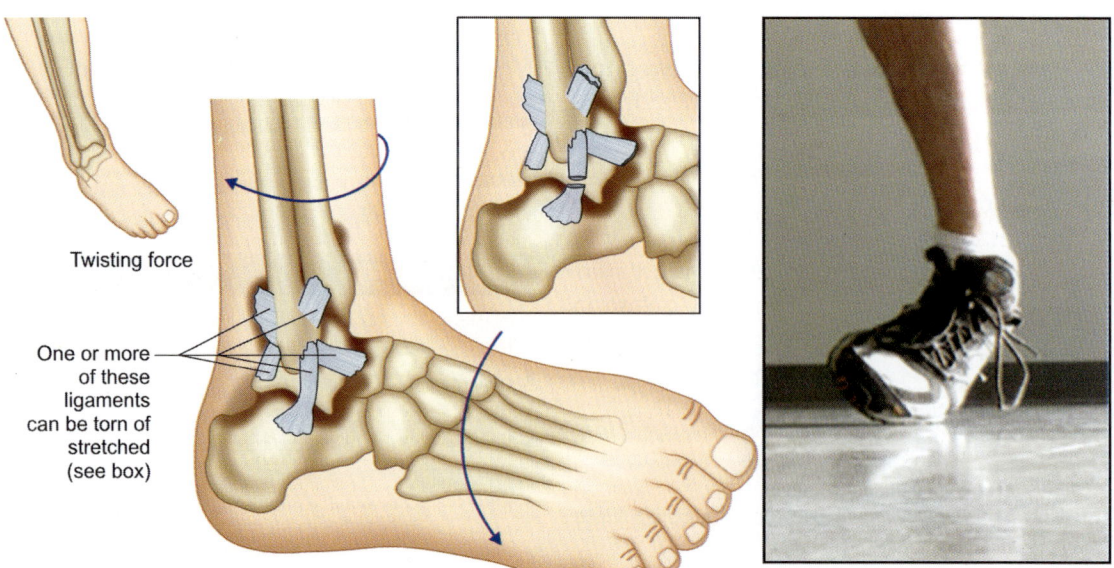

Twisting force

One or more of these ligaments can be torn of stretched (see box)

Fig. 43.1: Ankle sprain

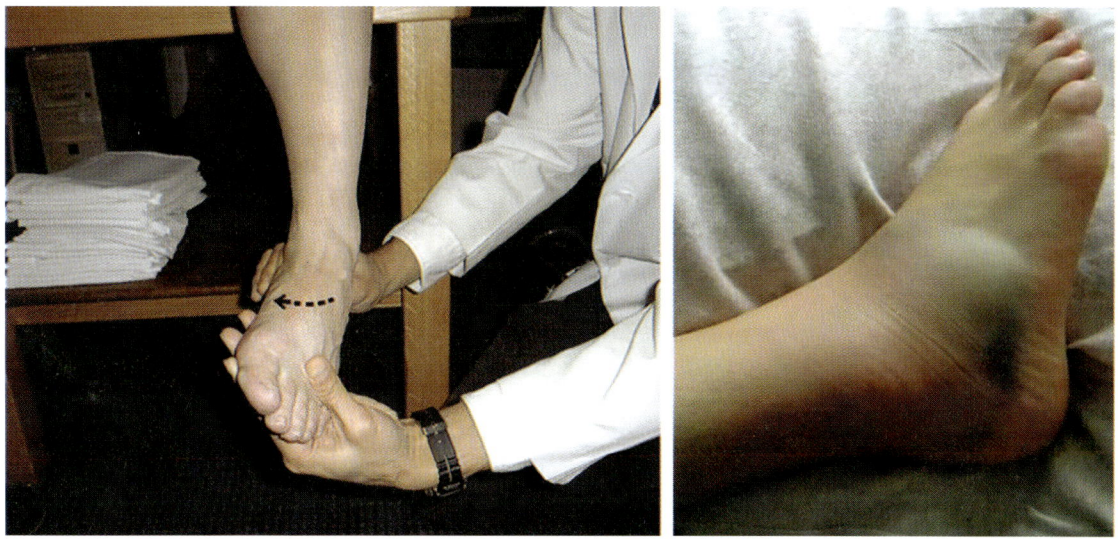

Fig. 43.2: Inversion injury of ankle

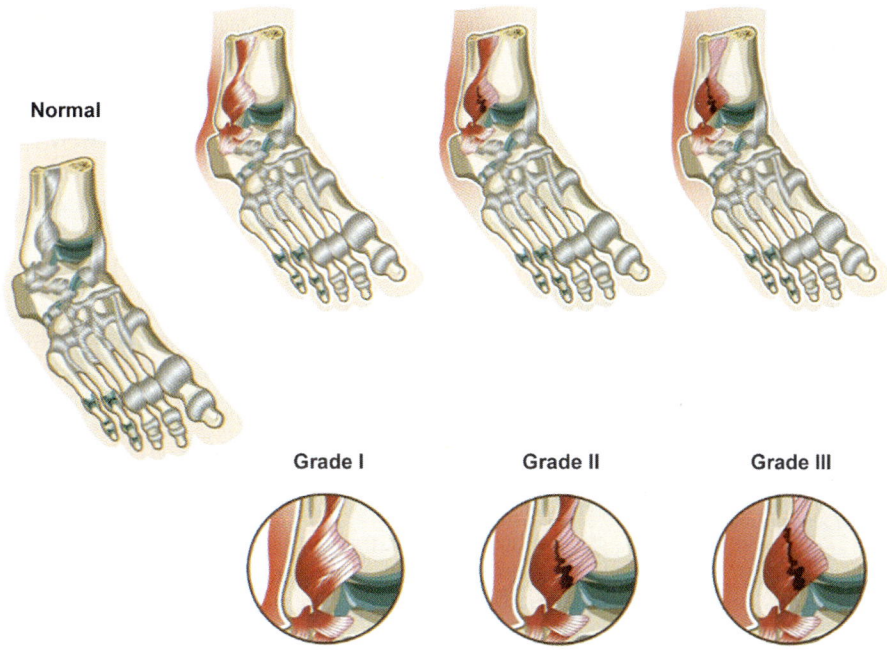

Fig. 43.3: Different grades ankle sprain

Patients usually have difficulty bearing weight.

• *Grade 3 injuries* involve complete rupture of the ligament, with immediate and severe swelling, ecchymosis, an inability to bear weight, and moderate-to-severe instability of the joint. Typically, patients cannot bear weight without experiencing severe pain.

CONSERVATIVE TREATMENT

Conservative therapy for acute ankle sprains may be described by the acronyms RICE (rest, ice, compression, and elevation) and PRICES (combination of protection, relative rest, ice, compression, elevation, and support). Protective devices include air splints or plastic and Velcro braces (Fig. 43.4). Ankle taping can also increase ankle stability, but its effectiveness is highly dependent on the expertise of the individual who performs the taping (Fig. 43.5).

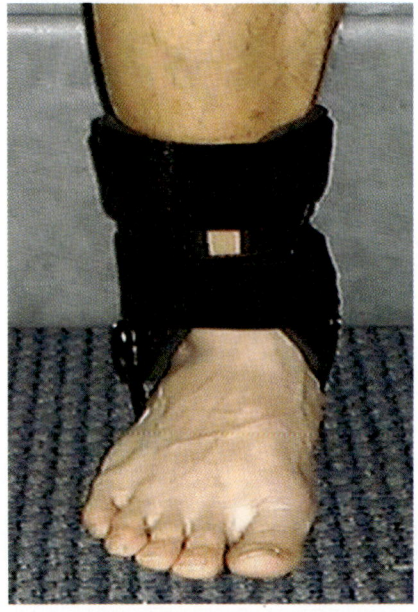

Fig. 43.4: Ankle brace

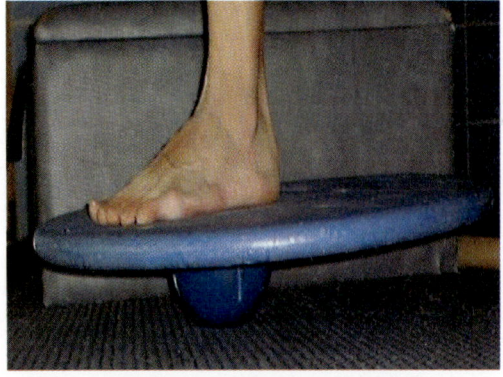

Fig. 43.5: Tilt board exercise

SURGERY

In most patients, there is no improved outcome with operative repair of third-degree anterior talofibular ligament tears and medial ankle ligament tears.

Indications for operative intervention in patients with an ankle sprain include the following:

- Distal talofibular ligament third-degree sprain that causes widening of the ankle mortise.
- Deltoid sprain with the deltoid ligament caught intra-articularly and with widening of the medial ankle mortise.
- In selected young patients with high athletic demands who have both anterior talofibular and calcaneofibular complete ruptures.

Surgical procedures for chronic ankle instability and sprains include the Watson-Jones procedure, the Evans procedure, and the Chrisman-Snook procedure.

PROGNOSIS

Studies have shown that at least 40% of acute ankle sprains result in residual ankle symptoms at 6 months. At least 10–20% of acute ankle sprains result in residual ankle instability, pain, or other chronic symptoms.

For the first 72 hours after a sprain or muscle strain, one should avoid HARM. This means one should avoid:

- Heat—such as hot baths, saunas or heat packs.
- Alcohol—drinking alcohol will increase bleeding and swelling, and slow healing.
- Running—or any other form of exercise that could cause more damage.
- Massage—which may increase bleeding and swelling.

The National Athletic Trainers' Association (NATA) has issued new guidelines for treating and preventing ankle sprains in athletes, including recommendations for the early use of nonsteroidal anti-inflammatory drugs (NSAIDs) post injury, functional rehabilitation rather than immobilization for grade I and II ankle sprains, and prophylactic ankle supports for athletes with a history of previous ankle sprains. Immobilization with a rigid stirrup brace or below-knee cast is recommended for grade III sprains for at least 10 days, followed by controlled therapeutic exercise.

BIBLIOGRAPHY

- http://emedicine.medscape.com/article/1907229-overview
- http://bcove.me/fe5b2psd
- https://www.youtube.com/watch?v=B0-n-ndTAX0

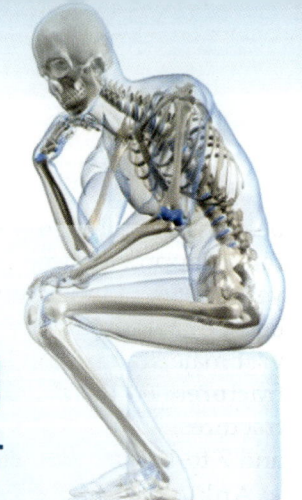

Chapter 44

Fractures Around the Ankle Joint

The tibia and fibula have specific parts that make up the ankle (Fig. 44.1):
• Medial malleolus—inside part of the tibia
• Posterior malleolus—back part of the tibia
• Lateral malleolus—end of the fibula

Ankle fractures account for 9% of fractures representing a significant portion of the trauma workload. Of all the ankle injuries evaluated in the ED, only 15% are ankle fractures. The frequency of ankle fractures has

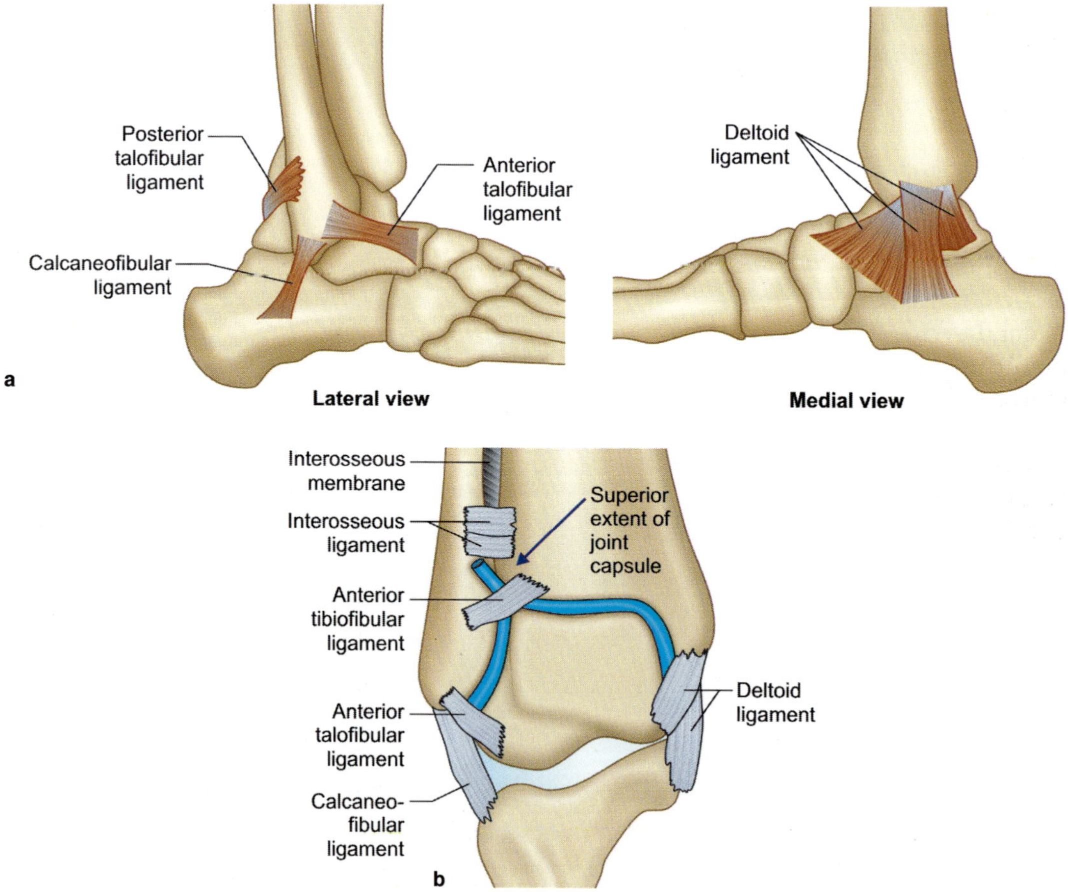

Lateral view

Posterior talofibular ligament
Anterior talofibular ligament
Calcaneofibular ligament

Medial view

Deltoid ligament

a

Interosseous membrane
Interosseous ligament
Anterior tibiofibular ligament
Anterior talofibular ligament
Calcaneofibular ligament
Superior extent of joint capsule
Deltoid ligament

b

Fig. 44.1a and b: Ligaments of the ankle joint

224

been increasing for the past 20 years, and the rate is approximately 187 in 100,000 person-years (USA). Over five million ankle injuries occur each year in the United States alone. The vast majority of ankle fractures are malleolar fractures: 60 to 70% occur as unimalleolar fractures, 15 to 20% as bimalleolar fractures, and 7 to 12% as trimalleolar fractures.

Ankle fractures have a bimodal age distribution with peaks in younger males and older females.

EXAMINATION (Fig. 44.2)

Initial examination should identify open injuries and any evidence of dislocation, both of which require urgent intervention. Dislocation with skin compromise necessitates immediate reduction on recognition to prevent skin necrosis.

- Palpation then proceeds in a logical sequence incorporating both medial and lateral sides, and including the whole length of the leg to the knee in order to avoid missing the high fibular (Maisonneuve) fracture. The neurovascular status of the limb should be checked before and after reduction.
  A standard radiological series of the ankle, including anteroposterior, lateral, and mortise radiographs, is generally sufficient to classify these injuries and plan treatment.
- Where a patient has more proximal leg tenderness or medial clear space widening with no obvious fibular fracture, full-length

radiographs of the tibia and fibula should be obtained to rule out the presence of a Maisonneuve injury.

Pott Fracture

Bimalleolar fractures, termed Pott fractures, involve at least two elements of the ankle ring. These fractures should be considered unstable and require urgent orthopedic attention.

Cotton Fracture

A trimalleolar or Cotton fracture involves the medial, lateral, and posterior malleoli. These fractures are considered unstable and require urgent orthopedic attention.

Tillaux Fracture

A Tillaux fracture describes a Salter-Harris (SH) type III injury of the anterolateral tibial epiphysis caused by extreme eversion and lateral rotation of the ankle. Incidence is highest in adolescents (Fig. 44.3).

Triplane Fracture

Triplane fracture is a combination of SH II and III fracture and is more likely than a Tillaux fracture to require open reduction and internal fixation (Fig. 44.4).

Maisonneuve Fracture

It is defined as a proximal fibular fracture coexisting with a medial malleolar fracture or disruption of the deltoid ligament. Maison-

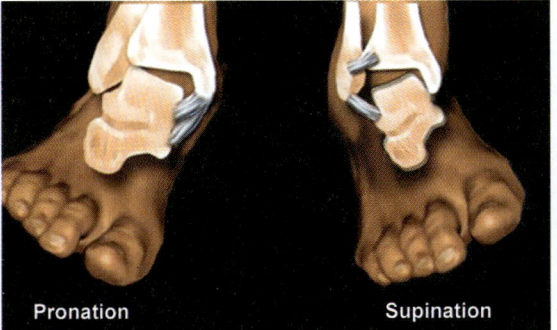
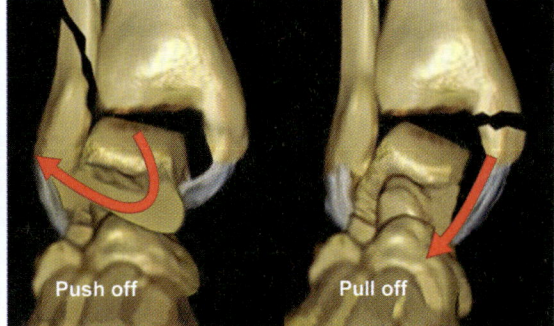

Fig. 44.2: Mechanism of ankle injury

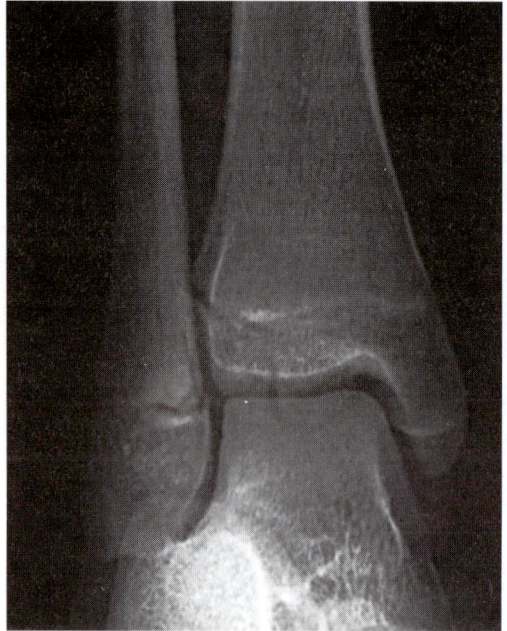

Fig. 44.3: Tillaux fracture

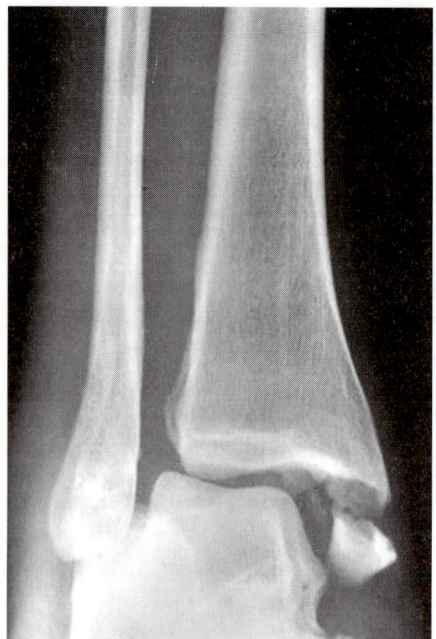

Fig. 44.5: Maisonneuve fracture

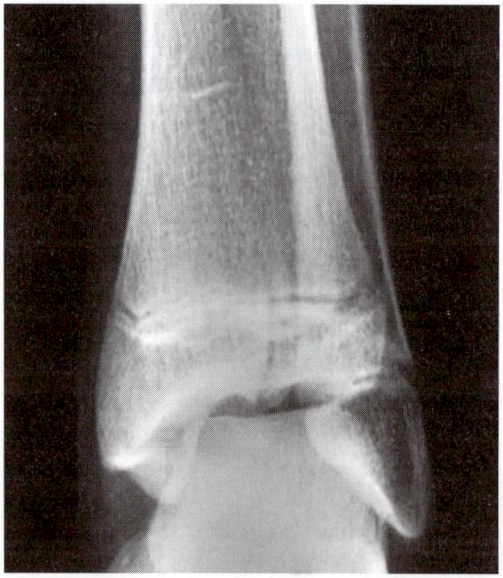

Fig. 44.4: Triplane fracture

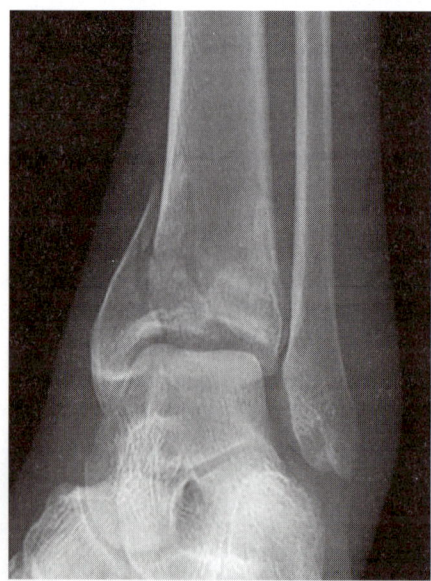

Fig. 44.6: Pilon fracture

neuve fractures are associated with partial or complete disruption of the syndesmosis (Fig. 44.5).

Pilon Fracture

A pilon fracture designates a fracture of the distal tibial metaphysis combined with disruption of the talar dome. An axial loading mechanism drives the talus into the tibial plafond (the distal articular surface of the tibia) (Fig. 44.6).

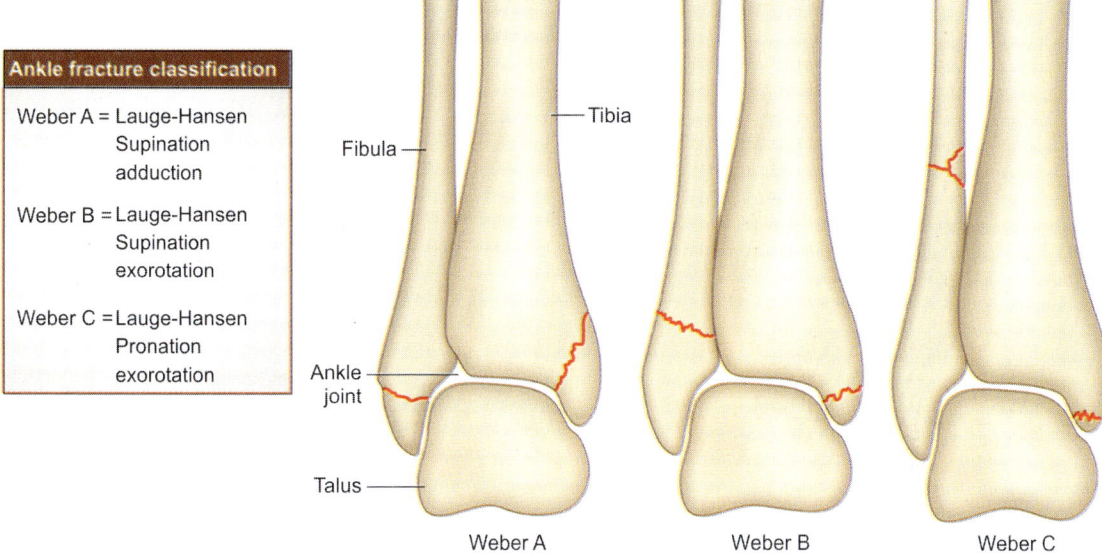

Fibula —

— Tibia

Ankle joint

Talus —

Weber A   Weber B   Weber C

Fig. 44.7: Ankle fracture classification

Ankle fracture classification

Weber A = Lauge-Hansen
          Supination
          adduction

Weber B = Lauge-Hansen
          Supination
          exorotation

Weber C = Lauge-Hansen
          Pronation
          exorotation

Classification of ankle fractures is important in order to estimate the extent of the ligamentous injury and the stability of the joint.

The Weber classification focuses on the integrity of the syndesmosis, which holds the ankle mortise together.

The Lauge-Hansen system focuses on the trauma mechanism.

DANIS WEBER'S CLASSIFICATION SYSTEM

- Type A depicts a transverse fibular avulsion fracture, occasionally with an oblique fracture of the medial malleolus. These result from internal rotation and adduction. These are usually stable fractures.
- Type B describes an oblique fracture of the lateral malleolus with or without rupture of the tibiofibular syndesmosis and medial injury (either medial malleolus fracture or deltoid rupture). These result from external rotation. These may be unstable.
- Type C designates a high fibular fracture with rupture of the tibiofibular ligament and transverse avulsion fracture of the medial malleolus. Usually, syndesmotic

injury is more extensive than in type B. These result from adduction or abduction with external rotation. These are usually unstable and require operative repair.

Weber classified them as (Fig. 44.7 to 44.9):

- Type A—infrasyndesmotic
- Type B—transsyndesmotic
- Type C—suprasyndesmotic

If an ankle fracture disrupts the ankle ring (formed by the ankle bones and ligaments) in one place, it often disrupts it in another; if ≥2 of the structures that stabilize the ankle ring are disrupted, the ankle is unstable.

MANAGEMENT

There are clinical criteria used to differentiate ankle fractures from ankle sprains. These guidelines, called the Ottawa criteria, help to determine, if X-rays should be done in people who have ankle pain.

There are many types of ankle fractures, and treatments vary significantly depending on the location and severity of the injury (Fig. 44.10).

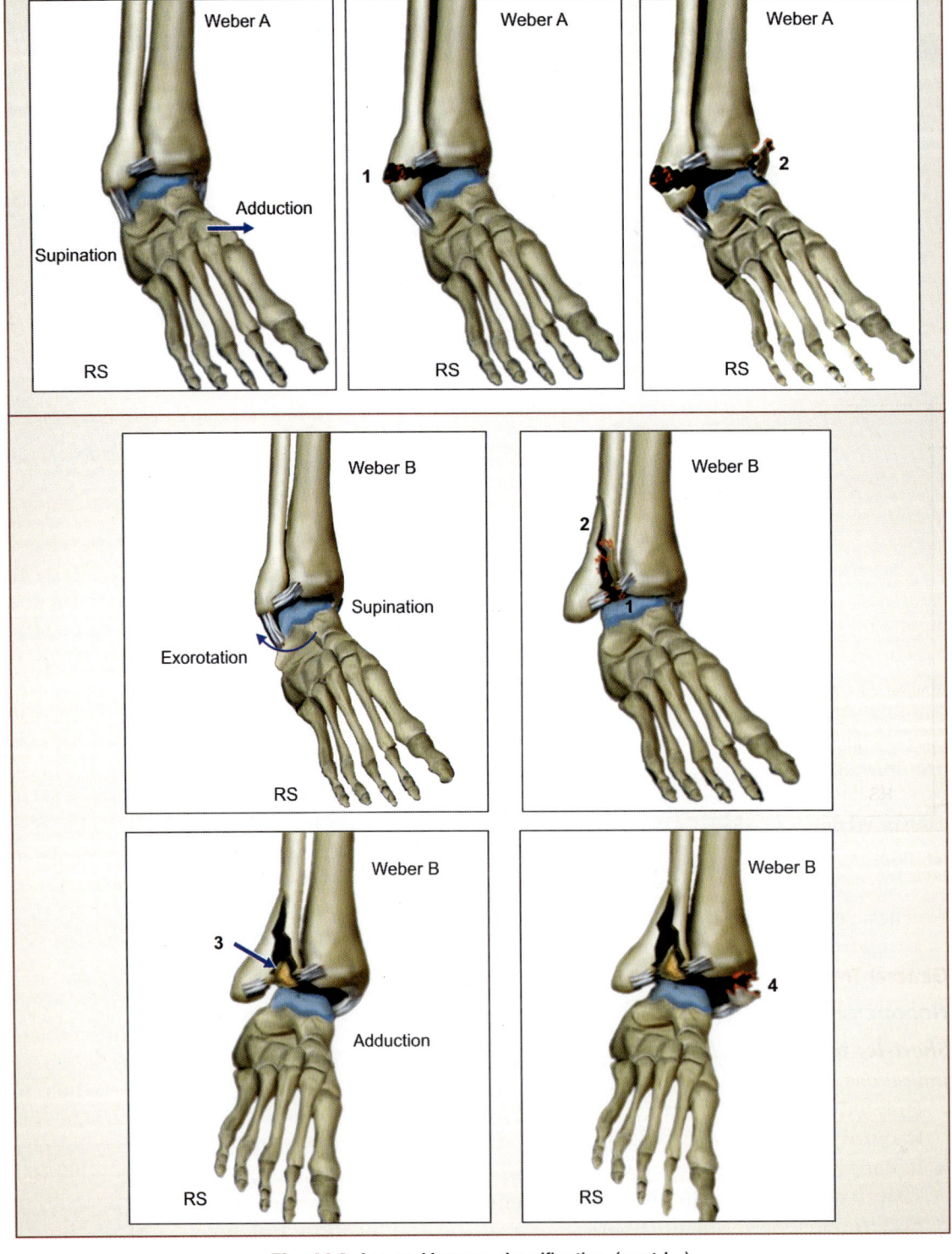

Fig. 44.8: Lauge-Hansen classification (contd...)

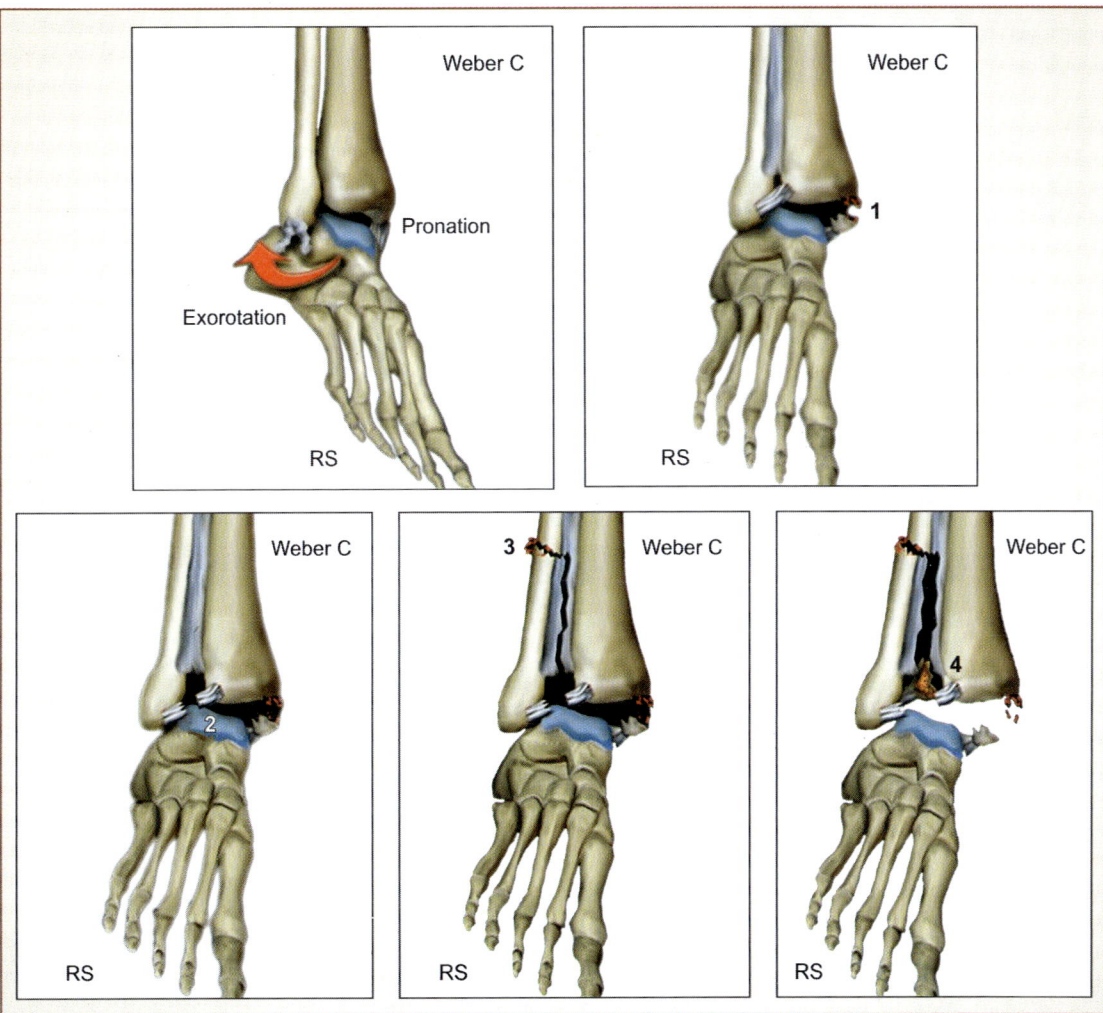

Fig. 44.8: Lauge-Hansen classification

General Treatment

Nonoperative

Short-leg walking cast/boot

Indications

- Isolated nondisplaced medial malleolus fracture or tip avulsions
- Isolated lateral malleolus fracture with <3 mm displacement and no talar shift
- Posterior malleolar fracture with <25% joint involvement or <2 mm step-off

Operative

Open reduction internal fixation (Fig. 44.11)
Indications

- Any talar displacement
- Displaced isolated medial malleolar fracture
- Displaced isolated lateral malleolar fracture
- Bimalleolar fracture and bimalleolar-equivalent fracture
- Posterior malleolar fracture with >25% or > 2 mm step-off

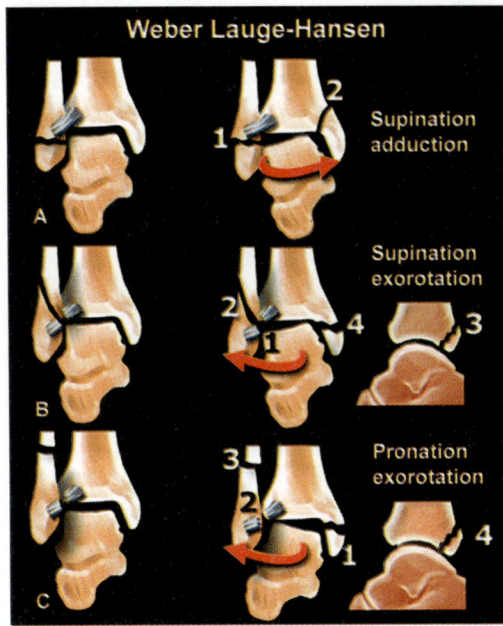

Fig. 44.9: Three grades of Weber

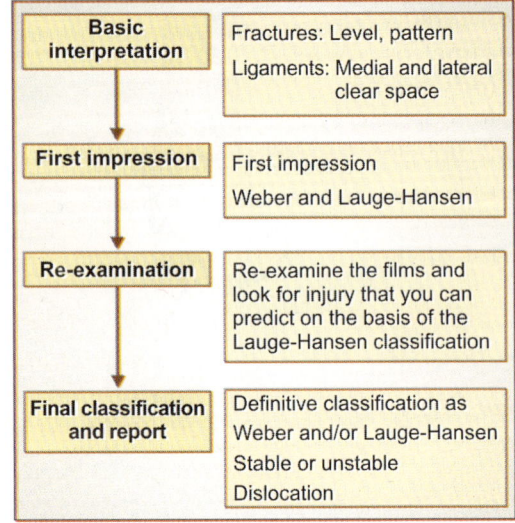

Fig. 44.10: Radiological assessment

- Bosworth fracture-dislocations
- Open fractures

Technique
- Goal of treatment is stable anatomic reduction of talus in the ankle mortise.
- 1 mm shift of talus leads to 42% decrease in tibiotalar contact area

Outcomes
- Overall success rate of 90%

  – Prolonged recovery expected (2 years to obtain final functional result)
- Significant functional impairment often noted.
- Worse outcomes with: Smoking, decreased education, alcohol use, increased age, presence of medial malleolar fracture.
- ORIF superior to closed treatment of bimalleolar fractures.
- In Lauge-Hansen supination-adduction fractures, restoration of marginal impaction of the anteromedial tibial plafond leads to optimal functional results after surgery.

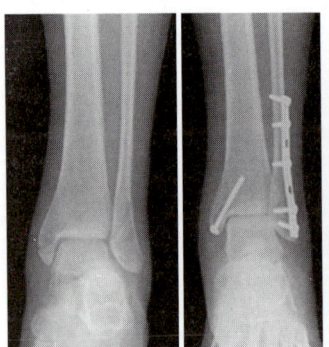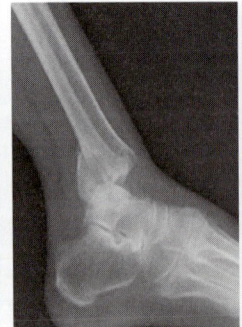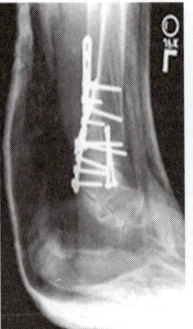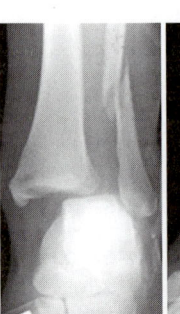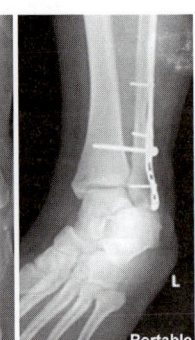

Fig. 44.11: Internal fixation

Postoperative rehabilitation
- Time for proper braking response time (driving) returns to baseline at nine weeks for operatively treated ankle fractures.
- Braking travel time is significantly reduced until 6 weeks after initiation of weight bearing in both long bone and periarticular fractures of the lower extremity.

Isolated Medial Malleolus Fracture

Nonoperative

Short leg walking cast or cast boot

Indications: Nondisplaced fracture and tip avulsions:
- Deep deltoid inserts on posterior colliculus
- Symptomatic treatment often appropriate

Operative

ORIF

Indications: Any displacement or talar shift

Technique
- Lag screw fixation: Lag screw fixation stronger, if placed perpendicular to fracture line
- Antiglide plate with lag screw: Best for vertical shear fractures
- Tension band fixation: Utilizing stainless steel wire

Isolated Lateral Malleolus Fracture

Nonoperative

Short leg walking cast vs cast boot

Indications
- If intact mortise, no talar shift, and <3 mm displacement
- Classically fractures with more than 4–5 mm of medial clear space widening on stress radiographs have been considered unstable and need to be treated surgically:
  - Recent studies have shown the deep deltoid may be intact with up to 8–10 mm of widening on stress radiographs

  - If the mortise is well reduced, results from operative and non-operative treatment are similar.

Operative

ORIF

Indications
- If talar shift or >3 mm of displacement
- Can be treated operatively, if also treating an ipsilateral syndesmosis injury

Technique
- Open reduction and plating
  - Plate placement
    - Lateral
      - Lag screw fixation with neutralization plating
      - Bridge plate technique
    - Posterior
      - Antiglide technique
      - Lag screw fixation with neutralization plating
      - Most common disadvantage of using posterior antiglide plating is peroneal irritation, if the plate is placed too distally
    - Posterior antiglide plating is biomechanically superior to lateral plate placement
- Intramedullary retrograde screw placement
- Isolated lag screw fixation: Possible, if fibula is a spiral pattern and screws can be placed at least 1 cm apart

Postoperative care
- Period of immobilization usually 4–6 weeks after ORIF
- Duration of immobilization should be doubled in diabetic patients

Medial and Lateral (Bimalleolar) Fracture

Operative

ORIF

Indications: Any lateral talar shift

Technique
- Fibula: Need to fix with one of the options listed in section above
- Medial malleolus
  - Fixation options
    - Cancellous lag screws
    - Bicortical screws
    - Tension band wiring
    - Antiglide plate to treat a vertical medial malleolus fracture
  - Orient screws parallel to joint for vertical medial malleolar fracture (Lauge-Hansen supination—adduction fracture pattern)

Functional Bimalleolar Fracture (deltoid ligament tear with fibular fracture)

Operative

ORIF of lateral malleolus

Indications
- Examination has been shown to be largely unreliable in predicting medial injury
- Can see significant lateral translation of the talus in this pattern

Technique
- Not necessary to repair medial deltoid ligament
- Only need to explore medially, if you are unable to reduce the mortise
- See isolated fibular fracture techniques above

Posterior Malleolar Fracture

Nonoperative

Short leg walking cast vs cast boot

Indications
- <25% of articular surface involved
- Evaluation of percentage should be done with CT, as plain radiology is unreliable.
- <2 mm articular step off
- Syndesmotic stability

Operative

ORIF

Indications
- >25% of articular surface involved
- >2 mm articular step off
- Syndesmosis injury

Technique
- Approach
  - Posterolateral approach
  - Posteromedial approach
  - Decision of approach will depend on fracture lines and need for fibular fixation
- Fixation
  - Anterior to posterior lag screws to capture fragment (if nondisplaced)
  - Posterior to anterior lag screw and buttress plate
  - Antiglide plate
- Syndesmosis injury
  - Stiffness of syndesmosis restored to 70% normal with isolated fixation of posterior malleolus (versus 40% with isolated syndesmosis fixation)
  - Stress examination of syndesmosis still required after posterior malleolar fixation
  - Posteroinferior tibiofibular ligament may remain attached to posterior malleolus and syndesmotic stability may be restored with isolated posterior malleolar fixation

Bosworth Fracture-Dislocation

Overview
- Rare fracture-dislocation of the ankle where the fibula becomes entrapped behind the tibia and becomes irreducible.
- Posterolateral ridge of the distal tibia hinders reduction of the fibula.

Operative
- Open reduction and fixation of the fibula in the incisura fibularis
  - Indicated in most cases.

Open Ankle Fracture

Operative

- Emergent operative debridement and ORIF: Indicated, if soft tissue conditions allow
- External fixation
  Indications: Soft tissue conditions and overall patient characteristics

ASSOCIATED SYNDESMOTIC INJURY (Fig. 44.12)

Overview

Suspect injury in all ankle fractures:
- Most common in Weber C fracture patterns
- Fixation usually not required when fibula fracture within 4.5 cm of plafond
- Up to 25% of tibial shaft fractures will have ankle injury

Evaluation

- Measure clear space 1 cm above joint
  - It has also been reported that there is no actual correlation between syndesmotic injury and tibiofibular clear space or overlap measurements.

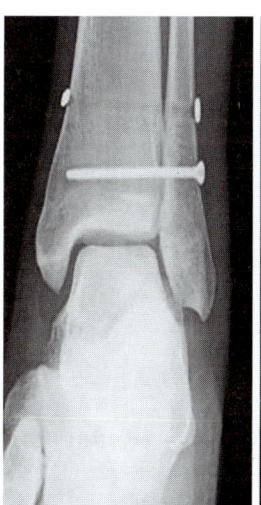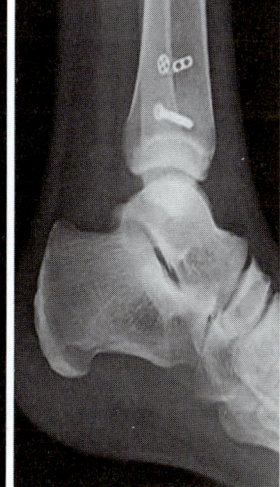

Fig. 44.12: Syndesmotic screws

- Lateral stress radiograph has more interobserver reliability than an AP/mortise stress film
- Best option is to assess stability intra-operatively with abduction/external rotation stress of dorsiflexed foot.
- Instability of the syndesmosis is greatest in the anterior-posterior direction.

COMPLICATIONS

Local blisters (Fig. 44.13), compartment syndrome, infection, malunion and secondary degenerative arthritis of the ankle joint are some important complications.

Post-traumatic arthritis has been described in 14% of patients despite an anatomic reduction, most likely as a result of chondral injury sustained at the time of initial injury.

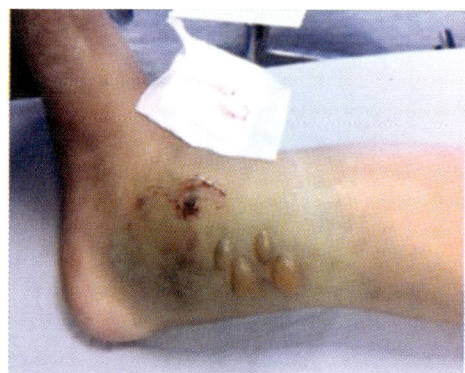

Fig. 44.13: Blisters

BIBLIOGRAPHY

- http://emedicine.medscape.com/article/824224-clinical#b5
- http://www.radiologyassistant.nl/
- http://radiologymasterclass.co.uk/
- https://www.youtube.com/watch?v=sKIyBsiI1Z4
- https://www.youtube.com/watch?v=fKDAhnwy0ec
- https://www.youtube.com/watch?v=-2A5yrS0tpg

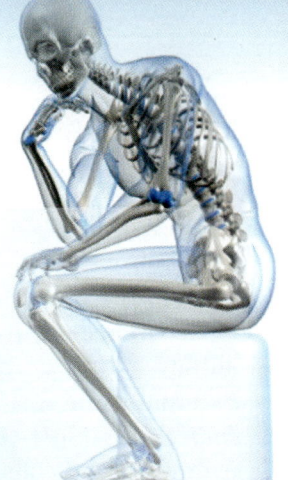

Fractures of Talus

The word *talus* is derived from the Latin word *taxillus*, which refers to the ankle bone of a horse. These bones were used as playing dice by Roman soldiers. Approximately 60% of its surface is covered by articular cartilage, and there are no muscular or tendinous attachments to this bone. Consequently, only a limited area of penetrable bone is available for vascular perforation. This feature, combined with small nutrient vessels, variations in intraosseous anastomoses, and a lack of collateral circulation, predispose the talus to osteonecrosis when its vascular supply is disturbed (Fig. 45.1).

Talus fractures are relatively uncommon, comprising less than 1% of all fractures.

Most talus fractures are the result of high-energy trauma such as a car collision or a fall from height. Injuries from sports, particularly from snowboarding, are another, less common, cause of talar injuries. There is an increased incidence of talus fracture among snowboarders due to the unique stress placed on the talus when landing from jumps on a snowboard.

Injuries of the talus are often surgical emergencies due to the tenuous blood supply to this bone. These fractures often require urgent treatment to realign the bone to maximize the body's ability to heal the bone and prevent dead bone (avascular necrosis) from developing.

Blood supply to the talus is derived from three arteries and in order of significance are:
1. Posterior tibial
2. Anterior tibial
3. Perforating peroneal

The main blood supply of the talar body enters the talar neck from the sinus tarsi (a fat-filled space between the talar neck and the calcaneus) and proceeds retrograde to supply the talar body (Fig. 45.2). Thus, fractures of the talar neck can compromise the vascularity of the body of the talus. The blood supply to the talus is very compromised with a fracture dislocation scenario. The posterior tibial artery has branches medially. The dorsalis pedis has branches anteriorly. The peroneal artery has branches laterally. They are all connected through a sling of vessels that lie within the sinus tarsi.

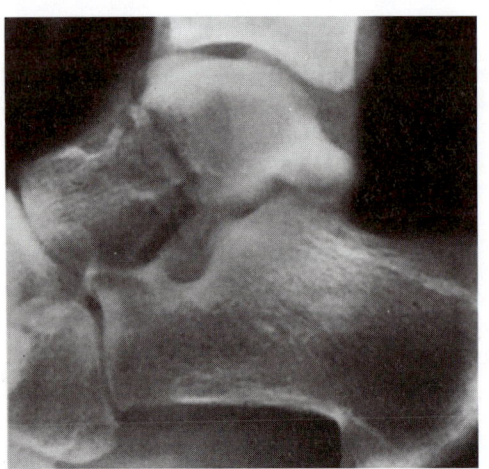

Fig. 45.1: Fracture of talus

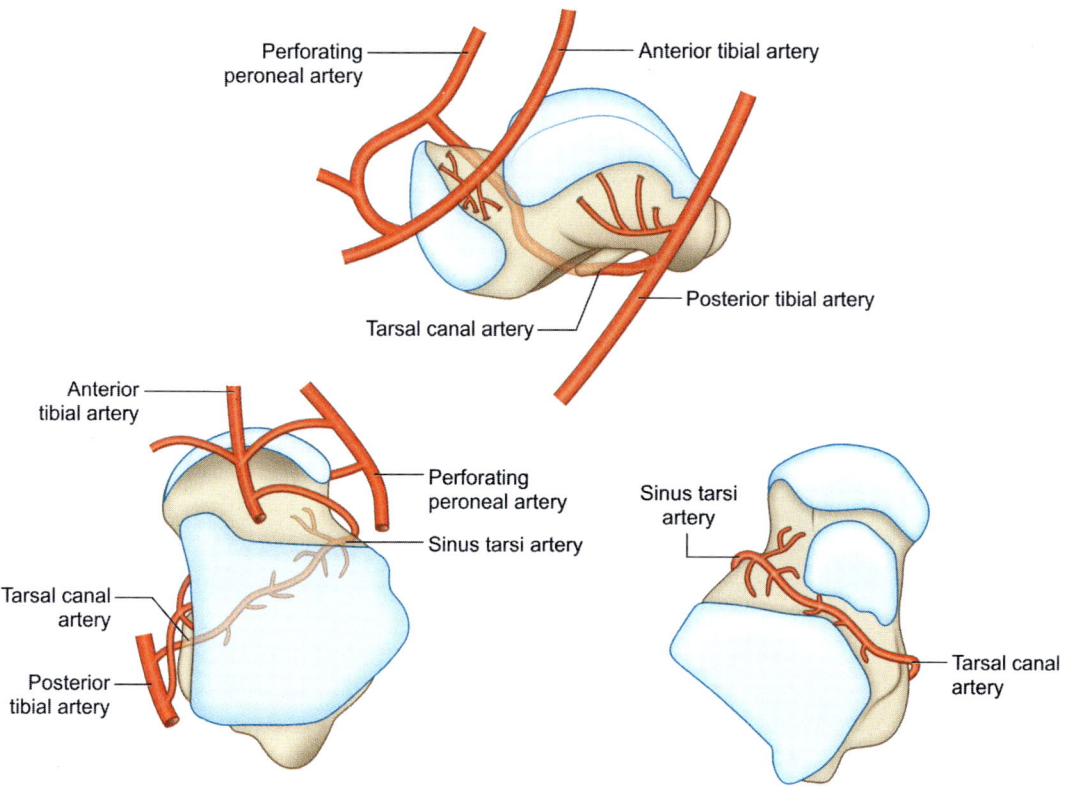

Fig. 45.2: Blood supply of talus

The deltoid branch of the posterior tibial artery must be protected. It is an important point for blood supply entry into the medial talus. This is the reason why a medial malleolar osteotomy is successful as it protects the talar blood supply.

The deltoid branches are important to supply blood to the medial talar neck and talar body. Branches from the dorsalis pedis supply the talar head and most of the dorsal talar neck. The artery of the tarsal canal coming from branches of the posterior tibial artery supply most of the talar body.

The peroneal artery has the least contribution laterally.

The talus has no muscular or tendinous attachments and thus relies on the integrity of its capsule for its blood supply. In a similar fashion to the scaphoid, the proximal body gets much of its blood supply from the distal head and, therefore, fractures can impair the blood supply and cause avascular necrosis.

HAWKINS CLASSIFICATION

(Table 45.1 and Figs 45.3, 45.4)

- Type I: Non-displaced fracture
- Type II: Displaced fracture with subluxation or dislocation of the subtalar joint and a normal ankle joint
- Type III: Displaced fracture with body of talus dislocated from both subtalar and ankle joint

Canale and Kelly described a rare type IV category which in addition to features describes in type III there is dislocation or subluxation of the head of the talus at the talonavicular joint.

CT scanning and magnetic resonance imaging (MRI) are used to diagnose clinically occult fractures.

Table 45.1: Hawkins classification of talar neck fracture (Hawkins 1970, revised by Canale 1978)

	Radiographic findings	Risk of AVN
Type I	Nondisplaced fracture line	0–13%
Type II	Displaced fracture, subluxation or dislocation of subtalar joint	20–50%
Type III	Displaced fracture, dislocation of subtalar and tibiotalar joints	69–100%
Type IV	Displaced fracture, disruption of talonavicular joint	High

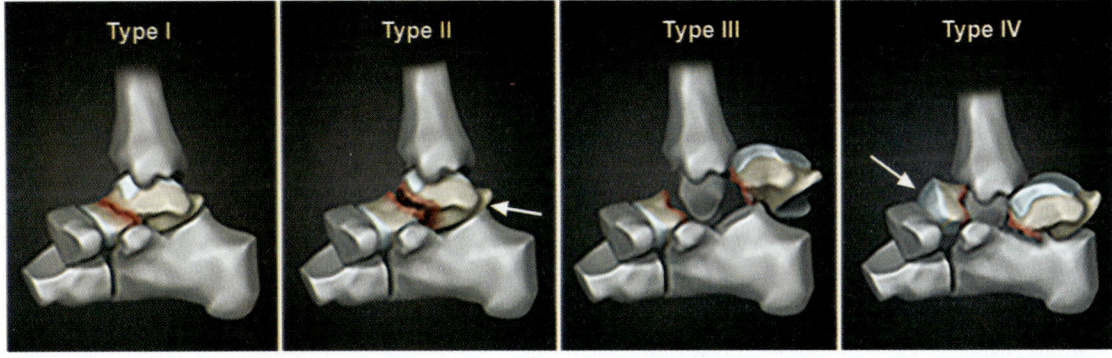

Fig. 45.3: Hawkins classification

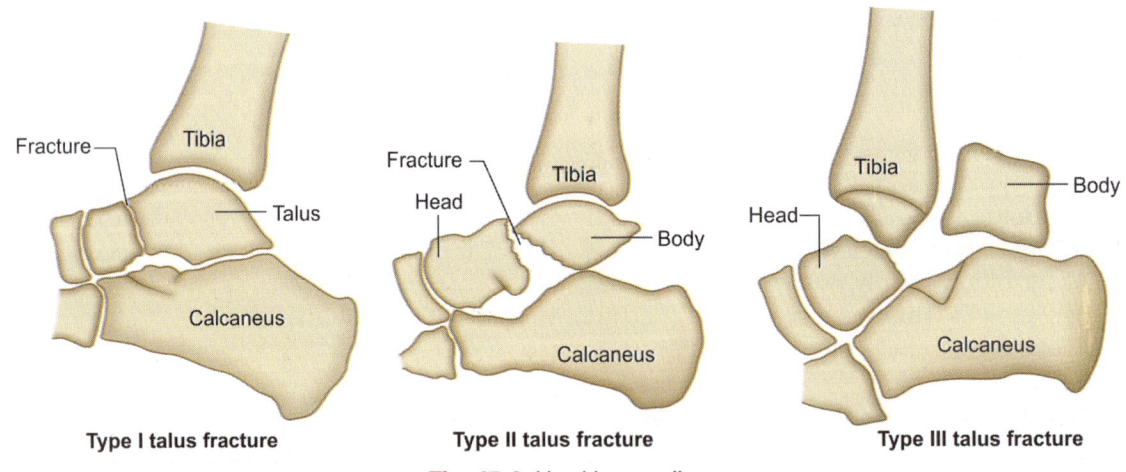

Fig. 45.4: Hawkins grading

Hawkins sign (Fig. 45.5) describes subchondral lucency of the talar dome that occurs secondary to subchondral atrophy 6–8 weeks after a talar neck fracture.

This indicates that there is sufficient vascularity in the talus, and is therefore unlikely to develop avascular necrosis later.

The os trigonum (Fig. 45.6) is an accessory bone (sesamoid) located posterior to the posterior tubercle of the talus. It is present in 5–14% of the population and is frequently unilateral. This accessory bone may be fused to the talus, calcaneus, or both. Patients with a fracture of the os trigonum often give a history of having sustained some ankle sprain weeks to months earlier, at which time radiographs were interpreted as normal. They give a history of persistent posterior and posterolateral ankle pain, swelling, and giving way of the ankle. All have a 25° decrease in

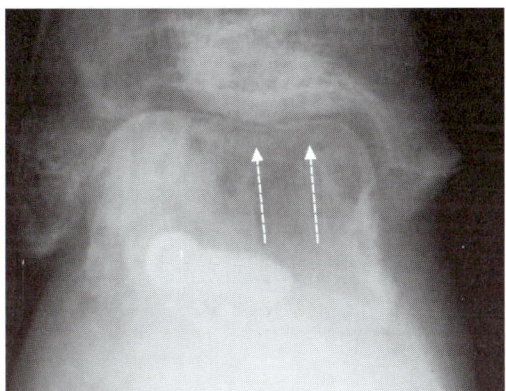

Fig. 45.5: Hawkins sign (indicates intact blood supply over talar dome)

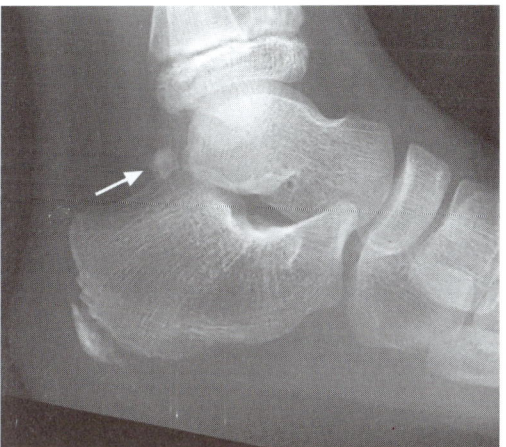

Fig. 45.6: Os trigonum

plantar flexion of the ankle and pain to palpation posterior to the tibia but anterior to the Achilles tendon. The pain is enhanced by forced plantar flexion of the ankle or resisted plantar flexion of the great toe.

TREATMENT

- *Type I fractures:* Short leg cast or boot and no weight bearing
- *Types II–IV fractures:* ORIF

The combined anteromedial and antero-lateral incisions are optimal for all talar neck fractures that are treated operatively. These two exposures ensure adequate visualization for reduction and fixation.

Helpful adjuncts in surgery when doing an open reduction include joysticks, external fixator, small distractor, or lamina spreader. A headlamp helps with visualization, and an image intensifier will guide the reduction of this difficult fracture (Fig. 45.7).

COMPLICATIONS

- Sloughing of skin and infection.
- Foot compartment syndrome.

Open fractures can occur in 15–25% of injuries, reflecting the high-energy mechanism of injury. The infection rate is up to 40% in open talus fractures.

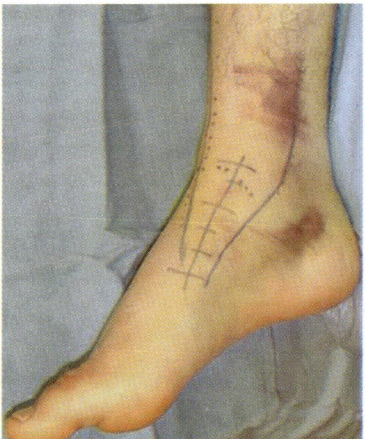
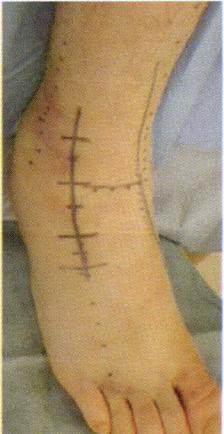
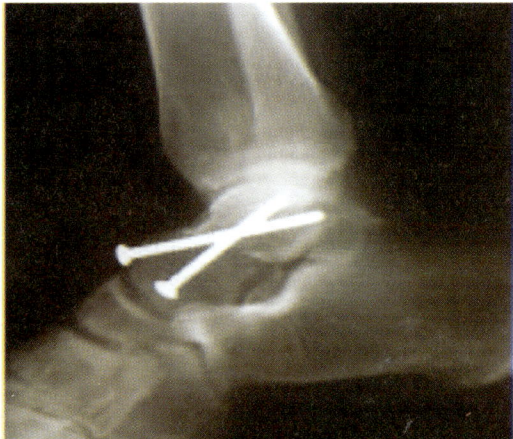

Fig. 45.7: Surgical incisions and screw fixation

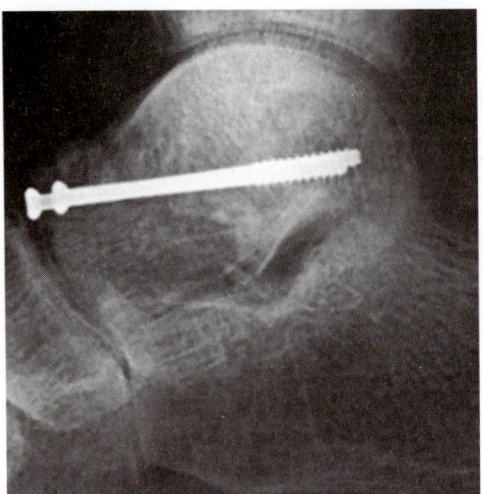

Fig. 45.8: AVN of talar body following fracture of talar neck

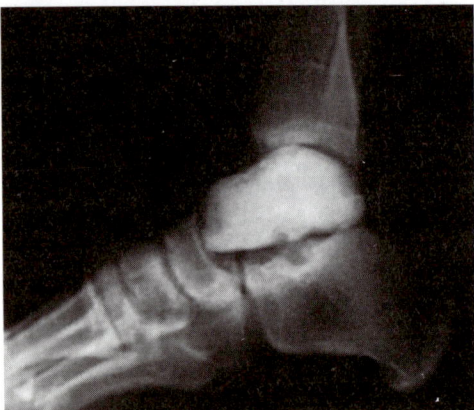

Fig. 45.9: Avascular necrosis

- Hardware complications
  - Loosening
  - Backing out
  - Hardware or peri-hardware fracture
- Tendon entrapment or injury
- Malunion
- Delayed union or nonunion occurs in approximately 15% of cases.
- Post-traumatic arthritis occurs in 40–90% of cases.
- Risk of avascular necrosis (AVN) increases with increase in classification type (Figs 45.8 and 45.9):
  - Type I fractures have 0–15% risk
  - Type II fractures have 20–50% risk
  - Type III fractures approach 100% risk
  - Type IV fractures have 100% risk

BIBLIOGRAPHY

- http://radiopaedia.org
- http://pubs.rsna.org/
- http://www.orthofracs.com/
- https://www.youtube.com/watch?v=OxehxKzWH88
- https://www.youtube.com/watch?v=GHuIEplufCE
- http://www.wisconsinfootandankleinstitute.com/

Fractures of Calcaneum

The calcaneus is the most commonly fractured tarsal bone and accounts for about 2% of all fractures and ~60% of all tarsal fractures. Calcaneal fracture is also known as *lover's fracture* and Don Juan fracture. The name lover's fracture is derived from the fact that a lover may jump from great heights while trying to escape from the lover's spouse.

They most often occur during high-energy collisions—such as a fall from height or a motor vehicle crash. Because of this, calcaneus fractures are often severe and may result in long-term problems. If bilateral calcaneal fractures are seen, then the spine should also be evaluated for fracture as the mechanism of injury is often a large load to the axial skeleton (Figs 46.1 and 46.2).

Calcaneal fractures can be divided broadly into two types:

1. *Extra-articular:* 25–30%

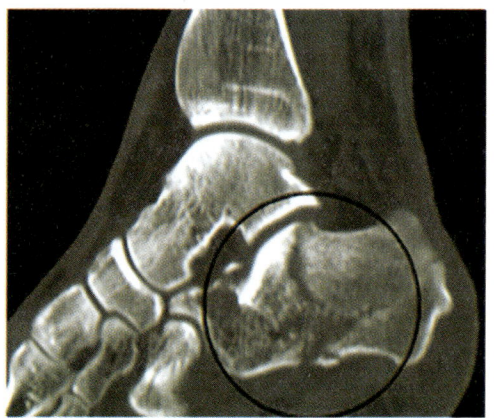

Fig. 46.1: Calcaneal fracture

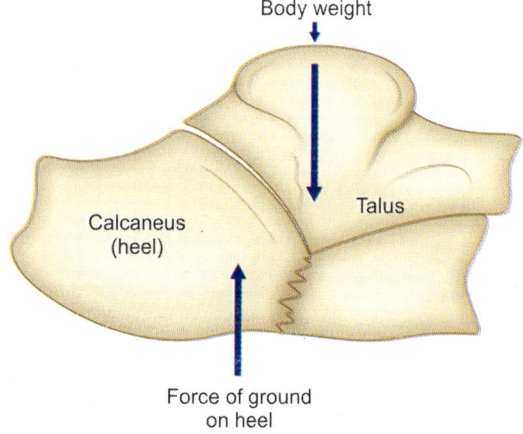

Fig. 46.2: Mechanism of injury

2. *Intra-articular:* 70–75%

A hematoma extending to the sole of the foot is called "Mondor sign", and is pathognomonic for calcaneal fracture.

RADIOGRAPHIC FEATURES

Plain Film

Plain radiographs of the foot are indicated for any suspected calcaneus injury. Also, consider imaging the contralateral ankle and foot for comparative purposes. Images should include anteroposterior (AP), lateral, oblique, axial, and Broden views (Fig. 46.3).

Lateral Radiograph

Bohler's angle is the angle between two tangent lines drawn across the anterior and posterior borders of calcaneus in the lateral

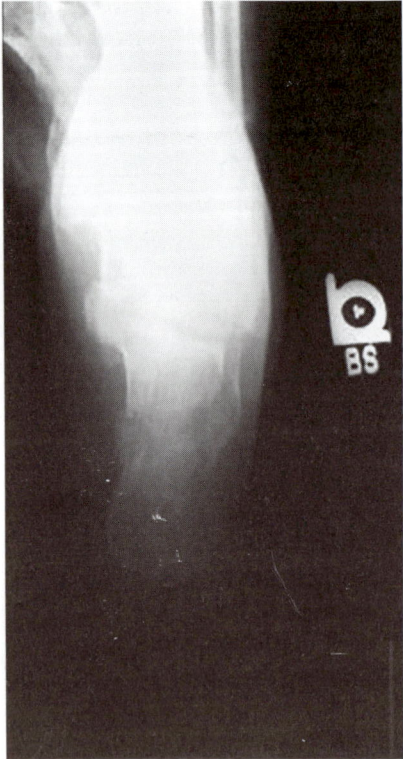

Fig. 46.3: Axial view

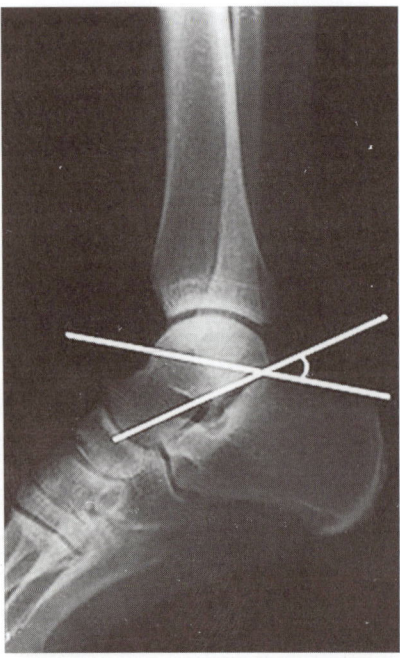

Fig. 46.4: Bohler's angle

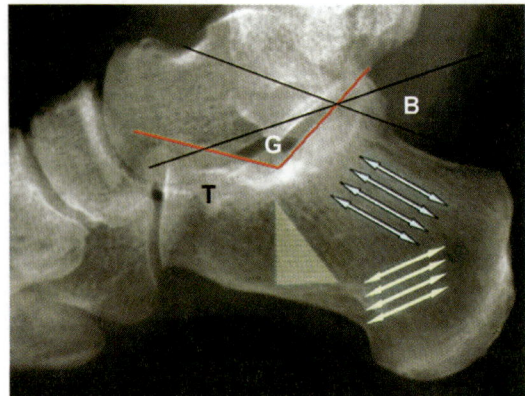

Fig. 46.4: G—critical angle of Gissane and B—Bohler's angle

view. When Bohler's angle becomes less than 20° it indicates a calcaneal fracture (Fig. 46.4).

The angle of Gissane, or "critical angle", is the angle formed by the downward and upward slopes of the calcaneal superior surface. On a lateral radiograph, an angle of Gissane of >130° suggests fracture of the posterior subtalar joint surface. Bohler's, or the "Tuber angle", is another normal anatomic landmark seen in lateral radiographs. It is formed by the intersection of: (1) A line from the highest point of the posterior articular facet to the highest point of the posterior tuberosity, and (2) a line from the former to the highest point on the anterior articular facet. An angle <20° suggests a depression of posterior facet and possible calcaneal fracture (Fig. 46.5).

CT

Intra-articular fractures are often classified using the Sander classification system, which is one of the systems that correlate well with patient outcome.

CLASSIFICATION

The Sanders classification system is the most commonly used system for categorizing intrarticular fractures. There are four types:

1. *Type I fractures* are non-displaced fractures (displacement <2 mm).

2. *Type II fractures* consist of a single intra-articular fracture that divides the calcaneus into two pieces.
   - Type IIA: Fracture occurs on lateral aspect of calcaneus.
   - Type IIB: Fracture occurs on central aspect of calcaneus.
   - Type IIC: Fracture occurs on medial aspect of calcaneus.
3. *Type III fractures* consist of two intra-articular fractures that divide the calcaneus into three articular pieces.
   - Type IIIAB: Two fracture lines are present, one lateral and one central.
   - Type IIIAC: Two fracture lines are present, one lateral and one medial.
   - Type IIIBC: Two fracture lines are present, one central and one medial.
4. *Type IV fractures* consist of fractures with more than three intra-articular fractures.

Extra-articular fractures include all fractures that do not involve the posterior facet of the subtalar joint.
- Type A involve the anterior calcaneus
- Type B involve the middle calcaneus. This includes the sustentaculum tali, trochlear process and lateral process.
- Type C involve the posterior calcaneus, the posterior tuberosity and medial tubercle included.

TREATMENT

The use of nonoperative versus operative interventions for calcaneus fractures is a controversial topic. Treatment goals of operative modalities include the following: (1) Restoration of heel height and length, (2) realignment of the posterior facet of the subtalar joint, and (3) restoration of the mechanical axis of the hindfoot.

Non-surgical treatment is indicated for extra-articular fractures and Sanders Type I intra-articular fractures, provided that the calcaneal weight-bearing surface and foot function are not compromised. Physicians may choose to perform closed reduction with or without fixation (casting), or fixation alone (without reduction), depending on the individual case.

Conservative, nonoperative care includes elevation, application of ice, early mobilization, and the use of a splint.

Many authors recommend short leg casting and no weight bearing for 2 weeks, followed by range-of-motion exercises. Progressive weight bearing should begin at 8 weeks, with full weight bearing by 12 weeks.

In the 1950s, operative treatment with a percutaneous "spike" became popular and was widely performed.

Displaced intra-articular fractures require surgical intervention within 3 weeks of fracture, before bone consolidation has occurred. Conservative surgery consists of closed reduction with percutaneous fixation. This technique is associated with less wound complications, better soft tissue healing (because of less soft tissue manipulation) and decreased intraoperative time. However, this procedure has increased risk of inadequate calcaneal bone fixation, compared to open procedures. Currently, open reduction with internal fixation (ORIF) is usually the preferred surgical approach when dealing with displaced intra-articular fractures.

Nonoperative

- *Cast immobilization with nonweight bearing for 6 weeks*
  - Indications: Calcaneal stress fractures
- *Cast immobilization with nonweight bearing for 10 to 12 weeks*
  - Indications
    - Small extra-articular fracture (<1 cm) with intact Achilles tendon and <2 mm displacement
    - Sanders Type I (nondisplaced)
    - Anterior process fracture involving <25% of calcaneocuboid joint
    - Comorbidities that preclude good surgical outcome (smoker, diabetes, PVD)

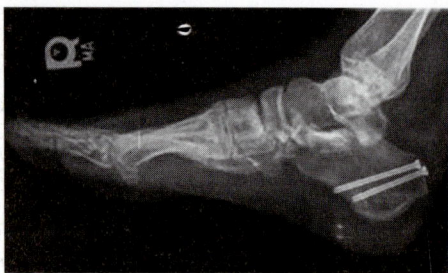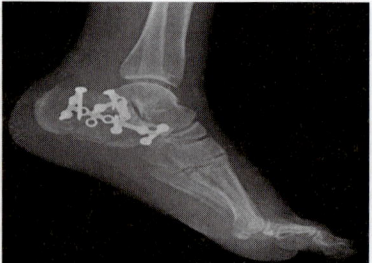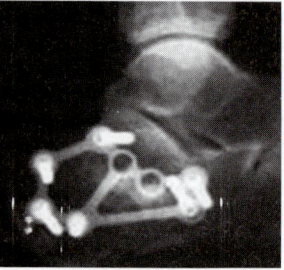

Fig. 46.6: Internal fixation

- Techniques: Begin early range of motion exercises once swelling allows.

Operative

- *Closed reduction with percutaneous pinning*
  - Indications:
    - Minimally displaced tongue-type fxs or those with mild shortening
    - Large extra-articular fractures (>1 cm)
    - Early reduction prevents skin sloughing and need for subsequent flap coverage
  - Techniques: Lag screws from posterior superior tuberosity directed inferior and distal
- *ORIF* (Fig. 46.6)
  - Indications:
    - Displaced tongue-type fractures
    - Large extra-articular fractures (>1 cm) with detachment of Achilles tendon and/or >2 mm displacement
    - Urgent, if skin is compromised
- *Sanders Type II and III:* Posterior facet displacement >2 to 3 mm, flattening of Bohler angle, or varus malalignment of the tuberosity
- Anterior process fracture with >25% involvement of calcaneocuboid joint
- Displaced sustentaculum fractures

Timing

- Wait 10–14 days until swelling and blisters resolve and wrinkle sign present 10–14 days.

- No benefit to early surgery due to significant soft tissue swelling.

Primary Subtalar Arthrodesis

Indications: Sanders Type IV

COMPLICATIONS

- Wound complications (10–25%): Increased risk in smokers, diabetics, and open injuries
- Subtalar arthritis: Increased with non-operative management
- Lateral impingement with peroneal irritation
- Damaged FHL:
  - At risk with placement of lateral to medial screws, especially at level of sustentaculum tali (constant fragment)
  - Damage to sural nerve, seen with lateral approach
- Compartment syndrome (10%): Results in claw toes
- Malunion

BIBLIOGRAPHY

- https://en.wikipedia.org/wiki/Calcaneal_fracture
- http://radiologymasterclass.co.uk/
- https://www.youtube.com/watch?v=5oNlURCSv0U
- https://www.youtube.com/watch?v=z3P0Zers6rM
- https://www.youtube.com/watch?v=h1NYDtrgdDs

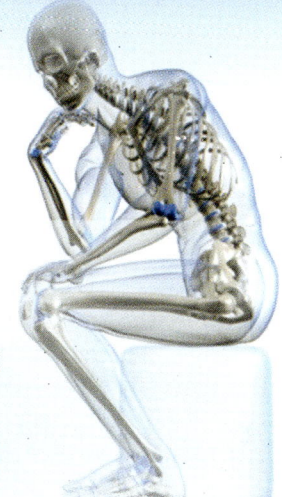

Fractures of Bones of Foot and Toes

The foot is divided into three sections:
- The forefoot contains the five toes (phalanges) and the five longer bones (metatarsals).
- The midfoot is a pyramid-like collection of bones that form the arches of the feet. These include the three cuneiform bones—the cuboid bone, and the navicular bone.
- The hindfoot forms the heel and ankle. The talus bone supports the leg bones (tibia and fibula), forming the ankle. The calcaneus (heel bone) is the largest bone in the foot.

Metatarsal fractures (Fig. 47.1) represent 5 to 6% of fractures encountered in primary care. They range from easily managed fractures to more complicated fractures that require surgical intervention. Professional football (soccer) players David Beckham, Wayne Rooney, Ashley Cole and Steve Gerrard have all sustained this foot injury in recent years.

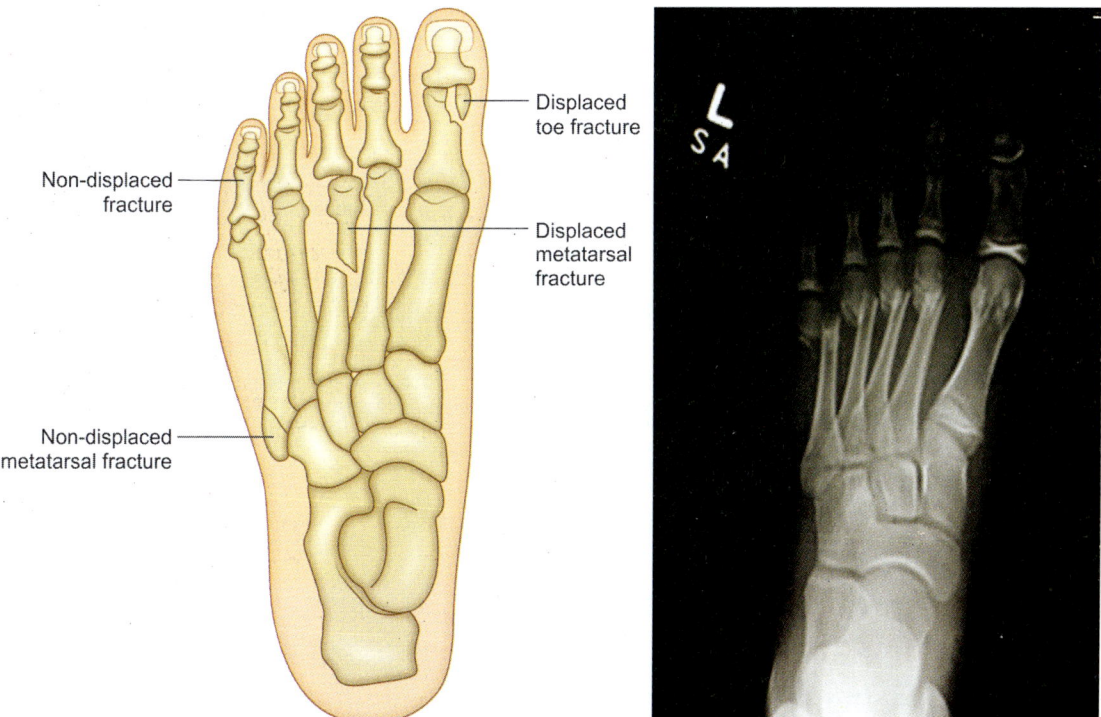

Fig. 47.1: Metatarsal fractures

Stress fractures are tiny, hairline breaks that are usually caused by repetitive stress. Stress fractures often afflict athletes who, for example, too rapidly increase their running mileage. They can also be caused by an abnormal foot structure, deformities, or osteoporosis. Improper footwear may also lead to stress fractures (Fig. 47.2).

TREATMENT (Fig. 47.3)

The ultimate treatment of metatarsal fractures varies depending on the type and location of the fracture. If the fracture is due to direct trauma and the fracture fragments are well aligned, then the treatment is immobilization in a removable plastic cast and non-weight bearing for 6–8 weeks (Fig. 47.4).

Nondisplaced fractures of the metatarsal shaft usually require only a soft dressing followed by a firm, supportive shoe and progressive weight-bearing.

Intra-articular or displaced metatarsal fractures, as well as most fractures that involve the first metatarsal or multiple metatarsals require better care and attention. Intra-

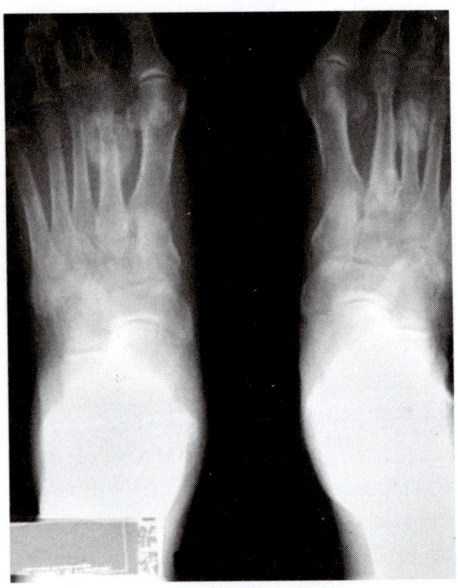

Fig. 47.2: Stress fracture of 2nd metatarsal with exuberant callus

operative treatment of metatarsal fracture can be treated with a variety of products including but not limited to cannulated screws, solid screws, trim-it bio-pins, locking and non-locking plates.

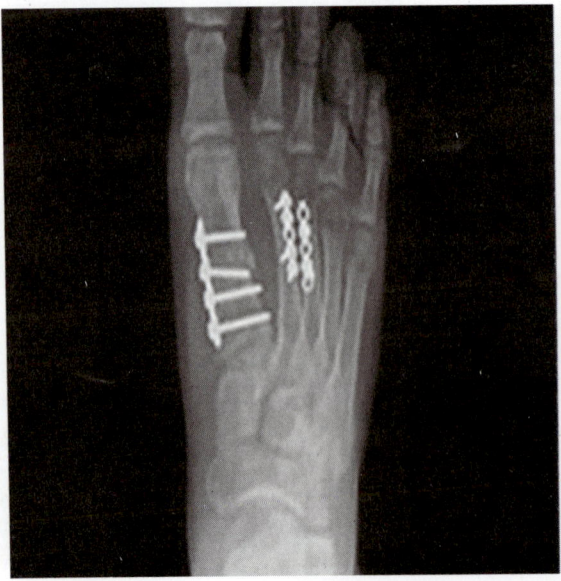
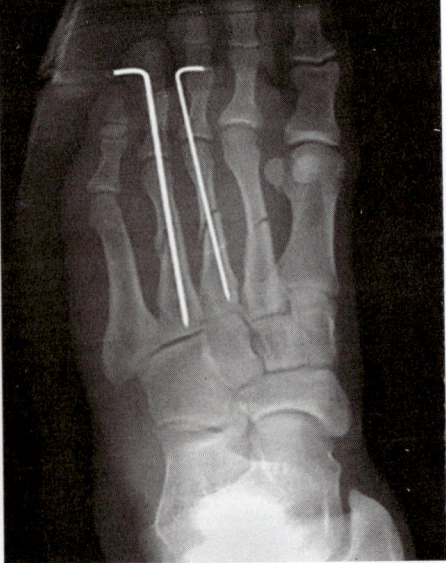

Fig. 47.3: Internal fixation of metatarsal fracture

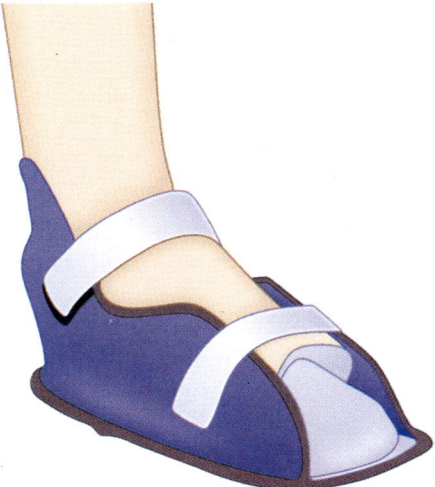

Fig. 47.4: A walking boot

COMPLICATIONS

- Nonunion
- Infection
- Painful hardware
- Compartment syndrome
- CRPS
- DVT/PE

FIFTH METATARSAL FRACTURE

The base of the fifth metatarsal is divided into three fracture zones (Fig. 47.5).

- *Zone 1 fractures* are avulsion or "chip" fractures that occur at the tip of the base of the fifth metatarsal. These fractures are typically treated without surgery using a

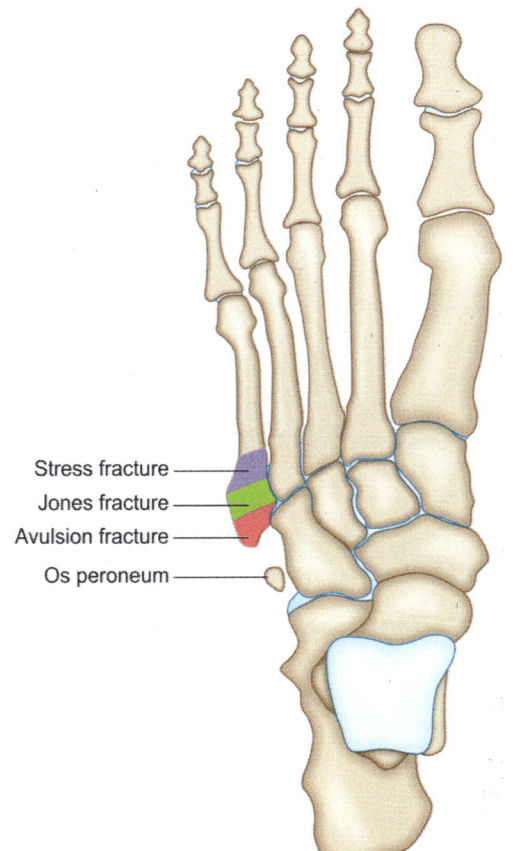

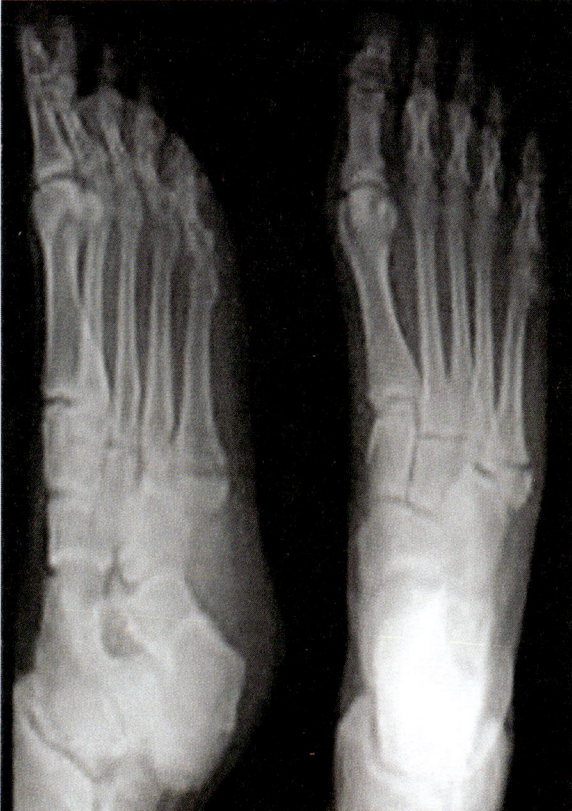

Stress fracture
Jones fracture
Avulsion fracture
Os peroneum

Fig. 47.5: Fractures at base of 5th metatarsal bone

cast, boot or hard-soled shoe. These fractures tend to heal within 6 to 8 weeks.

- *Zone 2 fractures* are typically known as Jones fractures. They occur at the intersection between the base and the shaft of the fifth metatarsal. These fractures are known to have a higher chance of not healing (nonunion). They are also at risk of refracture even after healing. Surgical treatment is commonly performed for these fractures.

- *Zone 3 fractures* happen along the shaft of the fifth metatarsal. These are typically stress fractures in athletes. Lengthy healing times and risk of refracture may be reasons for surgical repair in these fractures.

Avulsion fracture of the 5th metatarsal styloid, also known as a pseudo-Jones fracture, is one of the more common foot avulsion injuries, and accounts for over 90% of fractures of the base of the 5th metatarsal.

Stress Fractures of Metatarsals (Fig. 47.6)

Stress fractures can be considered an overuse injury of a bone. Briethaupt (Briethaupt, 1855), a military physician, first reported this injury in 1855. He presented the first description of a metatarsal stress fracture when he noted swelling and pain in the feet of Prussian military recruits. A March stress fracture is a small break in a metatarsal bone of the foot that occurs without a major traumatic episode. They were called March fractures because they were first seen in military recruits because of excess marching. These fractures still occur in that group.

They occur over time when repetitive forces result in microscopic damage to the bone. The repetitive force that causes a stress fracture is not great enough to cause an acute fracture. The most common cause of stress fractures is a sudden increase in physical activity. This increase can be in the frequency of activity—

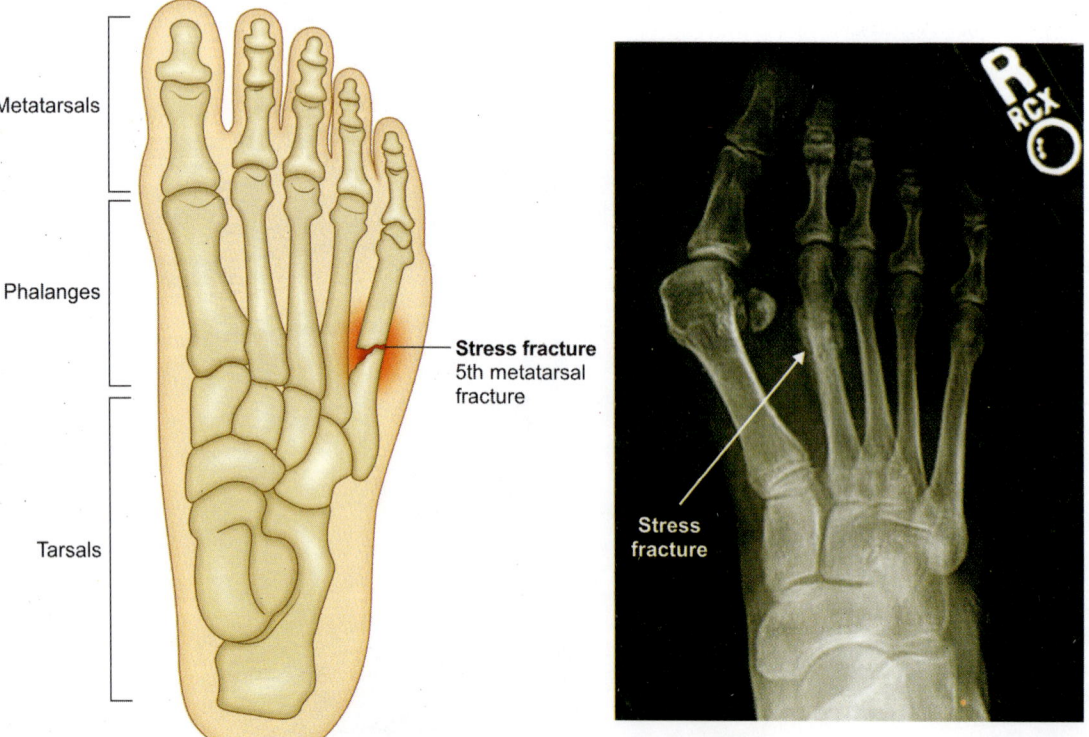

Fig. 47.6: Stress fracture

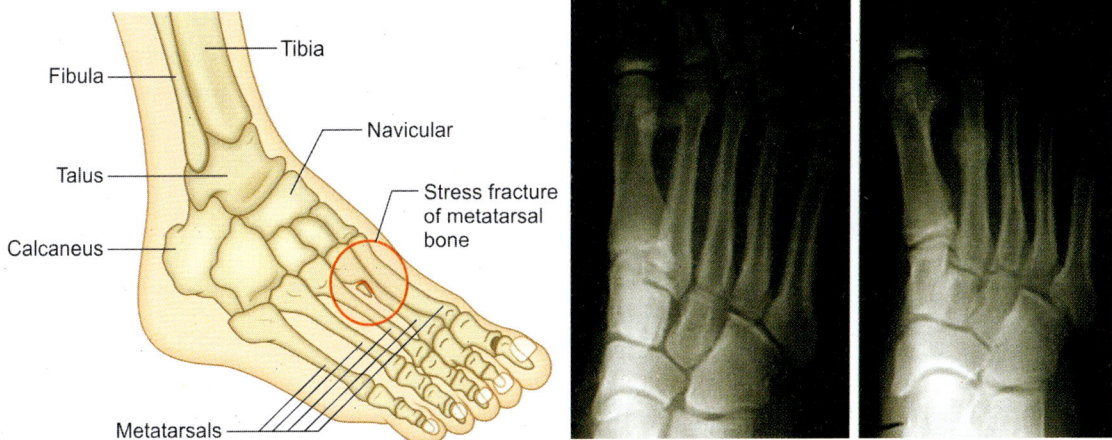

Fig. 47.7: Healing of stress fracture

such as exercising more days per week. It can also be in the duration or intensity of activity—such as running longer distances. Female athletes are about one-third more likely to develop stress fractures in the legs and feet.

Stress fractures typically result from one or more of the following:

- Hypermobile, pronated (flat) feet or high arched feet.
- Initiating a new activity too vigorously.
- An increase in training intensity.
- A change in activity surfaces.
- A return from a previous injury too quickly.
- An abrupt change of footwear.

In most cases, it takes from 6 to 8 weeks for a stress fracture to heal (Fig. 47.7).

Stress fractures of the second or third metatarsals rarely require surgical intervention. Most of these fractures heal uneventfully, and nonunion is rare. However, stress fractures of the fifth-metatarsal base are more problematic.

BIBLIOGRAPHY

- http://emedicine.medscape.com/article/85746-overview
- https://www.youtube.com/watch?v=_CItUTjO_jA
- https://www.youtube.com/watch?v=jWdP7JWhZbk

Lisfranc Injury of the Foot

The midfoot joint complex is also called the Lisfranc joint. It is named after French surgeon Jacques Lisfranc de St. Martin, who served in the Napoleonic army in the 1800s.

The Lisfranc joint complex has a specialized bony and ligamentous structure, providing stability to this joint.

It is an injury of the foot in which one or more of the metatarsal bones are displaced from the tarsus (Fig. 48.1).

The incidence of Lisfranc joint fracture: Dislocations in one case per 55,000 persons each year. Thus, these injuries account for less than 1% of all fractures. As many as 20% of Lisfranc joint injuries are missed on initial anteroposterior and oblique radiographs.

Injuries to the Lisfranc joint most commonly occur in automobile accident victims, military personnel, runners, horseback riders, football players and participants of other contact

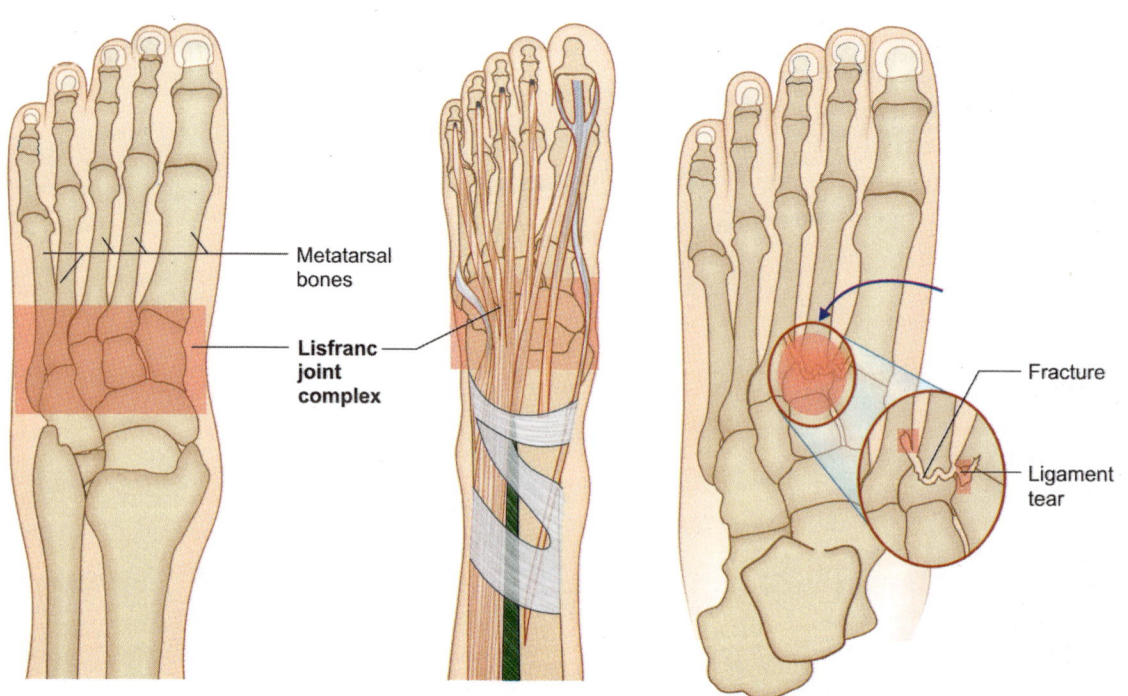

Fig. 48.1: Lisfranc injury

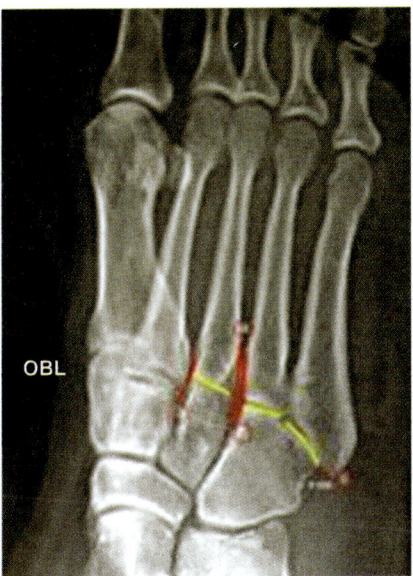

Fig. 48.2: Normal Lisfranc joint

means that the dorsal surface of the proximal second metatarsal is higher than the dorsal surface of the middle cuneiform.

CLASSIFICATION

1. *Homolateral* (Fig. 48.4): All five metatarsals are displaced in the same direction. Lateral

sports, or something as simple as missing a step on a staircase (Fig. 48.2).

Lisfranc joint injuries are rare, complex and often misdiagnosed. Typical signs and symptoms include pain, swelling and the inability to bear weight. Clinically, these injuries vary from mild sprains to fracture-dislocations (Fig. 48.3).

The initial radiographs of a suspected Lisfranc joint injury should include weight-bearing anteroposterior and lateral views, as well as a 30° oblique view.

On the radiographs, dislocation of the tarsometatarsal joint is indicated by the following: (1) Loss of in-line arrangement of the lateral margin of the first metatarsal base with the lateral edge of the medial (first) cuneiform; (2) loss of in-line arrangement of the medial margin of the second metatarsal base with the medial edge of the middle (second) cuneiform in the weight-bearing anteroposterior view and the presence of small avulsed fragments (fleck sign), which are further indications of ligamentous injury and probable joint disruption.

The lateral radiographic view of the foot may show a diagnostic "step-off," which

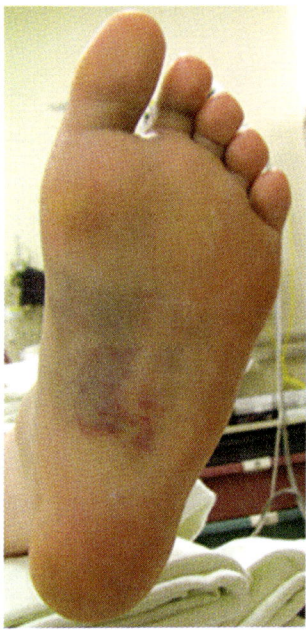

Fig. 48.3: The discoloration on the bottom of the foot is very suggestive of a Lisfranc injury

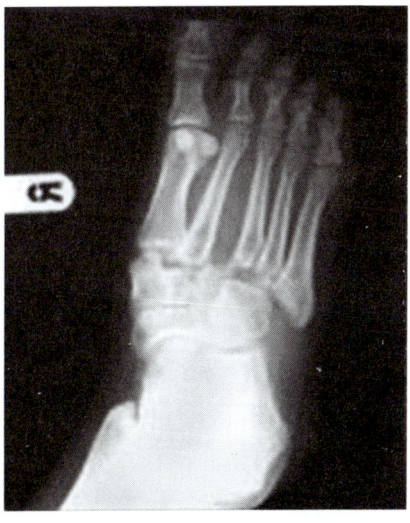

Fig. 48.4: Homolateral type

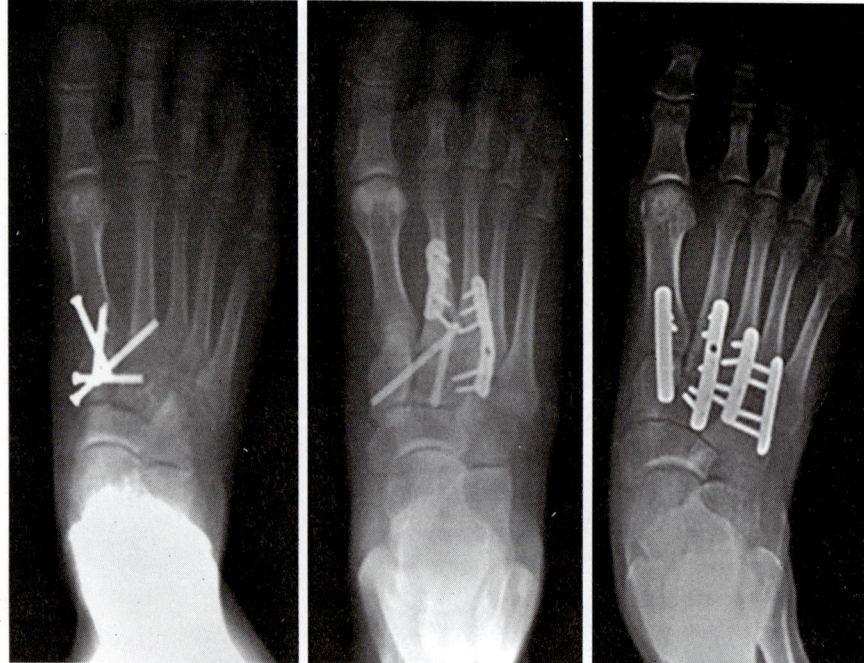

Fig. 48.5: Surgical treatment

displacement may also suggest cuboidal fracture.

2. *Isolated:* One or two metatarsals are displaced from the others.

3. *Divergent:* Metatarsals are displaced in a sagittal or coronal plane and may also involve the intercuneiform area and include a navicular fracture.

TREATMENT

Options include operative or non-operative treatment. If the dislocation is less than 2 mm, the fracture can be managed with casting for six weeks. For severe Lisfranc injuries, open reduction with internal fixation (ORIF) and temporary screw or Kirschner wire (K-wire) fixation is the treatment of choice.

If surgical repair is warranted, it should be done within the first 12 to 24 hours after the injury. Alternatively, surgery can be performed after seven to 10 days to allow the reduction of swelling (Fig. 48.5).

COMPLICATIONS

The three factors that appear to be most important in predicting the occurrence of complications with Lisfranc joint injuries are the extent of local trauma, a delay in injury recognition and the degree of displacement. Post-traumatic arthrosis is the most common complication of Lisfranc joint injury.

BIBLIOGRAPHY

- http://orthoinfo.aaos.org/topic.cfm?topic=A00162
- https://www.youtube.com/watch?v=WNifc7vHoq8
- https://www.youtube.com/watch?v=f26KukNYsWA

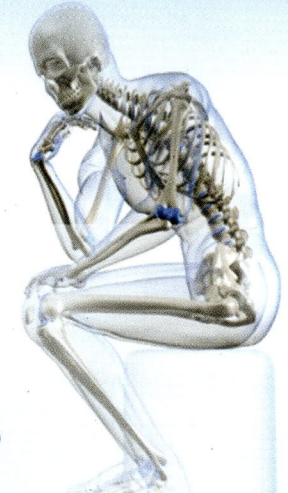

Peripheral Nerve Injuries

Acute peripheral nerve injuries are one of the complications of trauma affecting the extremities, and is present in 3–10% of patients, depending on the mechanism of trauma. Peripheral nerve injury or disease can cause symptoms of pain, dysesthesias, and either partial or complete loss of sensory and motor function. A thorough clinical history, physical examination, electrodiagnostic evaluation, and relevant radiographic studies should be performed to distinguish a peripheral nerve problem from one involving the spinal cord or brain, bone, or soft tissues (Fig. 49.1).

SIGNS AND SYMPTOMS OF A PERIPHERAL NERVE INJURY

They may include:
- Numbness
- Pain
- Burning or tingling sensation
- Muscle weakness
- Sensitivity to touch

CAUSES

Peripheral nerve injuries are caused mainly by trauma, either direct or indirect or repetitive movements that can damage the peripheral nerves. Other causes may include:
- Certain conditions (diabetes, carpal tunnel syndrome, ulnar entrapment at the elbow)
- Certain medications
- Injuries or tumors of the brachial plexus
- Exposure to toxins
- Fractures and dislocated bones
- Alcoholism

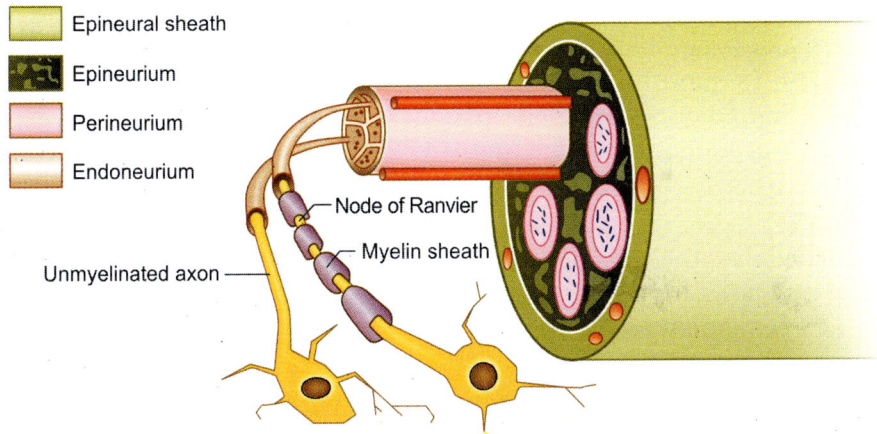

Fig. 49.1: Anatomy of peripheral nerve

Common etiologies of acute traumatic peripheral nerve injury (TPNI) include penetrating injury, crush, stretch, and ischemia.

PATHOPHYSIOLOGY

Regeneration Process after Transection

- Distal segment undergoes Wallerian degeneration (axoplasm and myelin are degraded distally by phagocytes).
- Existing Schwann cells proliferate and line up on basement membrane.
- Proximal budding (occurs after 1 month delay) leads to sprouting axons that migrate at 1 mm/day to connect to the distal tube.
- Under ideal conditions, axon regrowth from the proximal stump occurs at 1 mm/day. The time after which irreversible muscle atrophy has occurred and operation cannot provide benefit is 12–18 months. The Schwann cells and the endoneurial tubes remain viable for 18–24 months after injury. If they do not receive a regenerating axon within this span of time, the tubes degenerate. Reinnervation must occur not only before the muscle undergoes irreversible changes, but before the endoneurial tubes will no longer support nerve regrowth.
- The time distance equation has two primary variables: Irreversible changes in critical target structures (1958 WW Campbell/ Clinical Neurophysiology 119 (2008) 1951-1965) after 12–18 months, and axon regrowth at 1 mm/day from the site of injury or the site of surgical repair.

CLASSIFICATION

Classification of peripheral nerve injury assists in determining prognosis and management.

There are two commonly used classifications for peripheral nerve injury—Seddon's classification and the Sunderland's classification. Nerve injuries were classified into neuropraxia, axonotmesis and neurotmesis by Seddon et al. after his World War 2 experience of nerve injuries, in injured soldiers (Fig. 49.2). Sunderland expanded on this classification according to histological diagnosis.

Seddon classified nerve injuries into three major groups: Neuropraxia, axonotmesis, and neurotmesis whereas Sunderland expanded Seddon's classification to five degrees of peripheral nerve injury (Figs 49.3 and 49.4).

Neuropraxia

- Compression injury causing temporary disruption of nerve conduction.
- The whole nerve remains structurally intact.
- 8% elongation will diminish nerve's micro-circulation.
- 15% elongation will disrupt axons.
- Good prognosis with complete recovery of nerve function.

Axonotmesis

- The axon is damaged but the perineurium and epineurium remain intact.
- Leads to central chromatolysis
  - *Definition:* The reaction of a neuronal cell body in response to an axonal injury.
  - *Characteristics*
    - Swelling of the neuronal body
    - Dispersion of the Nissl bodies
    - Displacement of the nucleus to the periphery
  - *Function:* These changes reflect an increase in the protein synthesis in an effort to restore the integrity of the damaged axon.
- Results in Wallerian degeneration
  - *Definition:* An active neuronal degeneration process in response to axonal injury.
  - *Characteristics*
    - Initially retained electrical excitability of axon distal to the injury, lasting up to 36 hours
    - Progressive degeneration of distal segment cytoskeleton with dissolution of axonal membrane.

Grades of Nerve Injury (Seddon 1942)

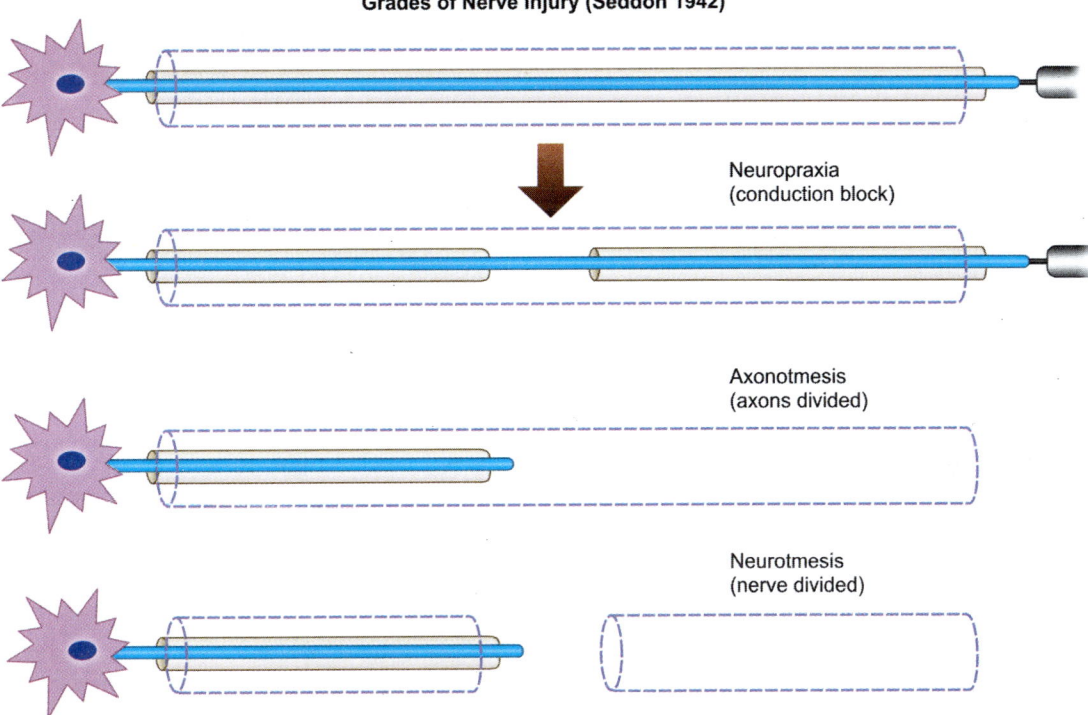

Neuropraxia
(conduction block)

Axonotmesis
(axons divided)

Neurotmesis
(nerve divided)

Fig. 49.2: Seddon's classification

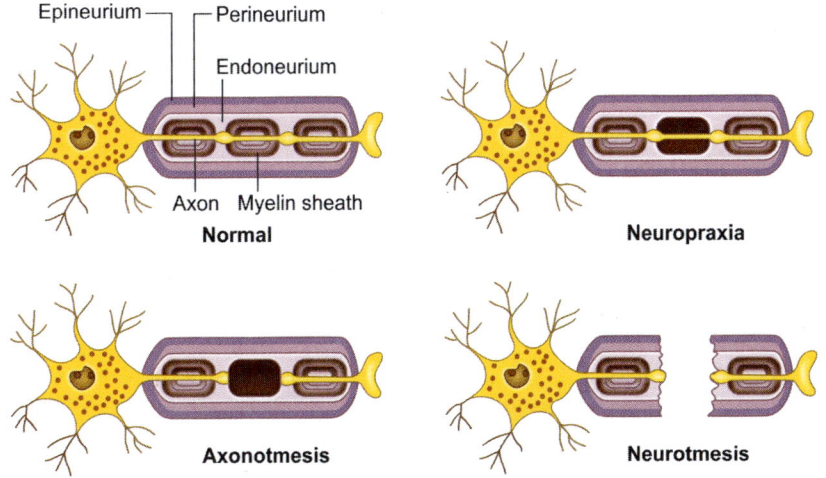

Fig. 49.3: Types of nerve injury

- Degradation of residual myelin sheath by macrophages and Schwann cells.
- Proximal stump either stays in place or retracts slightly; ultimately, the stump will sprout regenerative

nervous fibers that aim to reinnervate the distal tissues.
- Efficiency in the peripheral nervous system is significantly higher than in the central nervous system.

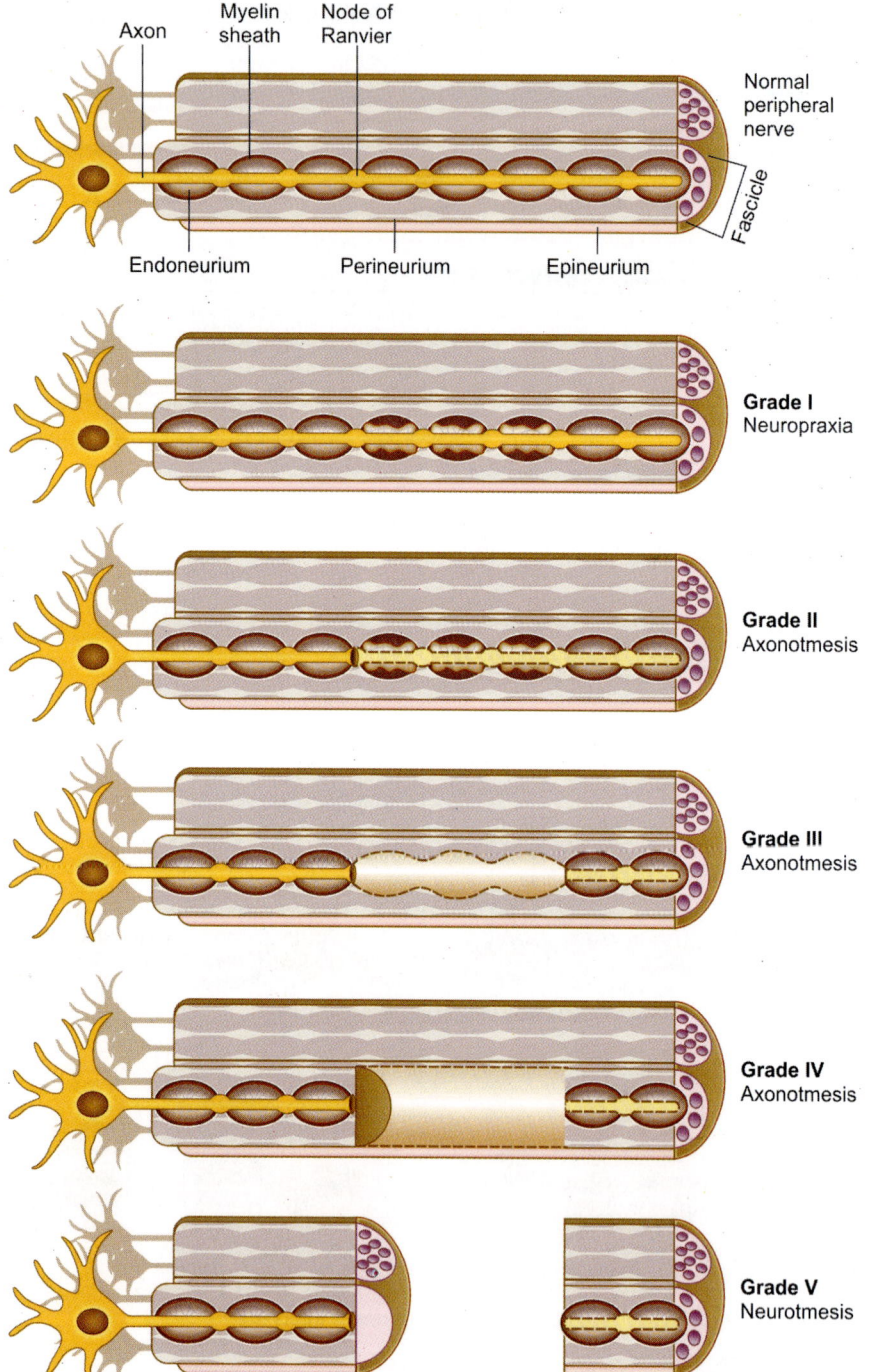

Fig. 49.4: Sunderland's classification

- *Functions:*
  - To clear axonal debris and prevent scarring.
  - Facilitate targeted reinnervation of tissues previously innervated by that axon before injury.
- Good chance of at least partial recovery

Neurotmesis

- Complete nerve transection
- Connective sheath damage
- Chances of recovery very poor without surgical repair

TRAUMATIC NEUROMA

Benign, painful nodular thickening caused by nerve regeneration at the site of different forms of nerve injury.

The diagnosis of peripheral nerve injuries is based on a thorough clinical history, neurological examination, and, in some cases, diagnostic tests (e.g. X-ray, if fracture is suspected).

Imaging

- *Plain X-rays:* Detection of compression or transection occurring due to dislocated bone or fracture segments.
- *CT/MRI:* Evaluation of causes like nerve tumors, avulsions, and focal soft tissue pathologies.

Electrodiagnostic studies

- Nerve conduction study/neurography
- Needle electromyography (EMG)

In neuropraxia, the compound muscle action potential (CMAP) and nerve action potential (NAP) elicited on stimulation distal to the lesion are maintained indefinitely. Stimulation proximal to the lesion reveals partial or complete conduction block, with varying degrees of loss of CMAP amplitude, change in CMAP configuration and slowing of conduction velocity, depending on the attributes of a particular lesion. These abnormalities should improve or disappear when remyelination is complete, provided there is no persistent pressure on the nerve. Some conduction slowing may persist permanently because remyelination characteristically leaves shorter, thinner internodes than were present originally, but this does not interfere with function. Late responses (F-waves and H-waves) are occasionally useful with extremely proximal lesions where it is not possible to directly stimulate proximal to the lesion, otherwise they are seldom of significant help. In a complete neural lesion, needle EMG will show no MUAPs under voluntary control, but fibrillations are not present.

The electrodiagnostic picture in axonotmesis and neurotmesis depends on the time that has passed between the injury and the evaluation. The CMAP and NAP distal to the injury decrease in amplitude in rough proportion to the degree of axon loss. This loss of amplitude is complete by day 9 for CMAPs and day 11 for NAPs. The earlier loss of the CMAP is related to changes in the neuromuscular junction. With any degree of injury, a study carried out in the first few days may show no conduction abnormality except for inability to conduct an impulse across the lesion on proximal stimulation.

CONSERVATIVE TREATMENT

- Observation and expectant management in closed injuries of the nerve with a high rate of spontaneous recovery.
- Activity modification (e.g. avoid sports or activities that increase likelihood of further nerve injury)
- *Splinting:* Prevents stiffness and contractures of joints, supports residual nerve functionality and reinnervation.
- *Electrical stimulation:* Supports the regeneration of the proximal axons and reinnervation of the denervated muscles after surgical nerve repair.
- *Drug therapy:* Treatment of chronic neuropathic pain following peripheral nerve

injury (e.g. gabapentin); in combination with surgical treatment to enhance remyelination and motor regeneration (e.g. lithium).

- *Analgesia:* Infiltration with local anesthetics.

SURGICAL REPAIR

Indications

- Open, non-contaminated, sharp injuries; concomitant vascular injuries → immediate surgical exploration and repair
- Open, contaminated injuries; postreduction palsy → early surgical exploration and repair (within 3 weeks)
- Patients without clinical or electromyographic signs of spontaneous recovery → delayed surgical exploration and repair (within 3 months)

Intraoperative eletrophysiologic evaluation has been accepted as an important tool in the management of lesions in continuity.

The "Rule of Three"

In summary, surgical timing in a traumatic peripheral nerve injury is defined by the "rule of three": Immediate surgery within 3 days for clean and sharp injuries; early surgery within 3 weeks for blunt/contusion injuries; and delayed surgery, performed 3 months after injury, for closed injuries.

Procedures

- *Nerve repair (neurorrhaphy):* Reconstruction of nerve continuity (Fig. 49.5)
- *Tendon transfer:* A tendon from a sufficiently powerful muscle is redirected towards another tendon in order to restore its motion and function.
- *Nerve transfer:* An intact healthy nerve is redirected towards a denervated nerve in order to restore the innervation of its target organ.

Primary repair is the optimal approach for peripheral nerve injuries taking place within

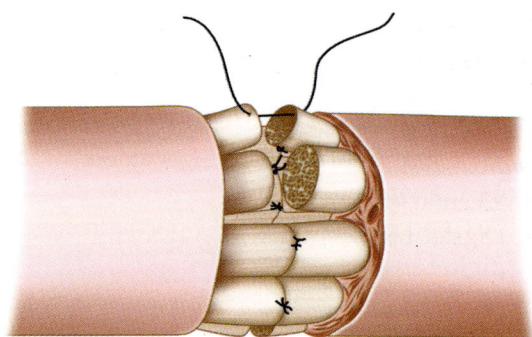

Fig. 49.5: Nerve repair

the first couple of days. Secondary repair takes place one week or more after the injury . Partial injuries (15% of injuries) as a consequence of stretch or contusions are commonly managed with secondary repair. For complete injuries, the method of repair depends on what is found during exploration. If the epineurium is found to be neatly divided, then primary repair without tension is usually undertaken, but if the ends are ragged, then a graft may be required.

Postoperatively nerve repairs should be protected by immobilization for 10–14 days and sometimes surgeons advocate up to 6 weeks depending on the nerve injury severity and cause. After this period, full passive and active range of motion is initiated for rehabilitation. Postoperatively, axons may take time to learn how to process new information especially following sensory nerves. Age is the most vital factor to determine the outcome of nerve repair and can account for 50% of the variance in success.

Nerve Grafting

In severe nerve injuries, the defect between the two nerve ends may be too large or cause inappropriate tension for end-to-end repair; then a bridge is indicated, by using a nerve graft. Typically donor grafts are autologous sensory nerves including the medial or lateral antebrachial cutaneous nerves, dorsal cutaneous nerve branch of the ulnar nerve, lateral femoral cutaneous nerve and superficial sensory branch of the radial nerve.

Autologous Graft

Indications
- ≥3 cm gap
- Digital nerve defects at wrist to common digital nerve bifurcation—use sural nerve
- At MCP to DIP level—use lateral antebrachial cutaneous nerve
- At DIP level—use AIN, PIN or medial antebrachial cutaneous nerve

Outcomes: Gold standard for segmental defects >5 cm

Collagen Conduit

- Tensioned closures inhibit Schwann cell activation and axon regeneration, compromise perfusion and lead to scarring
- Collagen conduits allow nutrient exchange and accessibility to neurotrophic factors to the axonal growth zone during regeneration

Indications: Defects ≤2 cm

Outcomes
- Equal results to autologous grafting when gap ≤5 mm
- Quality of nerve recovery drops with gaps >5 mm

Allograft

Off-the-shelf option for defects up to 5 cm.

PROGNOSIS
- Factors affecting success of recovery following repair are:
  - Age is single most important factor influencing success of nerve recovery.
  - Level of injury is second most important (the more distal the injury the better the chance of recovery).
  - Sharp transections have better prognosis than crush injuries.
  - Repair delay worsen prognosis of recovery (time limit for repair is 18 months).

Return of function: Pain is first modality to return.

BIBLIOGRAPHY
- https://www.ncbi.nlm.nih.gov/pmc/articles/PMC4408553
- https://en.wikipedia.org/wiki/Nerve_injury
- https://www.amboss.com/us/knowledge/Peripheral_nerve_injuries
- https://digitalcommons.unl.edu/cgi/viewcontent.cgi?article=1002&context=usuhs

Brachial Plexus Injuries

INTRODUCTION

The brachial plexus (Fig. 50.1) is a network of intertwined nerves that control movement and sensation in the arm and hand. A traumatic brachial plexus injury involves sudden damage to these nerves, and may cause weakness, loss of feeling, or loss of movement in the shoulder, arm, or hand. The brachial plexus has five anatomic sections, and injuries to the brachial plexus can occur in one or more of these areas (Fig. 50.2).

- Spinal nerves
- Trunks
- Divisions
- Cords
- Branches

A brachial plexus injury is found to occur in 1.5 of every 1,000 live births. Brachial plexus injuries can occur as a result of shoulder trauma, tumors, or inflammation.

ETIOLOGY

A list of common etiologies is given below.
- Vehicular accident (majority two wheelers) accounts for >90% of cases
- Industrial trauma-weight falling on shoulder from a height, being dragged inside a machine by the arm
- Heavy fall with stretching of neck
- Assault with a sharp object
- Bullet injury—rare in India

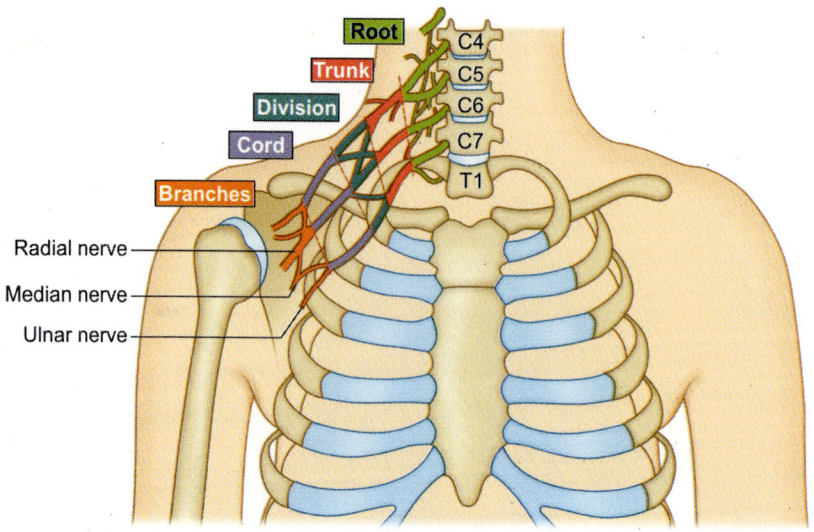

Fig. 50.1: Brachial plexus

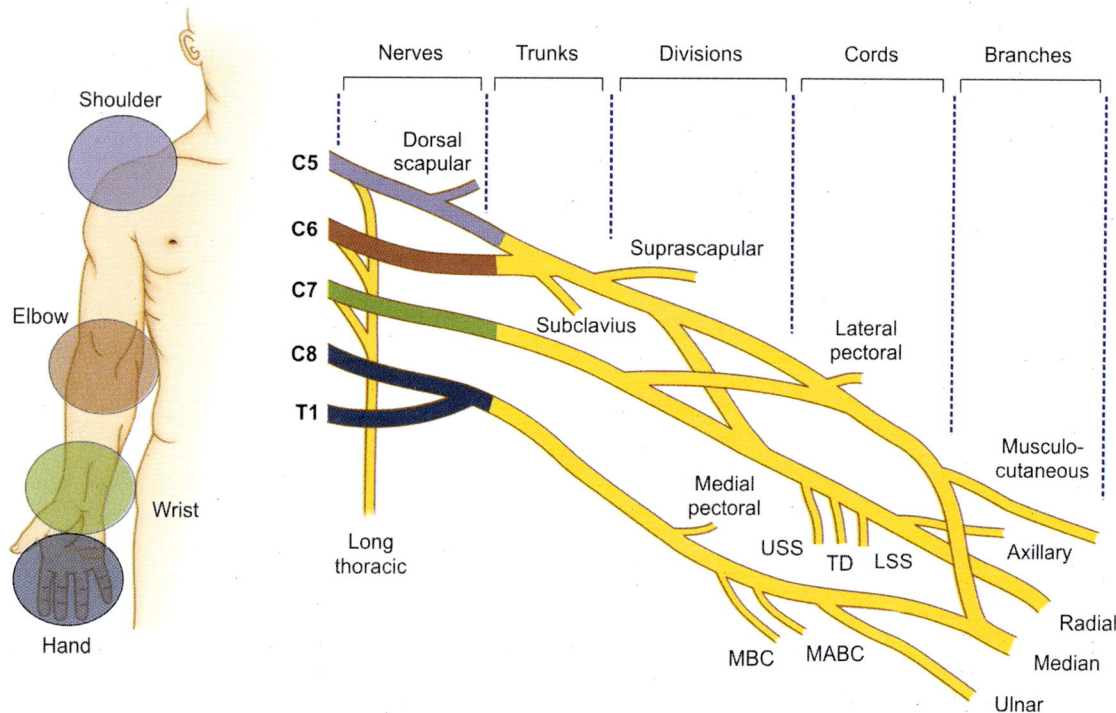

Fig. 50.2: Anatomy of brachial plexus

- Iatrogenic injury, either deliberate as in tumor surgery involving nerve roots or accidental while operating in the posterior triangle of the neck.

CLASSIFICATION

Brachial plexus injuries can be classified in various ways:

- As per site:
  a. Root
  b. Cord
  c. Trunk, or
  d. Nerve level injury
  e. Often a mixture of all
- Which roots:
  a. Upper plexus, i.e. C5, C6+/-C7 or
  b. Lower plexus C8, T1
  c. Global C5, C6, C7, C8, T1
- Relation to clavicle:
  a. Supraclavicular
  b. Retroclavicular
  c. Infraclavicular.

Brachial plexus injuries vary greatly in severity, depending upon the type of injury and the amount of force placed on the plexus. The same patient can injure several different nerves of the brachial plexus in varying severity.

- *Avulsion:* In this most severe brachial plexus injury, the nerve root has been torn from the spinal cord. These types of injuries may not be repairable with surgery.
- *Stretch (neuropraxia):* When the nerve is mildly stretched, it may heal on its own or require simple, nonsurgical treatment methods to return to normal function.
- *Rupture:* A more forceful stretch of the nerve may cause it to tear partially or fully. These types of injuries can sometimes be repaired with surgery.

UPPER TRUNK PALSY INJURY (Fig. 50.3)

- Upper trunk palsy occurs when the angle between the shoulder and the neck forcibly

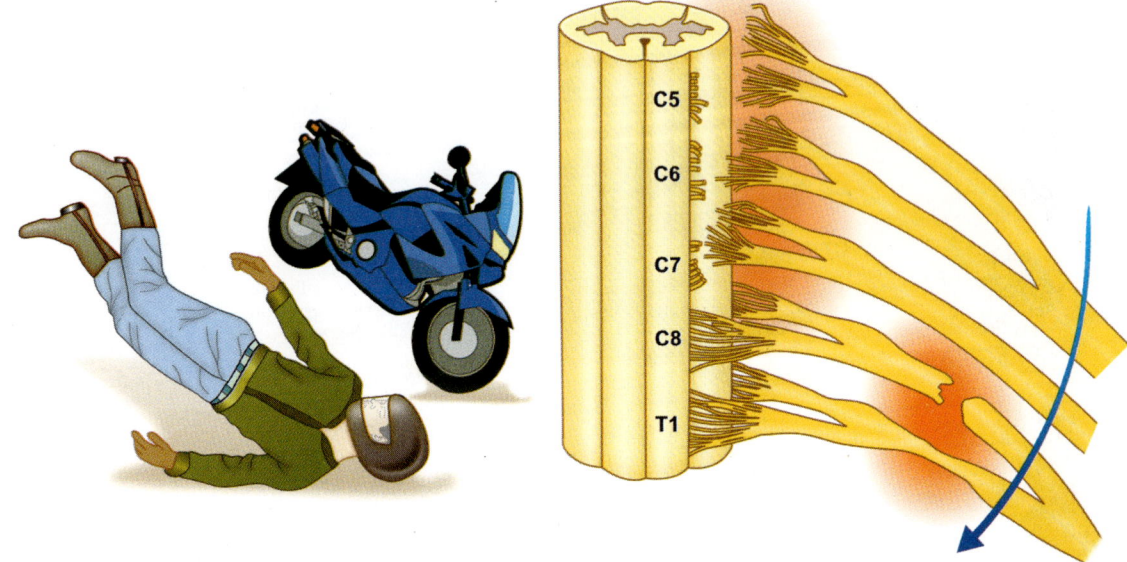

Fig. 50.3: Upper trunk injury

widens, such as when a fall forces the shoulder down and the head to the opposite side.

- Patients with upper trunk palsies are unable to use the shoulder to raise the arm away from the body, have weakness in the arm, and may be unable to bend the arm at the elbow. There may be loss of sensation in the shoulder, outside of the arm, and the thumb.
- A severe upper trunk injury may paralyze the shoulder muscles (deltoid muscle and rotator cuff), as well as the muscle in the upper arm (biceps.)

LOWER TRUNK PALSY INJURY (Fig. 50.4)

Lower trunk palsy occurs when the angle between the arm and the chest wall forcibly widens. This may damage the lower nerves and the lower trunks.

Patients with a lower trunk palsy will typically maintain shoulder and elbow strength, but will lose hand function. Over time, this will cause the fingers to contract into a claw position, and the patient will not be able to perform fine motor tasks. Patients also typically have hand numbness in at least the ring and small fingers.

TOTAL PLEXUS PALSY INJURY

Total plexus palsy may occur, if the force of the injury is extreme. In this palsy, all levels of the nerves and trunk are damaged. This results in complete paralysis of the arm and hand, which is often referred to as "flail limb".

Other mechanisms include gunshot and penetrating injuries and rare association with fractures of clavicle and injuries around shoulder or axillary region (Tables 50.1 and 50.2).

ELECTRODIAGNOSTIC STUDIES

The following things can be determined by electrodiagnostic studies:

- Type of lesion, i.e. pre- or post-ganglionic
- Localization of lesion to roots, trunks, cords and nerves
- Extent of the lesion
- Status of individual muscles—denervated, reinnervating, etc.
- Sequential study can point to recovery and help postoperative monitoring of results.

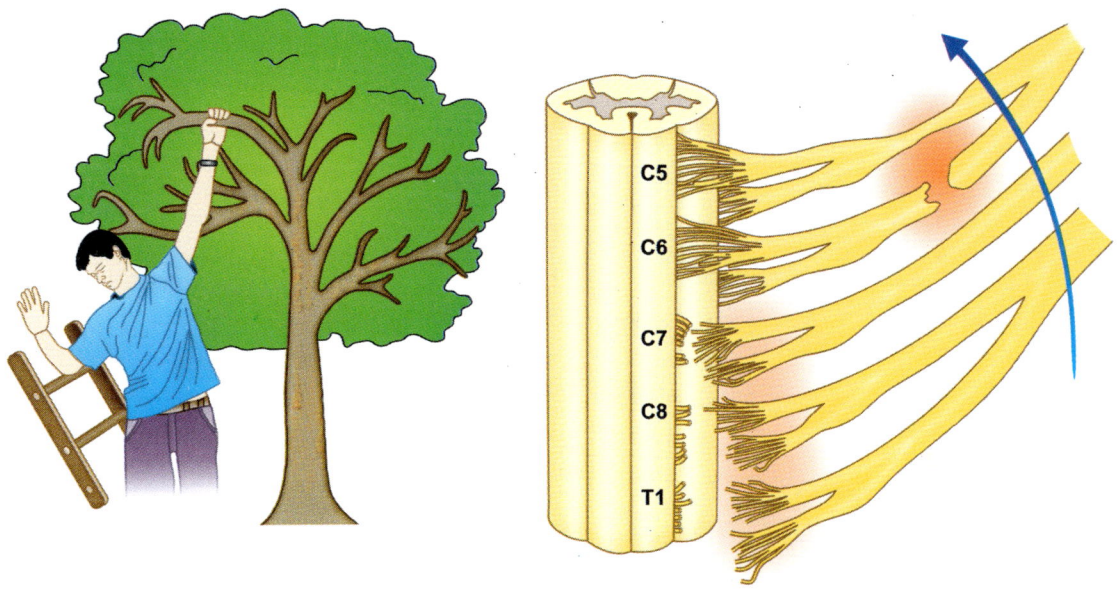

Fig. 50.4: Lower trunk injury

Table 50.1: Summary of root-wise motor function

Root value	Gross functions involved
C5, C6	Shoulder abduction and elbow flexion
C7	Triceps ± wrist extensor
C8, T1	Hand function
C5 to T1	Flail upper limb

Table 50.2: Summary of sensory innervation

Root value	Gross functions involved
C5	Skin over the deltoid
C6	Thumb and index finger
C7	Middle finger
C8	Ulnar two fingers but particularly little finger
T1	Medial forearm
T2	Inner arm

- Compound motor action potential (CMAP) of important nerves like the ulnar and median which are potential donor nerves in upper plexus injuries.

SURGICAL PROCEDURES (Fig. 50.5)

Any brachial plexus injury which has not shown substantial spontaneous recovery in 3 months deserves to be explored. Timing is crucial due to the eventual loss of neuromuscular end plates at 20 to 24 months after denervation. If there is global palsy with MRI proven pseudomeningoceles showing pre ganglionic avulsion type of injury, then no delay is justified.

Neurolysis

Removal of the constrictive scar tissue surrounding the nerve.

Neuroma Excision

When the neuroma is large it must be removed and the nerve is then reattached either with end-to-end techniques or with nerve grafts.

Nerve Grafting

When the gap between the nerve ends is so large that it is not possible to have a tension-free repair using the end-to-end technique, nerve grafting is used.

Neurotization

This is used generally in those cases where there is an avulsion. Donor nerves are used

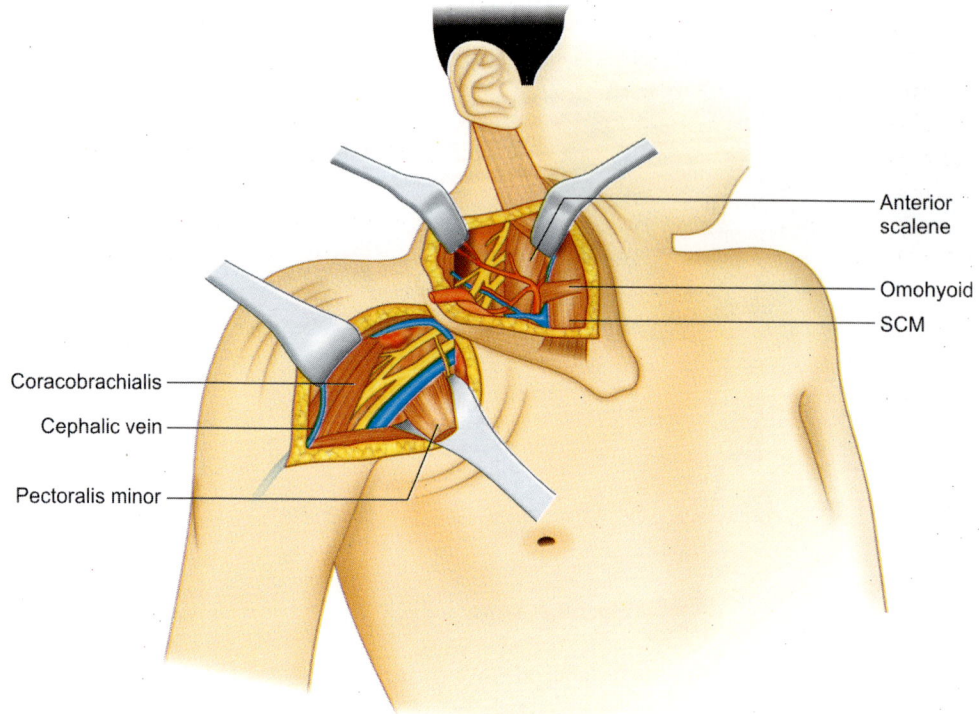

Fig. 50.5: Surgical exposure

for the repair. The parts of the roots still attached to the spinal cord can be used as donors for avulsed nerves.

Isolated Nerve Transfers

- Isolated transfer may be completed up to 12–18 months of age
- A nearby healthy nerve is attached to the damaged nerve, closer to the target muscle.

Additional procedures are available to improve the overall function of the affected limb.

Procedures include:
- Arthroscopic surgery and other minimally invasive techniques
- Tendon transfers
- Muscle transfers
- Shoulder reconstruction
- Rotational osteotomies
- Elbow reconstruction
- Botox injections

Nonsurgical management is also an important part of the treatment process.

Occupational and/or physical therapy is often recommended including range of motion, strengthening, neuromuscular electrical simulation, Kinesio taping, joint mobilization, aquatic therapy and use of orthoses.

NATURAL HISTORY AND PROGNOSIS

A mixed or incomplete recovery may occur, if the nerves do not fully reattach at their original motor and sensory targets.

Full recovery will occur, only if sensory fibers reach their sensory end targets and motor fibers reach their muscle targets.

The ability to bend the elbow (biceps function) by the third month of life is an indicator of probable recovery. In addition to bicep function, active movement of the wrist in upward motion as well as thumb and fingers straightening is an even stronger indicator of excellent spontaneous improvement.

About two-thirds of children with brachial plexus palsy get better on their own with minimal treatment.

The timeframe of surgical repair is an important factor in recovery. Within 18 months, the muscles that have not already connected to nerves may have weakened to the point where it is no longer possible.

Age impacts results of surgery. Young patients at or around 20 years show rapid recovery with higher gain of strength. People over 40 are thought to show reduced results; however, they still show adequately good results to justify surgery at any age unless medical factors make the person unfit for reconstruction.

Horner's sign indicates a very proximal (usually pre-ganglionic) type of lesion and signals the need for aggressive early management of the plexus injury with multi-staged reconstruction including FFMT amongst other things.

For avulsion and rupture injuries, there is no potential for full recovery unless surgical repair is done in a timely manner. For neuroma and neuropraxia injuries, the potential for improvement varies. Most patients with neuropraxia injuries have a fair prognosis of recovering spontaneously with a 90–100% return of function. If surgery is needed, microsurgical nerve repair may be undertaken as early as 3 months. Primary nerve repair is typically completed by approximately 6 months of age.

BIBLIOGRAPHY

- https://www.mayoclinic.org/diseases
- https://www.orthobullets.com/trauma/1008/brachial-plexus-injuries
- https://www.cincinnatichildrens.org/health/b/brachial-plexus
- https://www.youtube.com/watch?v=JfsjQwCL0xU
- https://www.youtube.com/watch?v=Mh4Neyyzc5c

Axillary Nerve Injury

The axillary nerve innervates all the portions of the deltoid muscle and teres minor muscle. It also provides a sensory branch named the upper lateral cutaneous nerve of the arm that innervates the skin over the lateral aspect of the shoulder.

The axillary nerve originates from the posterior cord of the brachial plexus and contains fibers that originate from C5 and C6 nerve roots that travel via the upper trunk of the brachial plexus and then into the posterior cord. It passes through the quadrilateral space around the posterior and lateral surface of the proximal humerus (Figs 51.1 and 51.2).

The axillary nerve terminates into anterior and posterior muscular branches, both of which innervate the deltoid muscle. The upper lateral cutaneous nerve of the arm arises from the posterior branch.

- *Spinal roots:* C5 and C6.
- *Sensory functions* (Fig. 51.3): Gives rise to upper lateral cutaneous nerve of arm, which innervates the skin over the lower deltoid (regimental badge area).
- *Motor functions:* Innervates the teres minor and deltoid muscles.

In 65% of cases, the axillary nerve splits into anterior and posterior branches within the quadrangular space, and in the remaining 35%

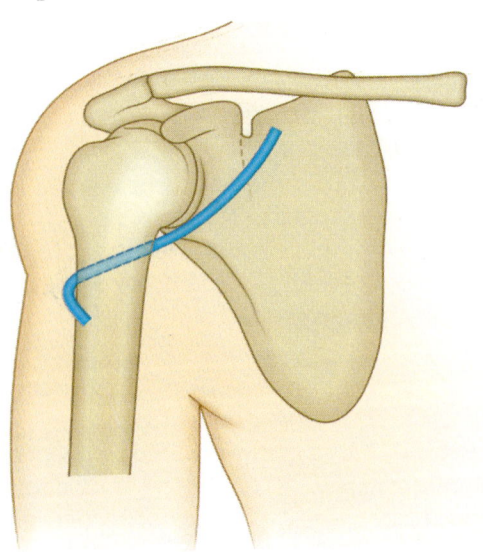

Fig. 51.1: Anatomy of axillary nerve

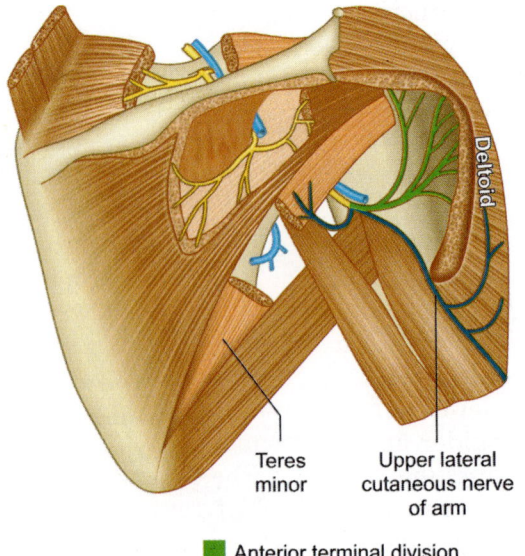

Teres minor

Upper lateral cutaneous nerve of arm

■ Anterior terminal division

■ Posterior terminal division

Fig. 51.2: Axillary nerve

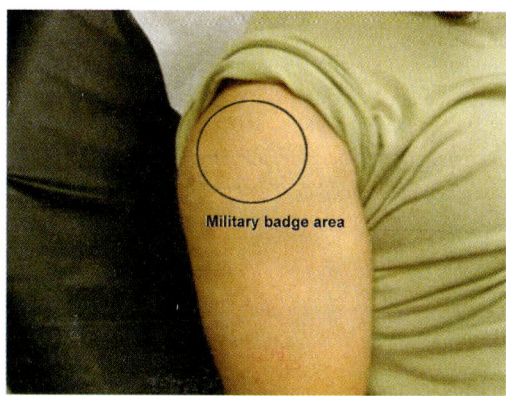

Fig. 51.3: Sensory supply of axillary nerve

splits within the deltoid muscle. The anterior branch ascends around the surgical neck of humerus with the posterior circumflex humeral artery and its branches distributed anteriorly to the deltoid muscle. In 100% of cases, the posterior branch innervates the teres minor muscle and gives off a branch for the superior lateral brachial cutaneous nerve. The anterior branch innervates the joint capsule and the anterior and middle parts of deltoid.

The axillary nerve is one of the most common peripheral nerves injured in athletes who participate in contact sports. It can occur from glenohumeral dislocation, proximal humerus fracture or from a direct blow to the anterolateral deltoid muscle. Compression neuropathy has been reported to occur in quadrilateral space syndrome.

The clinical history is important in evaluating patients with suspected axillary nerve palsy. History of distinct trauma to the shoulder, either blunt trauma, traction injury or penetrating trauma should raise suspicion for an axillary nerve injury. Classically, patients will present with trauma to the shoulder and they will report inability to abduct the shoulder. The patient will also report pain in the shoulder due to the original injury. Loss of deltoid muscle bulk and inability to abduct the shoulder is observed in axillary nerve injuries. Some associated sensory loss over the lateral aspect of the deltoid area can be also present but the sensation may be spared despite significant weakness.

The diagnostic workup includes electro-diagnostic studies, X-rays and MRI of the shoulder. Clinically suspected axillary nerve injuries should be confirmed by electrophysiological testing, including nerve conduction studies and needle electromyography. The nerve conduction study is performed with recording of the compound muscle action potential (CMAP) from the deltoid muscle using surface electrodes. The stimulation is at the Erb's point. The contralateral side should be also tested with the nerve conduction study for comparison. The needle electromyography of the deltoid muscle will help to evaluate for any preserved motor units, will help to determine the timing of the injury and will also help to determine early reinnervation process, which may not be obvious on the clinical exam.

Many axillary nerve injures are mild and can be subclinical. Most injuries are due to closed trauma and they are probably due to neuropraxia or axonotmesis. Both of these types of injures have good overall prognosis for spontaneous recovery of deltoid muscle function. Most patients with axillary nerve injury will have an excellent response to non-operative treatment. Physical therapy should be initiated including passive and active range of motion. The physical therapy will help to preserve the maximum range of motion and will help to prevent joint contracture. Excellent functional recovery of the shoulder can be seen even in cases in which only partial reinnervation of the deltoid muscle occurs after significant axillary nerve injury.

The indication for operative treatment of axillary neuropathy due to trauma will be determined based on the evidence of recovery and nature of the injury. If there is no clinical or electrodiagnostic evidence of recovery by 3 months after the injury, it is a reasonable time-frame to consider operative treatment.

However, if the cause of the axillary nerve injury is penetrating trauma or other trauma that is highly suspicious for neurotmesis, operative exploration should be performed much sooner.

The results of operative repair are best, if surgery is performed within 3 to 6 months from the injury. Surgical options include neurolysis, nerve grafting, and neurotization.

The results of repair of axillary nerve injuries have been good compared with treatment of other peripheral nerve lesions, due to the monofascicular composition of the nerve and the relatively short distance between the zone of injury and the motor end-plate.

Traditionally, nerve autografts have been used to reconstruct peripheral nerve defects not amenable to primary repair. Autograft alternatives include allografts and artificial nerve conduits. The cadaveric nerve allograft provides an unlimited graft source without the comorbidities associated with autograft reconstruction while retaining the elements that promote cell migration into the graft.

BIBLIOGRAPHY

- https://www.cancertherapyadvisor.com
- https://www.youtube.com/watch?v=meUFZb8Lw5M
- https://teachmeanatomy.info/upper-limb/nerves/axillary-nerve/
- https://uoftorthopaedics.ca/.../3.2-Hand-UE_Unit-5_Axillary-Nerve-Injury-Diagnosis-

Ulnar Nerve Injury

Ulnar nerve lacerations have been identified as the most common major upper extremity peripheral nerve injury when compared with the median, radial, and brachial plexus nerves. They can occur directly from a penetrating injury or secondary to a forearm fracture, and most are seen either at or distal to the elbow. The complete transection of the ulnar nerve remains a challenging problem for hand surgeons and their patients, and outcomes are typically worse than those seen after other peripheral nerve lacerations. Despite advances in microsurgical nerve repair, repairs often leave patients with functional deficits, especially in adults.

The ulnar nerve is an extension of the medial cord of the brachial plexus. It is a mixed nerve that supplies innervation to muscles in the forearm and hand and provides sensation over the medial half of the fourth digit and the entire fifth digit (the ulnar aspect of the palm) and the ulnar portion of the posterior aspect of the hand (dorsal ulnar cutaneous distribution) (Fig. 52.1).

The ulnar nerve and its branches innervate the following muscles in the forearm and hand:

- An articular branch that passes to the elbow joint while the ulnar nerve is passing between the olecranon and medial epicondyle of the humerus
- In the forearm, via the muscular branches of ulnar nerve:
  - Flexor carpi ulnaris

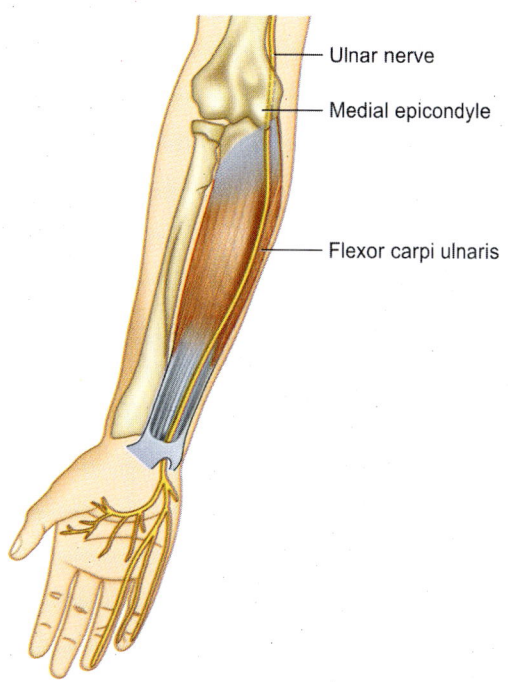

Fig. 52.1: Anatomy of ulnar nerve

  - Flexor digitorum profundus (medial half)
- In the hand, via the deep branch of ulnar nerve:
  - Hypothenar muscles
    - Opponens digiti minimi
    - Abductor digiti minimi
    - Flexor digiti minimi brevis
  - The third and fourth lumbrical muscles
  - Dorsal interossei
  - Palmar interossei

- Adductor pollicis
- Flexor pollicis brevis (deep head)
- In the hand, via the superficial branch of ulnar nerve:
  - Palmaris brevis

The ulnar nerve also provides sensory innervation to the fifth digit and the medial half of the fourth digit, and the corresponding part of the palm:

- Palmar branch of ulnar nerve—supplies cutaneous innervation to the anterior skin and nails.
- Dorsal cutaneous branch of ulnar nerve—supplies cutaneous innervation to the dorsal medial hand and the dorsum of the medial 1½ fingers.

CAUSES OF ULNAR NERVE INJURY

- Traction injuries
- There may be progressive compression because of inflammation and adhesions due to repetitive strain.
- Direct trauma.
- Bony growths in the ulnar groove.
- Individuals involved in contact sports such as football, soccer or rugby suffer more from this injury.

The ulnar nerve in children is not commonly injured. The most common causes of trauma to the ulnar nerve in children involve fractures around the elbow and their treatment, namely, supracondylar humerus and medial epicondylar fractures.

NEURO EXAMINATION

Weakness

- Wrist flexion
- Flexion of the little finger
- Abduction of the index and little fingers
- Adduction of the thumb

Diminished Sensation (Fig. 52.2)

- Palmar surface of the medial 1½ fingers
- Dorsal surface of the medial 1½ fingers

CLINICAL EXAMINATION

Compression at the Elbow

- Paraesthesia within the distribution of the ulnar nerve:
  - 4th and 5th digit
  - Hypothenar eminence
- Paresis of the following muscle groups:
  - Flexor carpi ulnaris

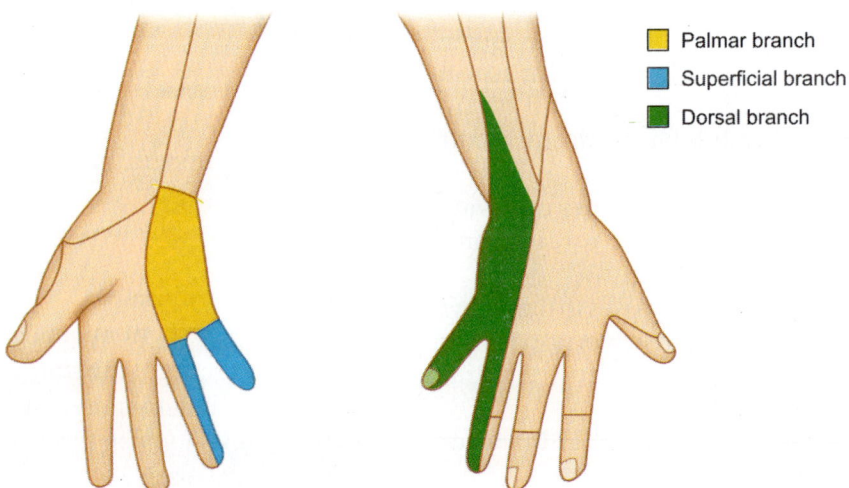

Palmar branch
Superficial branch
Dorsal branch

Fig. 52.2: Sensory supply of hand by ulnar nerve

– Flexor digitorum profundus
– Small intrinsic muscles of the hand

Compression at the Wrist Proximal to the Flexor Retinaculum

• Paraesthesia within the distribution of the ulnar nerve:
 – 4th and 5th digit
 – Hypothenar eminence
• Paresis of small intrinsic muscles of the hand

Compression at the Wrist Distal to the Flexor Retinaculum

• Motor features only: Paresis of small intrinsic muscles of the hand
• No sensory symptoms

Proximal as well as distal lesions lead to claw hand deformity.

Ulnar claw (Fig. 52.3) consists of hyper-extension of the metacarpophalangeal joints (due to the lack of innervation to the medial two lumbricals) and flexion of the inter-phalangeal joints of 4th and 5th finger. This depends on the location of the injury, as higher injuries may de-innervate the ulnar part of flexor digitorum profundus, so the flexed appearance may not be apparent.

The Ulnar Paradox

Usually, the more proximal a nerve injury, the worse it is. The opposite is true when we consider the ulnar nerve. This is because one of the muscles that flexes the fingers (flexor digitorum profundus, which lies in the forearm) is partially innervated by it. Hence, a proximal injury will remove innervation to the forearm muscles and the hand muscles.

A distal injury only takes out the hand muscles; hence the still functioning finger flexors give the patient a clawed appearance in the ring and little finger. With a proximal injury leading to an open palm, there is more capacity for hand function.

• *EMG:* Main confirmatory diagnostic test; it identifies the level of nerve compression.
• *Ultrasound and MRI:* Used to support the EMG findings and to detect possible causes of compression (e.g. space-occupying lesions).

TREATMENT OPTIONS

Treatment Goals

• Identify the presence of a complete ulnar nerve laceration, a partial ulnar nerve laceration, or a ulnar nerve neuropraxia.
• Repair the complete or partial nerve laceration.
• Carefully follow the patient with a ulnar nerve stretch injury; a few patients with neuropraxia will require neurolysis.
• Improve function of injured upper extremity with an ulnar nerve laceration.

Conservative

• Nonoperative treatment of ulnar nerve complete or partial lacerations is appropriate when the patient's associated injuries or medical comorbidities prevent anesthesia and a lengthy microsurgical repair.
• Isolated ulnar nerve complete and partial lacerations should be repaired early, but repair is not an emergency.
• Irrigation, debridement, and closure of the skin laceration with a scheduled operative nerve repair 1–3 weeks is reasonable.

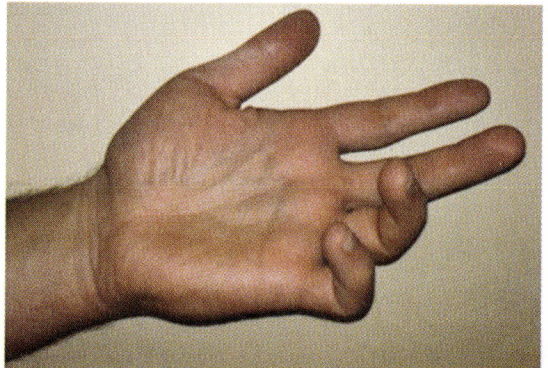

Fig. 52.3: Ulnar claw

- Neuropraxia of the ulnar nerve secondary to a stretch injury is rare, but a stretch injury could be watched for signs of spontaneous recovery.

Operative

- Complete ulnar nerve lacerations in civilian practice are usually seen acutely and are usually caused by sharp lacerations from broken glass, knives, saws, or vehicular accidents.
- Complete nerve lacerations should be repaired with microsurgical procedures.
- Choices for microsurgical repair include:
  1. Epineural repair
  2. Group fascicular repair
  3. Nerve repair with nerve grafts
  4. Nerve repair with nerve conduit
  5. Nerve transfers
- For transected nerves or in cases in which a segment not transmitting, nerve action potential (NAP) requires resection, end-to-end epineurial repair can sometimes be achieved. Sharp dissection is necessary to mobilize proximal and distal stumps with adequate cross-sections to healthy epineurial and fascicular structure before suture or graft repairs can be made.
- Partial nerve lacerations can be repaired by dissecting the internal epineurium and isolating the transected fascicular groups, gently looping the intact fascicular groups and then repairing the cut fascicular groups by suturing the internal epineurial sheaths.
- If there is a significant true defect, e.g. after a bullet wound, then repairing the cut fascicular groups with nerve grafts between the cut fascicular groups is indicated.
- Neurolysis of the ulnar nerve for a neuropraxia is uncommon.
- Ulnar nerve lacerations should be repaired as quickly as possible, and the ulnar artery should also be repaired regardless of the apparent vascular supply to the hand.

- Compared with the median nerve, in which it is difficult to regain lost nerve length, the ulnar nerve can be transposed anterior to the elbow, usually deep with respect to the pronator and the flexor carpi ulnaris muscles. This maneuver typically gains 2.5–3.8 cm of length.

The primary goals of tendon transfer procedures for ulnar nerve palsy are restoration of small and ring finger DIPJ flexion (in cases of high ulnar nerve palsy), restoration of key pinch, correction of clawing, integration of MCPJ and IPJ flexion, and improvement in grip strength. Both the ECRB (Smith) and brachioradialis (Boyes) are strong donor MTUs that can be used to restore key pinch, and that do not leave a functional deficit when harvested. They must be lengthened by tendon grafts and then passed between the 2nd and 3rd metacarpals into the palm. Here they are routed towards the thumb, using the 2nd metacarpal as a pulley, and inserted on the adductor pollicis insertion (Fig. 52.4).

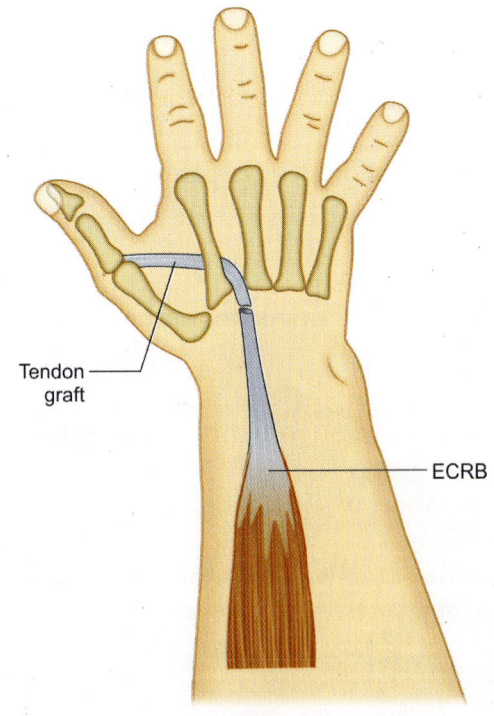

Tendon graft

ECRB

Fig. 52.4: Tendon transfer surgery

Correction of clawing is another primary goal in the treatment of ulnar nerve palsy. This requires correction of MCPJ hyperextension, the problem that initiates clawing. Procedures can be categorized as static or dynamic.

Osseous blocks on the dorsum of the metacarpal head have been described. Zancolli described an MCPJ capsulodesis, in which a distally based flap of the volar plate was advanced proximally and sutured to the metacarpal neck, effectively limiting MCPJ extension. Bunnell described a partial release of the A1 and A2 pulleys to allow bowstringing of the flexor tendons. This results in increasing the moment arm of the flexor tendons at the MCPJ, thereby preventing MCPJ hyperextension. Static tenodesis with a tendon graft can also be performed. The tendon graft is sutured to the deep transverse intermetacarpal ligament, passed through the lumbrical canal, and sutured to the extensor apparatus or to the lateral band. This type of static tendon graft effectively limits the amount of MCPJ extension.

Dynamic tenodesis can also be performed, as popularized by Fowler and Tsuge. A tendon graft is looped through the extensor retinaculum at the wrist. The two free ends of the tendon graft are passed through the intermetacarpal spaces into the palm, along the course of the lumbricals, and out to the fingers where they are inserted to the lateral bands. When the wrist is flexed, an active tenodesis effect occurs, resulting in MCPJ flexion and IPJ extension. Both the static procedures and the active tenodesis procedure are most useful in patients with simple clawing (Fig. 52.5).

There are a number of tendon transfer procedures available that provide dynamic correction of clawing, integrate MCPJ and IPJ flexion, and in some cases augment grip strength. These can be divided into superficialis transfers and transfers powered by wrist motors. In the modified Stiles-Bunnell

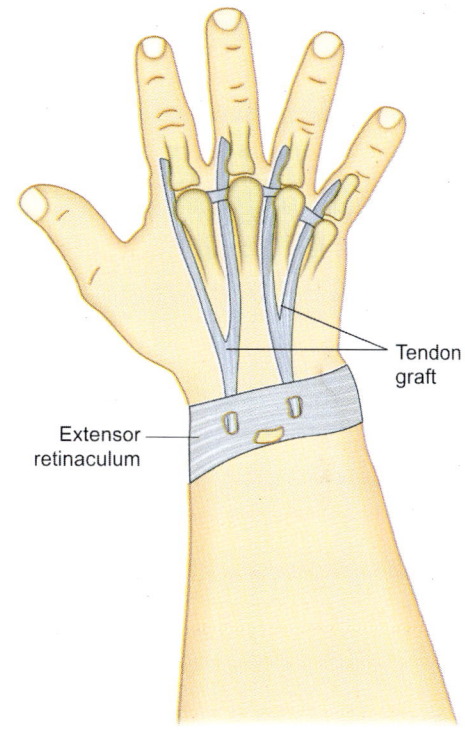

Tendon graft

Extensor retinaculum

Fig. 52.5: Tendon transfer

procedure, the middle finger superficialis tendon is divided distally in the finger and retrieved into the palm. It is then split into four slips. Each slip is then passed along the path of the lumbrical, volar to the deep transverse metacarpal ligament, and back into the finger, where it is inserted on the lateral band.

Brand, Riordan and others described the use of wrist-level motors to treat clawing and integrate finger flexion as well as augment grip strength. The FCR, ECRL, ECRB, or brachioradialis may be used.

TREATMENT

In acute open ulnar nerve injury, immediate exploration and primary neurorrhaphy is recommended as long as the repair can be achieved under minimal tension. For contaminated wounds, for which immediate repair would be imprudent, a delayed repair can be performed ideally in less than 72 hours, but up to 7 days without detriment to outcome. Delays in repair increase the likelihood for nerve grafting, neuron loss, and fibrosis of the distal stump.

High ulnar nerve injuries traditionally have had poor outcomes with regard to intrinsic muscle recovery. Once the nerve has been injured, the motor end plates begin the process of degeneration. Functional recovery is determined by the time required for the motor end plate to be reinnervated and by the number of regenerated motor axons that can reach target muscle.

BIBLIOGRAPHY

- gradestack.com/Dr.../Nerve-Injuries/Ulnar-Nerve-Injury
- https://www.aafp.org/afp/2010/0115/p147.html
- cme.uthscsa.edu/Courses/TSHT/2017
- https://www.physio-pedia.com/Ulnar_Nerve
- https://geekymedics.com/nerve-supply-to-the-upper-limb

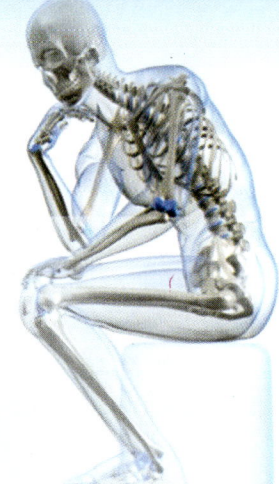

Radial Nerve Injuries

INTRODUCTION

The radial nerve is the terminal continuation of the posterior cord of the brachial plexus. It, therefore, contains fibers from nerve roots C5–T1. The nerve terminates by dividing into two branches:

- *Deep branch* (motor)—innervates the muscles in the posterior compartment of the forearm.
- *Superficial branch* (sensory)— contributes to the cutaneous innervation of the dorsal hand and fingers.
    - The radial nerve innervates the muscles located in the posterior arm and posterior forearm.
    - In the arm, it innervates the three heads of the triceps brachii, which acts to extend the arm at the elbow. The radial nerve also gives rise to branches that supply the brachioradialis and extensor carpi radialis longus (muscles of the posterior forearm).
    - A terminal branch of the radial nerve, the deep branch, innervates the remaining muscles of the posterior forearm. As a generalisation, these muscles act to extend at the wrist and finger joints, and supinate the forearm.

As a result of its proximity to the humeral shaft, as well as its long and tortuous course, the radial nerve is the most frequently injured major nerve in the upper limb, with its close proximity to the bone making it vulnerable when fractures occur. The radial nerve gets injured or damaged due to its anatomical positioning as this nerve is fixed and near the humerus bone.

Radial nerve injuries can occur after trauma. Common forms of radial nerve injuries occur with the following:

- After fractures of the humerus, especially spiral fracture patterns along the distal third of the humerus (Holstein-Lewis fracture) with a known associated incidence of radial nerve neuropraxia in the range of 15 to 25%.
- Improper use of crutches.
- Overuse of the arm (secondary to manual labor, chronic overuse, or sport-related participation)
- Work-related accidents

With the hand supinated, and the extensors aided by gravity, hand function may appear normal. However, when the hand is pronated, the wrist and hand will drop. This is also referred to as "wrist drop." If damaged at the axilla, there will be a loss of extension of the forearm, hand, and fingers.

Injuring the radial nerve distal to the elbow joint can occur from:

- Elbow dislocations
- Elbow fractures
- Tight casts/compressive bandages

This causes weakness in extension of the hand and fingers and presence of finger drop and partial wrist drop (Fig. 53.1).

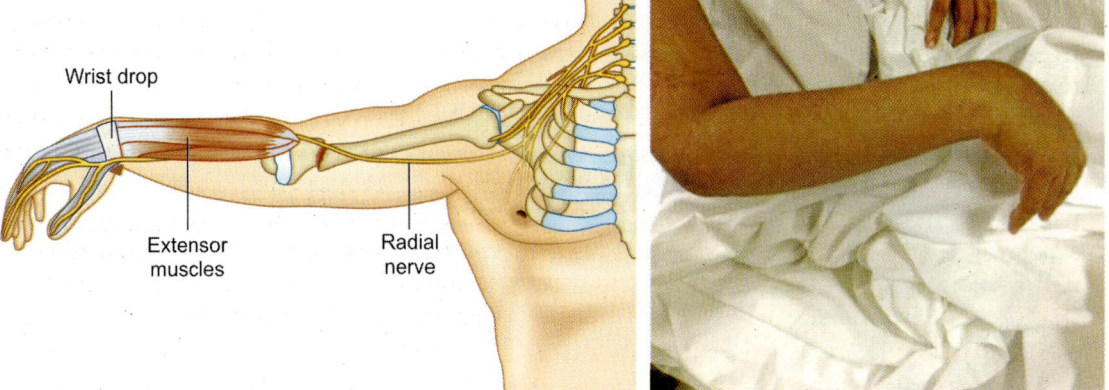

Fig. 53.1: Wrist drop

The clinical examination is the fundamental diagnostic tool. All the muscles innervated by the radial nerve can be tested for strength and function, including the triceps, forearm supinator, and wrist and finger extensors. For the upper lesions of radial nerve, loss of elbow extension should be evaluated with gravity eliminated. The examiner should be aware that with digital flexion, some extension of the wrist is possible with tight passive extensors. Digital extension is an area where most errors in diagnosis can occur. Extension of interphalangeal (IP) joints is accomplished by the interossei and lumbrical muscles innervated by the ulnar nerve. With radial nerve injury, only extension in the MCP joints is affected. One can also test the sensation on the dorsum of the hand and lateral 3½ fingers as well as the arm and forearm.

Radial nerve palsy in the middle third of the arm is characterized by palsy or paralysis of all extensors of the wrist and digits, as well as the forearm supinators. Very proximal lesions also may affect the triceps. Numbness occurs on the dorsoradial aspect of the hand and the dorsal aspect of the radial 3½ digits.

The importance in the difference in high and low radial nerve palsies is in the presence or absence of active wrist extension. The radial nerve proper will innervate the brachioradialis (BR), extensor carpi radialis longus (ECRL), and extensor carpi radialis brevis (ECRB) prior to dividing into the PIN and the radial sensory nerve and thus, a patient with the high radial nerve palsy will lack wrist extension, thumb extension, and digital extension.

With radial nerve injuries, three functions are lost and must be replaced:

a. Thumb extension

b. Finger extension

c. In high nerve palsies, wrist extension.

Electromyograms or nerve conduction studies (EMG/NCS) can help differentiate nerve versus muscle injury, measuring the speed at which the impulses travel along the nerve. EMG/NCS is also utilized for follow-up management in serial observations for the return of nerve function. It is important to note that more than 90% of radial nerve palsies will resolve in 3 to 4 months with observation alone.

The return of function following radial nerve palsy follows a predictable clinical pattern. Brachioradialis followed by ECRL are the first to return; whereas, EPL and EIP are last to return.

Radial nerve palsy occurs in 6 to 18% of humeral shaft fractures. The majority of radial nerve palsies represents neuropraxic injuries and will improve with observation alone (>90%). Splinting and range of motion exercises of the hand are encouraged to prevent contracture formation. Electromyography and nerve conduction tests are performed after 3 months, if failure of improvement of the palsy is noted clinically. Exploration and neurolysis or repair of the nerve is performed, if no signs of recovery are seen after 3 to 4 months. Indications for acute nerve exploration include penetrating open fractures, high-grade soft tissue injuries, or secondary nerve palsies (in some cases).

Treatment of radial nerve palsy can be either non-operative or operative. One of the most important aspects of this treatment is to maintain a full passive range of motion in all the affected joints through exercise programs and the use of dynamic splints. Surgical treatment is indicated in cases when nerve transection is obvious, as in open injuries or when there is no clinical improvement after a period of conservative treatment. The nerve can be repaired by direct suturing or nerve grafting. Other reconstructive procedures, such as tendon transfers, may also become necessary to overcome any permanent nerve dysfunction. Nerve transfers and functional free muscle transfers are currently gaining in popularity.

Treatment for radial nerve palsy is usually a brace or cockup splint as well as physical therapy to help maintain muscle strength and to avoid contracture. EMG and nerve studies. The brachioradialis muscle is the first to recover and can be done as early as three weeks, but follow the progress. Nerve exploration is indicated in open humeral fractures with radial nerve palsy or in conditions that have had sufficient time without nerve recovery. A tendon transfer may be necessary, if the nerve cannot be repaired or the function cannot be restored.

Tendon transfer is essential in irreparable or long-standing radial nerve palsies in order to restore hand function. Tendon transfer is still the most commonly used techique for motor reconstruction in chronic cases. A waiting period of one year is usually sufficient to see any evidence of nerve regeneration. Following a radial nerve injury, the extrinsic extensor function of the hand and wrist is lost. This results in an inability to extend the fingers and wrist and affects grip strength and finger flexion, and has a large influence on thumb usage. Tendon transfer surgery must restore finger, thumb and wrist function without inflicting other motor deficits on the hand. With over 50 described techniques, the surgeon must choose the most suitable for the individual patient. Most often we use the pronator teres to extensor carpi radialis brevis transfer to restore wrist extension, the flexor carpi radialis for finger extension (Brand technique) and the palmaris longus to extensor pollicis longus (EPL) transfer for thumb extension. The flexor carpi radialis tendon can also be used to restore thumb abduction and extension, where it is transferred to the tendons of the first extensor compartment.

The breadth of surgical intervention ranges from direct nerve repair to tendon transfer, with a wide variety of options supported in the literature. New frontiers in nerve regeneration with stem cells have yielded preliminarily promising results, and future developments in this field are anticipated.

The Holstein-Lewis humeral shaft fracture, that is, a simple spiral fracture in the distal third of the shaft with the distal bone fragment displaced and the proximal end deviated toward the radial side, was originally described by Arthur Holstein and Gwilym Lewis in the American Journal of Bone and Joint Surgery in 1963. This fracture type accounts for 7.5% of all the humeral shaft fractures and is associated with a significantly increased risk of acute radial nerve palsy compared with patients with other types of humeral shaft fractures. The overall outcome regarding fracture healing, radial nerve recovery, and function is very good regardless of the primary treatment modality, i.e. operative or nonoperative treatment.

The main treatment of wrist drop is to provide dorsal wrist cock-up splints with or without dynamic finger extensions. This maintains some hand function, especially ulnar-innervated finger abduction and adduction. Splinting remains the most important intervention, especially because most radial palsies have a good prognosis.

Currently, priority is given to re-innervation of the extensor carpi radialis brevis (ECRB) for wrist extension and the posterior interosseous nerve (PIN) for finger and thumb extension.

The branch to the flexor digitorum superficialis (FDS) muscle (median nerve) is rotated to the ECRB and branches to the palmaris longus (PL) and flexor carpi radialis (FCR) (median nerve) are coaptated to the PIN.

BIBLIOGRAPHY

- https://depts.washington.edu
- https://neuromuscular.wustl.edu
- https://geekymedics.com/nerve-supply-to-the-upper-limb
- https://www.ncbi.nlm.nih.gov

Median Nerve Injuries

The median nerve originates from the medial and lateral cords of the brachial plexus. It runs down the arm and enters the forearm with the brachial artery. Any sort of damage or injury to the median nerve in the elbow results in symptoms in the forearm, wrist, and hand. The injuries to median nerve comprise conditions where there is partial or complete tear of the nerve or compression of the nerve due to a displacement fracture or due to additional fluid after an injury. Due to its length, there are various places where the nerve can get damaged. The nerve is susceptible to injury at the elbow, forearm, wrist, and hand. The lesions of median nerve may take place at the following four sites: (a) At elbow, (b) at mid-forearm, (c) at wrist (distal forearm), and (d) in the carpal tunnel.

At elbow, the median nerve can be injured due to supracondylar fracture of humerus, application of tight tourniquet during venipuncture, and entrapment of nerve between two heads of pronator teres or underneath the fibrous arch linking the two heads of flexor digitorum superficialis.

Median nerve palsy is caused by deep, penetrating injuries to the arm, forearm, or wrist area, and occasionally from blunt force trauma or neuropathy.

Median nerve palsy is perhaps the most devastating single nerve injury of the upper extremity. Not only is there a loss of fine motor control and opposition, but sensibility is lost over the area of the hand used for precision movements and prehensile functioning.

Injuries to the median nerve can be separated into high and low median nerve palsies, depending on the level of injury (Fig. 54.1).

Patients with low median nerve palsy—for example, because of a lesion at the wrist—lack the ability to abduct and oppose the thumb due to paralysis of the thenar muscles. They will also have sensory loss in the thumb, index finger, long finger, and the radial aspect of the ring finger. In contrast, patients with high median nerve palsy (lesion at the elbow and above) have weakness in forearm pronation and wrist and finger flexion, in addition to lack of thumb opposition (Fig. 54.2).

Signs of a median nerve lesion include weak pronation of the forearm, weak flexion and radial deviation of wrist, with thenar atrophy and inability to oppose or flex the thumb; sensory distribution includes thumb, radial 2½

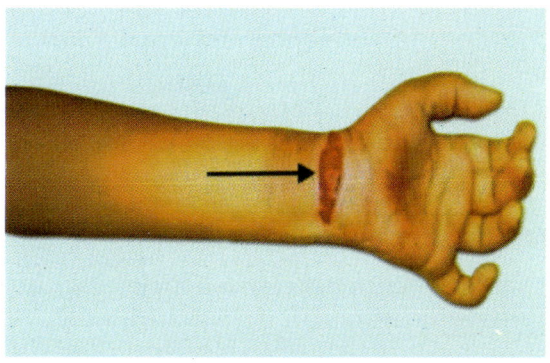

Fig. 54.1: Wrist laceration

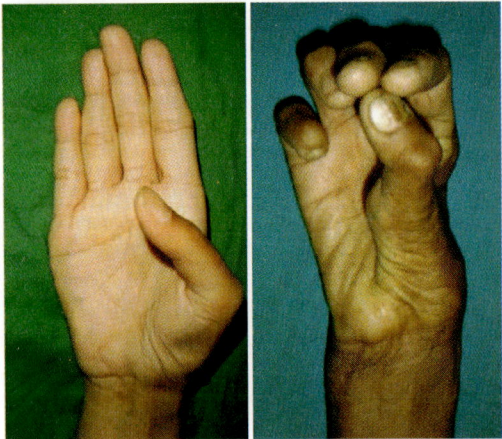

Fig. 54.2: Signs of median nerve injury

fingers, and corresponding portion of palm (Fig. 54.3).

Lesions above the Elbow

- *Motor deficit:*
  - Loss of pronation of forearm.
  - Weakness in flexion of the hand at the wrist.
  - Loss of flexion of thumb, 2nd and 3rd digits.

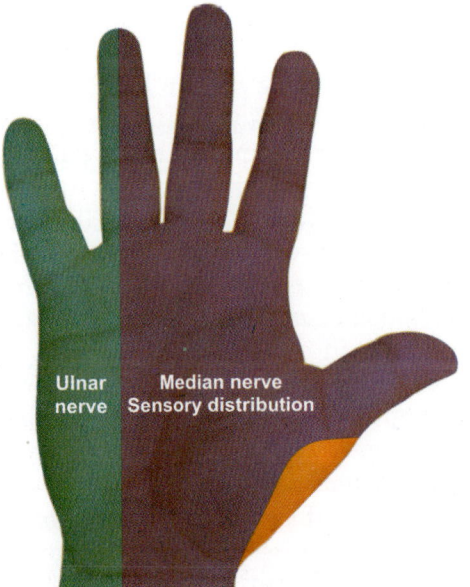

Ulnar nerve   Median nerve Sensory distribution

Fig. 54.3: Sensory supply in hand

- Loss of abduction and opposition of thumb.
- Fixed hyperextension of index finger, middle finger and thumb.
- *Sensory deficit:* Loss of sensation in the thumb, 2nd and 3rd digits, and the thenar area.

Lesions between Elbow and Wrist

- *Motor deficit:*
  - Loss of pronation of forearm.
  - Loss of flexion of thumb, 2nd and 3rd digits.
  - Loss of abduction and opposition of thumb.
- *Sensory deficit:* Loss of sensation in the thumb, 2nd and 3rd digits, and the thenar area.

Lesions Proximal to the Carpal Tunnel

- *Motor deficit:*
  - Loss of flexion of thumb, 2nd and 3rd digits.
  - Loss of abduction and opposition of thumb.
- *Sensory deficit:* Loss of sensation in the thumb, 2nd and 3rd digits, and the thenar area.

Lesions within the Carpal Tunnel

- *Motor deficit:*
  - Loss of flexion of thumb, 2nd and 3rd digits.
  - Loss of abduction and opposition of thumb.
- *Sensory deficit:* Loss of sensation in the thumb, 2nd and 3rd digits, but excluding the thenar eminence.

TREATMENT GOALS

- Identify the presence of a complete median nerve laceration, a partial median nerve laceration, or a median nerve neuropraxia.

- Repair the complete or partial nerve laceration.
- Carefully follow the patient with a median nerve stretch injury; some patients with neuropraxia will require neurolysis.
- Improve function of injured upper extremity with a median nerve laceration.

Conservative

- Nonoperative treatment of median nerve complete or partial lacerations is appropriate when the patient's associated injuries or medical comorbidities prevent anesthesia and a lengthy microsurgical repair.
- Isolated median nerve complete and partial lacerations should be repaired early, but repair is not an emergency.
- Irrigation, debridement, and closure of the skin laceration with a scheduled operative nerve repair 1–3 weeks is reasonable.
- Neuropraxia of the median nerve secondary to a stretch injury is rare, but a stretch injury could be watched for signs of spontaneous recovery.
- An exception to the watch-and-wait plan for a median nerve neuropraxia includes acute carpal tunnel syndrome associated with a distal radius fracture, which does not resolve soon after fracture reduction and splinting.
- Another exception is the patient with severe compartment syndrome type median nerve pain that continues or worsens with fracture reduction.
- This patient with severe nerve pain may have the median nerve caught in the fracture.

Operative

- Complete median nerve lacerations in civilian practice are usually seen acutely and are caused by sharp lacerations from broken glass, knives, saws, or vehicular accidents.

- Complete nerve lacerations should be repaired with microsurgical procedures.
- Choices for microsurgical repair include:
  1. Epineural repair
  2. Group fascicular repair
  3. Nerve repair with nerve grafts
  4. Nerve repair with nerve conduit
  5. Nerve transfers
- Partial nerve lacerations can be repaired by dissecting the internal epineurium and isolating the transected fascicular groups, gently looping the intact fascicular groups and then repairing the cut fascicular groups by suturing the internal epineurial sheaths.
- If there is a significant true defect, e.g. after a bullet wound, then repairing the cut fascicular groups with nerve grafts between the cut fascicular groups is indicated.
- Neurolysis of the median nerve for a neuropraxia is uncommon.
- Nerve transfer for brachial plexus reconstruction are well defined in the literature; however, their usefulness for reconstructing median nerve lacerations is not well defined.

Tendon Transfer Procedures

The most devastating loss of movement following high or low median nerve injury is the loss of thumb opposition. This can be restored with an opponens plasty, or opposition transfer. The superficialis opponens plasty, described by Royle in 1938, involves dividing the ring finger FDS distally in the finger, retrieving the FDS proximal to the carpal tunnel, redirecting the tendon distally through the FPL sheath, and inserting it into the thumb. This transfer was later modified by Thompson by redirecting the tendon subcutaneously to the thumb, instead of through the FPL tendon sheath. Bunnell recommended rerouting the tendon around a looped strip of FCU to achieve a more effective line of pull.

In cases of high median nerve injury, thumb IPJ flexion and index finger DIPJ flexion can be restored with transfer of the BR, the ECRL, or ECU.

Opposition Transfers

- *Royle-Thompson:* Flexor digitorum superficialis 4 through palmar fascia sling to abductor pollicis brevis or extensor pollicis brevis
- *Bunnell:* FDS 4 through flexor carpi ulnaris sling to abductor pollicis brevis or extensor pollicis brevis
- *Burkhalter:* Extensor indicis around ulnar wrist to abductor pollicis brevis or extensor pollicis brevis
- *Camitz transfer:* Palmaris longus with palmar fascia to abductor pollicis brevis
- *Huber transfer:* Abductor digiti minimi to abductor pollicis brevis or extensor pollicis brevis
- Extensor digiti minimi around ulnar border wrist to abductor pollicis brevis, extensor expansion, and extensor pollicis longus

Transfers for Thumb Flexion

- Brachioradialis to flexor pollicis longus
- Extensor carpi radialis longus/extensor carpi radialis brevis to flexor pollicis longus

Transfers for Index and Middle Finger Flexion

- Intact ulnar flexor digitorum profundus side-to-side
- Extensor carpi radialis longus to flexor digitorum profundus

Transfers for Forearm Pronation

- Zancolli rerouting of the biceps tendon

PROGNOSIS

Following nerve bruising, recovery should be full.

Following mild nerve stretching/crushing, again recovery should be full although there may be some residual stiffness and sometimes aching especially in cold weather. This may improve for up to 3–4 years from injury.

Following more severe stretching/crushing, recovery is rarely complete. In almost all cases, there will be some numbness and stiffness and aching especially in cold weather. This may improve for up to 3–4 years from injury but rarely recovers fully.

If a nerve has been cut and repaired then full recovery can occur in patients under 10 but this is not guaranteed. Full recovery is very rare in adults. If the nerve is small, the loss of function may be small although cut nerves have a tendency to give significant long-term pain in some cases. The severity of the long-term problems is dependent on a number of factors: Which nerve is injured; the severity of the injury (crushes are worse than clean cuts); and the age of the patient (older patients do less well). Recovery in feeling and muscle power may improve for up to 2 years from injury. Cold intolerance, i.e. stiffness and pain in the cold may improve for up to 3–4 years from injury.

In median nerve injury, the loss of sensibility is of critical importance. Complete median nerve distribution sensory loss is considered by some to be a contraindication to tendon transfer. A hand in which median nerve sensibility is present, or in which a return of sensation is expected, will have a much better outcome following the tendon transfer procedures.

BIBLIOGRAPHY

- https://www.handsurgeryresource.com/median-nerve-laceration
- https://www.slideshare.net/benthungoe/median-nerve-palsy-and-tendon-transfers
- https://www.youtube.com/watch?v=HPD_IeefAGI
- https://www.youtube.com/watch?v=Vv78MFi-HRY
- https://www.youtube.com/watch?v=EFRpTUJuWCY

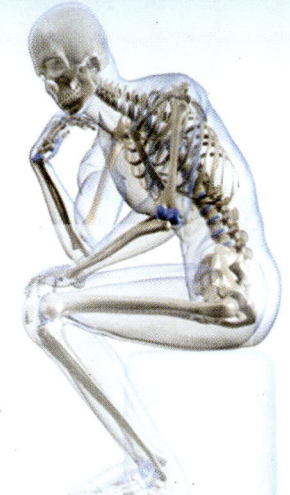

Sciatic Nerve Injury

INTRODUCTION

The sciatic nerve is the largest nerve in the body and begins from nerve roots in the lumbar spinal cord in the low back and extends through the buttock area to send nerve endings down the lower limb.

The sciatic nerve arises from lumbrosacral plexus—L4, L5, S1, S2, S3 (Fig. 55.1):

- Nerve emerges from pelvis below piriformis and enters thigh between ischial tuberosity and greater trochanter.
- In 10% of patients, the sciatic nerve is separated in greater sciatic foramen by all or part of the piriformis.
- Nerve enters thigh beneath lower border of gluteus maximus.
- Descends near middle of thigh, lying on adductor magnus muscle and being crossed obliquely by long head of biceps femoris.

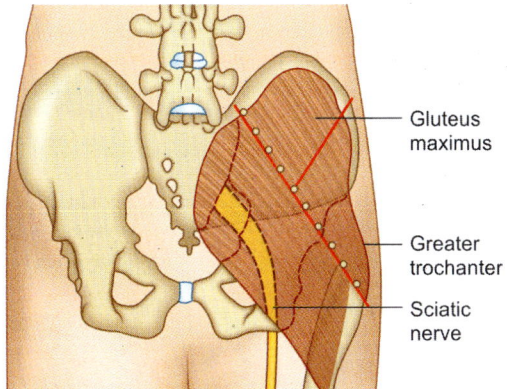

Fig. 55.1: Anatomy of sciatic nerve

- Nerve usually separates in upper part of popliteal space; then, it divides into tibial nerve and common peroneal nerve.

The sciatic nerve also provides sensation to the back of the thigh, part of the lower leg, and the sole of the foot. Partial damage to the nerve may demonstrate weakness of knee flexion, weakness of foot and ankle movements. A person's reflexes may be abnormal, with weak or absent ankle-jerk reflex.

CAUSES

Sciatic nerve injury may occur due to: Stab wounds, fractures of the pelvis, posterior dislocation of the hip joint or badly-placed intramuscular injection in the gluteal region.

When injury occurs to the sciatic nerve due to posterior hip dislocation (incidence is 8–20%), the common peroneal nerve is usually affected, causing weakness in dorsiflexion of the ankle and loss of toe extension can also occur.

Sciatic nerve injury leads to foot drop deformity, wasting of the calf muscles and loss of Achilles tendon reflex. There will be paralysis of muscles of the extensor and peroneal compartments. Sensory loss below the knee may lead to trophic ulcer except for the area supplied by the saphenous nerve.

MANAGEMENT

Ankle-foot orthoses (AFO) are helpful in the treatment of paralyzed extensor muscles of the foot (Fig. 55.2).

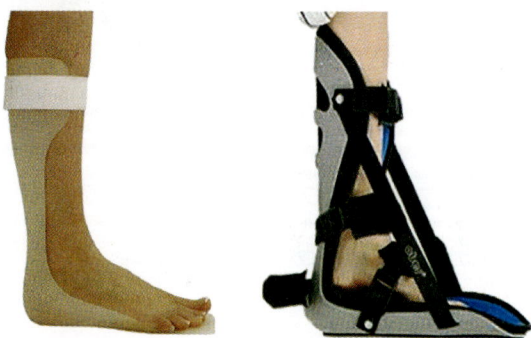

Fig. 55.2: Ankle-foot orthosis

Bracing with an AFO and physical therapy is useful in all causes of drop foot to assist in ambulation and prevent contracture of the ankle plantar flexors. The primary purpose of the AFO is to increase dorsiflexion during swing phase, provide medial and lateral stability at stance, and possibly increase pushoff stimulation at the late phase of stance.

When nerve injury is the cause of drop foot, treatment focuses on restoring the nerve continuity by nerve grafting (transfer of functional fascicles, nerve repair or removal of the nerve insult).

The surgical treatment should be connected with the etiology of the foot drop and can include: Neurolysis of the nerve, "end to end" repair, autogenous nerve graft procedures, nerve transfers, and direct neuromuscular neurotization and tendon transfers. In proximal sciatic nerve lesions, nerve transfers and one-stage nerve repair with concomitant tendon transfer are valuable methods of the treatment of drop foot. Surgical options in the lower extremity include ankle arthrodesis and tendon transfer.

BIBLIOGRAPHY

- https://www.youtube.com/watch?v=fJ6sFqV4pkQ
- https://www.ncbi.nlm.nih.gov/pubmed/23289258
- https://www.youtube.com/watch?v=J7-L9MFRXD8

Common Peroneal Nerve Injury

My foot has fallen and it can't get up!

Common peroneal nerve palsy has been reported to be the most frequent lower extremity palsy characterized by a supinated equinovarus foot deformity and foot drop.

Common peroneal nerve (Fig. 56.1) comes off the sciatic nerve in the thigh. It then courses around the fibular neck and bifurcates into:

- **Deep peroneal nerve**
  - Innervates the anterior compartment of the leg → dorsiflexes ankle and extends toes
  - Provides sensation to the first dorsal webspace
- **Superficial peroneal nerve**
  - Innervates the lateral (peroneal) compartment of the leg → everts foot and plantarflexes ankle
  - Provides sensation to anterolateral distal third of the leg and the majority of dorsum of the foot (except the first webspace)

Common peroneal nerve palsy may be due to:
- **Traumatic causes**
  - Knee dislocation
  - Direct impact or cut on the fibular neck
  - Following surgery to the knee

Taking a look at foot nerve anatomy, the peroneal nerve is a branch of the sciatic nerve that extends from the low back and controls the muscles responsible for lifting the foot. It wraps around the leg from the back of the knee to the front of the shin and lies pretty close to

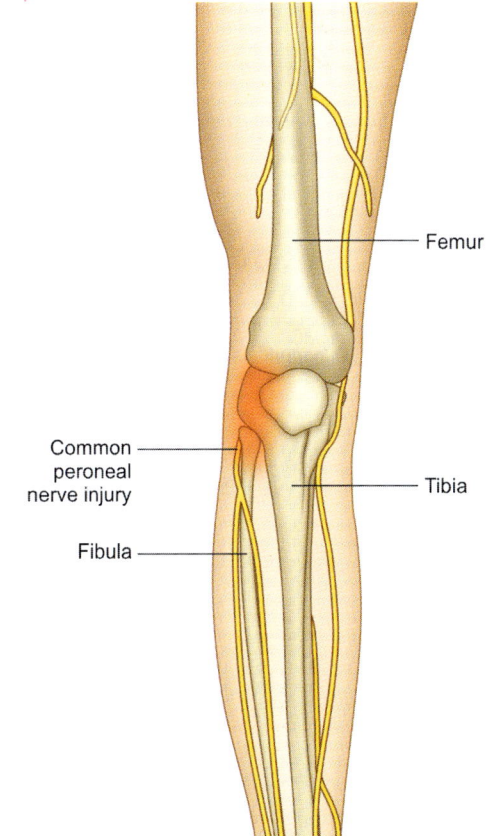

Fig. 56.1: Common peroneal nerve

the surface of the skin. This makes it vulnerable to being pinched in quite a few scenarios, including:
- Trauma to the knee or shin
- A dislocated knee or fractured fibula
- Knee or hip replacement surgery

- Long hours kneeling or in a squatted position
- Habitual leg crossing
- Wearing a leg cast
- Childbirth

Foot drop is defined as a weakness or failure of function in the tibialis anterior, causing restricted functional movement, a slowing down of walking speed and an increased risk of falling. The most common symptom of foot drop, high steppage gait, is often characterized by raising the thigh up in an exaggerated fashion while walking, as if climbing the stairs.

MANAGEMENT

Surgical options include tenodesis, arthrodesis, and tendon transfers.

The goal of surgery for drop foot is a stable plantigrade foot that is shoeable, brace free and prevents tripping (Fig. 56.2).

It has been suggested that a tendon transfer may be considered, if there is no significant neural recovery at 1 year (Table 56.1).

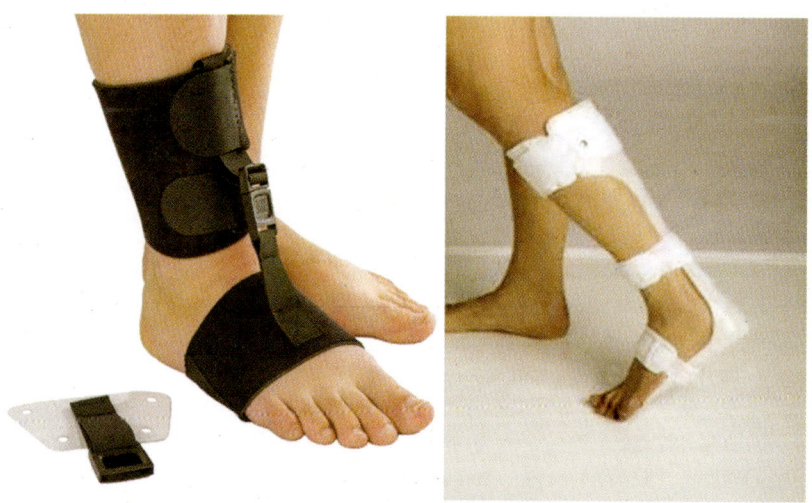

Fig. 56.2: Foot drop splint

Table 56.1: Surgical options for foot drop

	Tendon transfer	Nerve transfer
What is it?	Tibialis posterior tendon is transferred via the interosseous membrane to reach the dorsum of the foot	Fascicle of the tibial nerve (to FHL/FDL) is transferred to the tibialis anterior nerve branch of deep peroneal nerve
Effect	A plantar flexor is converted into a dorsiflexor	Nerve for toes flexor is used to reinnervate the tibialis anterior muscle
Tendon/muscle biomechanics	Altered	Preserve
Timescale to perform procedure	May be performed even in late cases	Ideally not later than 3–6 months since injury
Likely outcome	Foot may be brought up to neutral without orthosis power is about 30% of the opposite ankle	Potential of restoring near normal ankle dorsiflexion but result is not consistent

The transfer of the tibialis posterior tendon to the paralysed tendons on the anterior aspect of the ankle not only restores the function of the paralyzed muscles, but also removes the deforming force on the medial aspect of the foot.

During the operation, the tendon of the posterior tibial muscle is transected as far distally as possible. It is then re-routed above the medial malleolus and around the tibia (circum tibial route), or the interosseous membrane is incised and the tendon of the tibialis posterior is pulled anteriorly (interosseous route). The tendon is split into two slips and then sutured to the tendons of the anterior tibial muscle medially and the peroneus brevis or tertius laterally, while the foot is resting in a splint in dorsiflexion. Postoperatively, the foot remains in plaster for about 6 weeks.

Dynamic tendon transposition represents the gold standard for surgical restoration of dorsiflexion of a permanently paralyzed foot.

The objectives of tendon transfer for treatment of post-traumatic foot drop are: (1) To improve functional deficit by restoring or reinforcing lost functions; (2) to neutralize deforming forces; and (3) to gain stability eliminating the need for bracing during gait. These objectives can be achieved by static and dynamic surgical procedures. The former (arthrodesis, osteotomy, tenodesis) changes uncorrected fixed and nonfunctional postures into more functional postures and results in better overall function but does not restore lost movements. Generally, static procedures are used as a support or after failure of dynamic procedures and/or when dynamic procedures are not indicated (severe articular incongruence, wide traumatic palsy, cerebropathy, neuropathy, etc.). Dynamic surgical procedures act by transferring functional muscles or changing their osseous insertions, improving function, and, most of all, restoring lost movement. For common peroneal nerve palsy, the functions that must be restored are foot dorsiflexion, supination, hallux and toe dorsiflexion, avoiding a steppage gait, correcting equinus and varus deformities, and digit drop.

Posterior tibial tendon transfer has long been the mainstay to combating drop foot. Watkins, et al. first reported on this tendon transfer in 1954. Classically, the surgeon transfers the posterior tibial tendon through the interosseous membrane and inserts the tendon to the third cuneiform. There have been many modifications since the induction of this procedure. Perhaps most common is the split posterior tibial tendon transfer. In this procedure, one splits the tendon longitudinally to the musculotendinous junction and inserts the lateral half into the peroneus brevis just proximal to its insertion. This technique balances the hindfoot and restores dorsiflexor power without weakening posterior tibial tendon function. When the surgeon cannot sacrifice the posterior tibial tendon, he or she can utilize the peroneal longus tendon in a similar fashion.

For treatment of complete nerve palsy, transosseous rerouting to the third cuneiform of the tibialis anterior tendon and dual transfer of tibialis posterior and flexor digitorum longus tendons is a reliable method to restore balanced foot and toe dorsiflexion producing a normal gait without the need for orthoses.

The posterior tibial transfer procedure can either involve transfer of the posterior tibial tendon alone or transfer with attachment to two other tendons—the peroneus longus and the anterior tibialis. When all three tendons are used it is called a Bridle procedure because the three tendons are attached in a bridle configuration (Fig. 56.3).

In the surgery of foot drop, the common method of correction is by transfer of tibialis posterior muscle, either to the joint capsule in the middle of the foot (Selvapandian's method) or a double transfer to the toe extensor tendons (Srinivasan's method).

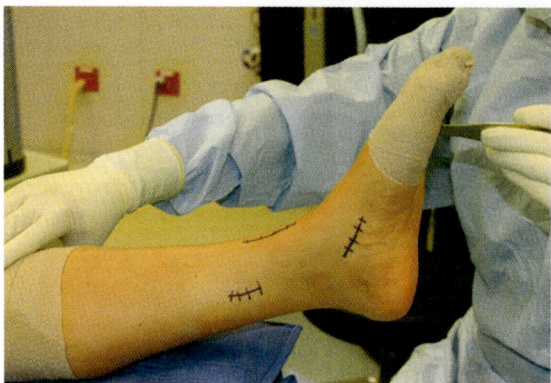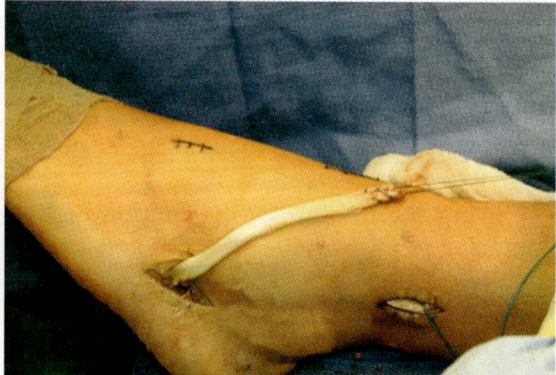

Fig. 56.3: Tendon transfer for foot drop

BIBLIOGRAPHY

- http://www.nerveclinic.co.uk
- https://www.podiatrytoday.com
- http://mcmasterpa.weebly.com/ortho---msk-videos.html

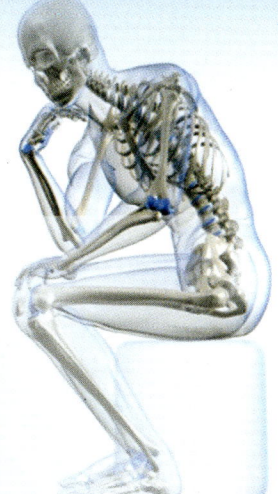

General Principles of Fracture Management

A break in the structural continuity of bone is called fracture.

Fracture is a soft tissue injury where the bone is broken (AO definition).

A fracture is a partial or complete interruption in the continuity of bone (Fig. 57.1).

How Fractures Happen?

- *A single traumatic incident:* Post-traumatic fracture
- *Repetitive stress:* Stress fracture
- *Abnormal weakening of the bone:* Pathological fracture

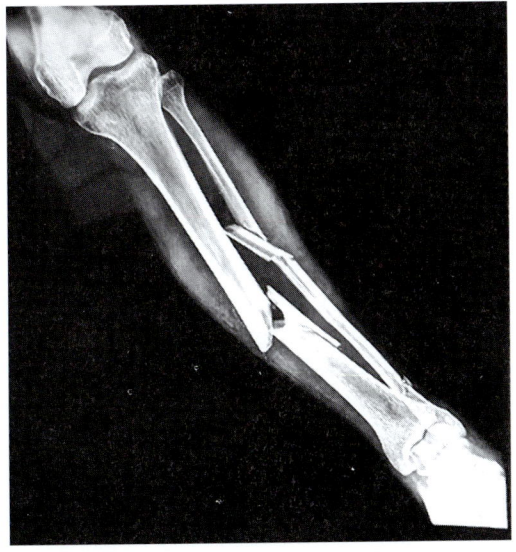

Fig. 57.1: Fractures of tibia and fibula

CLINICAL FEATURES

- Pain, redness, and swelling at the site of injury
- Deformity and axis deviation
- Bone fragments penetrating the skin
- Palpable step-off or gap
- Bone crepitus
- Concomitant soft tissue injuries
- Neurovascular compromise below site of injury

BIOLOGY OF BONE HEALING

Bone is a composite structure with mineral and organic components. The mineral component contains calcium, phosphate, and hydroxyl ions which are organized into a compound called hydroxyapatite [$Ca_5(PO_4)_3$ (OH)]. This mineral skeleton provides the strength, stiffness, and rigidity characteristic of bone. The organic or protein component consists primarily of type I collagen, which lends tensile strength and resiliency. The outer covering of bone, the periosteum, provides the vascular supply that plays an essential role in fracture healing. The periosteum in children is substantially thicker and more robust than in adults, accounting in part for the more rapid healing of pediatric fractures.

Bone healing is usually divided into three slightly overlapping stages: Inflammatory, reparative, and remodeling (Fig. 57.2).

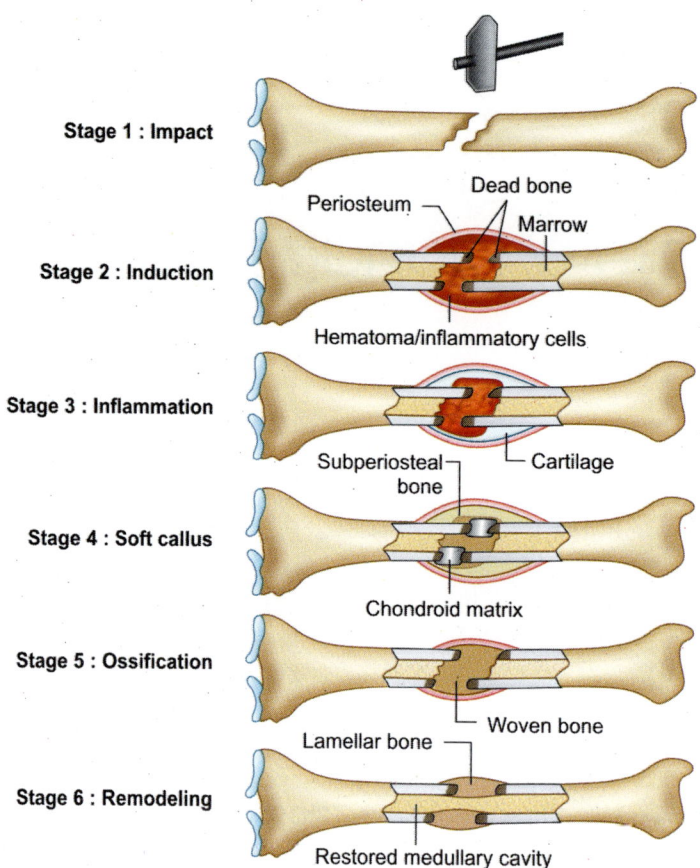

Stage 1 : Impact

Stage 2 : Induction

Periosteum

Dead bone

Marrow

Hematoma/inflammatory cells

Stage 3 : Inflammation

Subperiosteal bone

Cartilage

Stage 4 : Soft callus

Chondroid matrix

Stage 5 : Ossification

Woven bone

Lamellar bone

Stage 6 : Remodeling

Restored medullary cavity

Fig. 57.2: Various steps in healing of a fracture

Stages of Fracture Healing (Fig. 57.3)

The initial inflammatory phase is dominated by vascular events. Following a fracture, a hematoma forms which provides the building blocks for healing. Subsequently, reabsorption occurs of the 1 to 2 mm of bone at the fracture edges that have lost their blood supply. It is this bone reabsorption that makes fracture lines become radiographically distinct 5 to 10 days after injury. Next, multipotent cells are transformed into osteoprogenitor cells, which begin to form new bone.

In the reparative phase, new blood vessels develop from outside the bone that supplies nutrients to the cartilage, which begins to form across the fracture site. Nearly complete immobilization is desirable during both the inflammatory phase and the early reparative phase to allow for the growth of these new vessels. However, once neovascularization is complete, progressive loading and stress across the fracture site are desirable to augment callus formation.

Callus typically forms as a collar of new, endochondral bone around the fractured area. This callus is initially highly cartilaginous, but hardens as mineralization and endochondral calcification occur during the remodeling phase. Late in the reparative phase, clinical union of the fracture occurs. Clinical union occurs when the fractured bone does not shift on clinical examination, the fracture site is nontender, and the patient can use the injured limb without significant pain. Because the

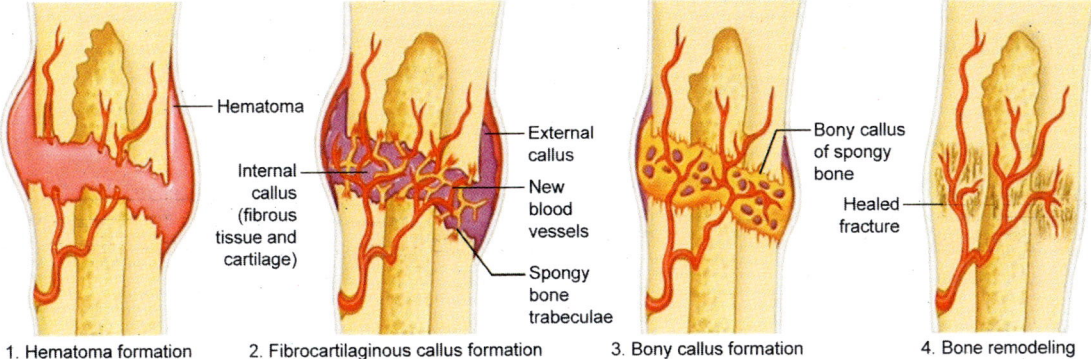

1. Hematoma formation 2. Fibrocartilaginous callus formation 3. Bony callus formation 4. Bone remodeling

Fig. 57.3: Stages of fracture healing

initial callus is cartilaginous, clinical union may occur before evidence of radiographic union is appreciable on radiographs. Clinical union classically marks the end of the reparative phase of fracture healing.

In the remodeling phase, the endochondral callus becomes completely ossified and the bone undergoes structural remodeling. The process of remodeling occurs quickly in young children, who remodel their entire skeleton every year. By late childhood, the rate of skeletal remodeling is approximately 10% per year and continues near this level throughout life.

In addition to patient age, other factors affecting the rate of bone remodeling include thyroid and growth hormone levels, calcitonin, glucocorticoids, and nutritional status. Common conditions that impair fracture healing include diabetes mellitus, arterio-vascular disease, anemia, hypothyroidism, malnutrition (e.g. vitamin C or D deficiencies, inadequate protein intake), excessive chronic alcohol use, and tobacco use. Specific medications may also impair fracture healing, including nonsteroidal anti-inflammatory drugs, glucocorticoids, and certain antibiotics (e.g. ciprofloxacin).

CLINICAL DIAGNOSIS OF A FRACTURE

• History of trauma

• Symptoms and signs (Fig. 57.4):
  1. Pain and tenderness
  2. Swelling
  3. Deformity
  4. Bony crepitus
  5. Loss of function
  6. Nerve and vascular injury

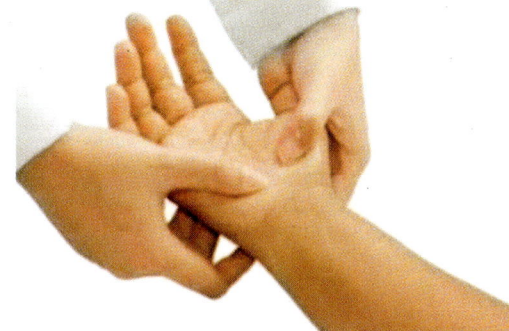

Fig. 57.4: Clinical examination of a fracture

FRACTURE DESCRIPTION

Overview

The essential first step of fracture treatment is to identify precisely the type of fracture present. At a minimum, a fracture should be identified using the following (Figs 57.5 and 57.6):

• Name of the injured bone
• Location of the injury (e.g. dorsal or volar; metaphysis, diaphysis, or epiphysis)

- Orientation of the fracture (e.g. transverse, oblique, spiral)
- Condition of the overlying tissues (e.g. open or closed fracture).

Other important descriptors include fracture angulation, comminution, and displacement.

The Rules for Orthopedic

X-ray requests → Two views → Two joints → Two limbs → Two injuries → Two occasions.

Rule of two should always be followed:

- *Two views* (in two orthogonal planes: AP or PA view and lateral view. The view from one plane may miss certain findings.)
- *Two joints* (distal and proximal joint: Because bones are joined in the fashion of parallelogram)
- *Two limbs* (especially in children to get an idea about the ossification center)
- *Two injuries*

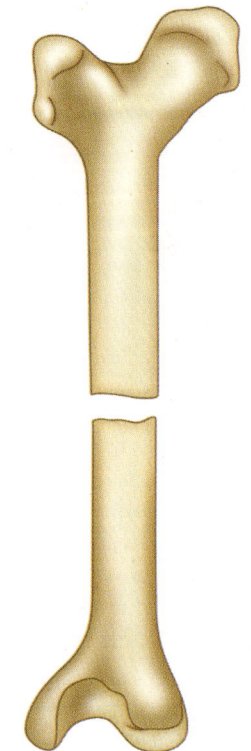

Fig. 57.6: Transverse fracture

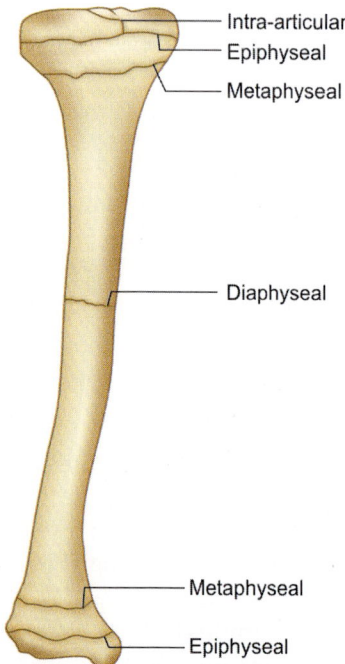

Fig. 57.5: Anatomic location of a fracture in long bone

- *Two occasions* (first at the time of diagnosis, i.e. before the reduction, and the second one is taken after the reduction)

CLASSIFICATION

Fracture classification is based on the following:

Anatomy

- Location: Affected bone (proximal, distal)
- *Position:* Diaphysis, metaphysis, epiphysis

Extent

- Complete
- Incomplete
- *Orientation:* Transverse, oblique, spiral (Fig. 57.8)
- *Displacement:* Nondisplaced, displaced, angulated
- Fragmentation
- Comminuted fracture
- Segmental fracture
- Soft tissue involvement

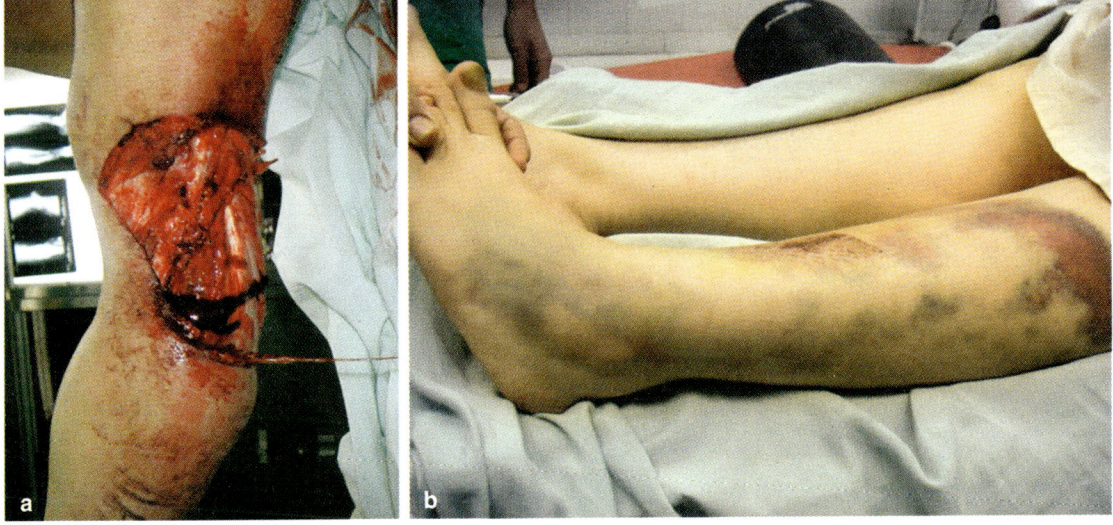

Fig. 57.7: (a) Open fracture; (b) Closed fracture

- Closed fracture (simple fracture)
- Open fracture
- *Growth plate involvement (pediatric fractures):* Salter-Harris fractures (Fig. 57.7)

MANAGEMENT OF FRACTURES

The goal of fracture management is bony union of the fracture without further bone or soft-tissue damage that enables early restoration of maximal function.

Treatment of Closed Fractures

- Emergency care (splinting)
- Odefinitive fracture treatment
- Rehabilitation (muscle activity and early weight bearing are encouraged.

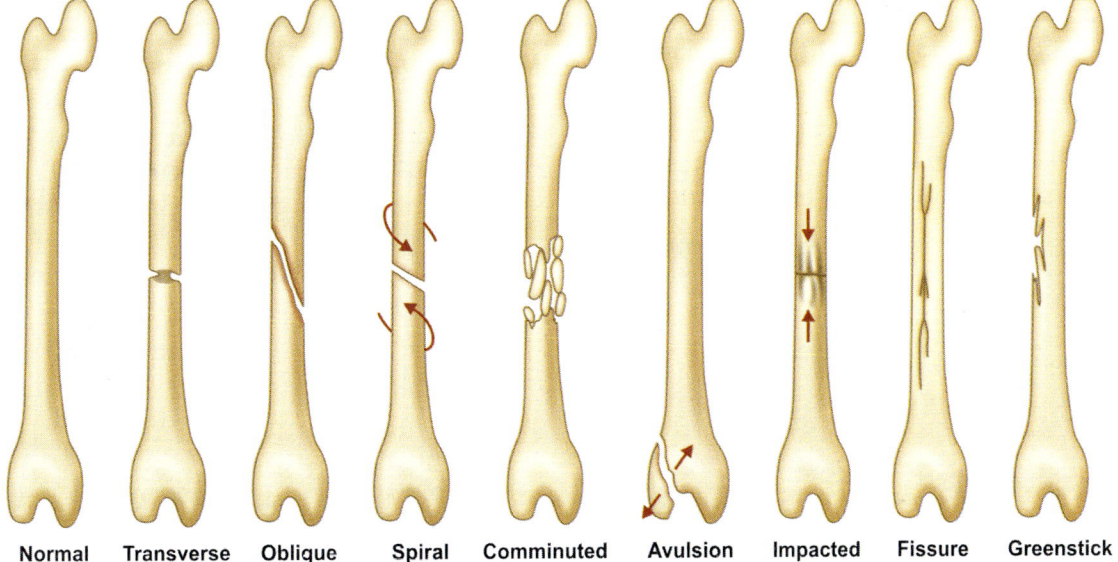

| Normal | Transverse | Oblique | Spiral | Comminuted | Avulsion | Impacted | Fissure | Greenstick |

Fig. 57.8: Radiological types of fracture

General Approach

- Wound care
- Pain management (e.g. non-opioid analgesics, opioids)
- Fracture care (conservative or surgical)
  1. Anatomic reduction
  2. Fixation
  3. Immobilization (Fig. 57.9)

Principles of treatment

- Anatomical reduction
- Stable internal fixation
- Preservation of blood supply
- Early mobilization

Open fractures

- Wound debridement
- Antibiotic prophylaxis
- Stabilization of the fracture
- Early wound cover

The goal of fracture treatment is to obtain union of the fracture in the most anatomical position compatible with maximal functional return of the extremity:

- Conservative
- Operative

Conservative Fracture Management

- *Indications:* Stable fractures
- Mainstay management of pediatric fractures
- *Procedure:* Closed reduction and, if necessary, immobilization of the fractured bone and adjacent joints with a cast or splint

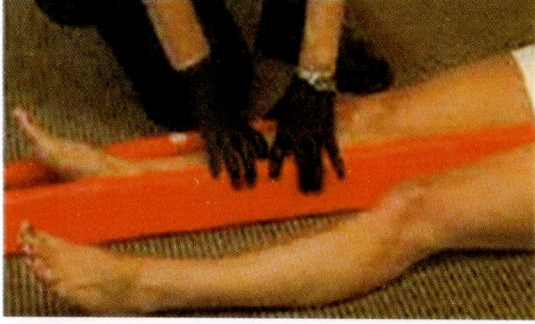

Fig. 57.9: Emergency splinting of a fracture

Fracture management can be divided into: nonoperative (also known as "conservative") and operative techniques. The nonoperative approach consists of a closed reduction, if required, followed by a period of immobilization with casting or splinting. Closed reduction is needed, if the fracture is significantly displaced or angulated.

Surgical Fracture Management

Indications

- Open fractures
- Unstable fractures
- Severe displacements (e.g. rotational deformities) and displaced fragments
- Inadequate manual reduction and fixation

Procedure: Anatomic reduction of the fracture and subsequent fixation and immobilization using:

- *External fixation:* Immobilizing a fracture using pins or screws that are secured outside the skin, or
- *Internal fixation:* Immobilizing a fracture using implants (e.g. plates, screws, wires)
- *Open reduction and internal fixation:* Realignment of the ends of a fracture, and stabilization of the fracture using implants (e.g. plates, screws, wires)

Absolute indications for ORIF of fractures include:

- Unable to obtain an adequate reduction
- Displaced intra-articular fractures
- Certain types of displaced epiphyseal fractures
- Major avulsion fractures where there is loss of function of a joint or muscle group
- Non-unions

Relative indications for ORIF of fractures include:

- Delayed unions
- Multiple fractures to assist in care and general management
- Unable to maintain a reduction
- Pathological fractures

- To assist in nursing care
- *Operative treatment:* The four AO [Arbeits-geme in Schaftfür Osteosynthese fragen) (Association for Osteosynthesis)] principles:
  - Anatomic reduction of the fracture fragments.
  - Stable fixation, absolute or relative, to fulfill biomechanical demands.
  - Preservation of blood supply to the injured area of the extremity and respect for the soft tissues.
  - Early range of motion (ROM) and rehabilitation.

The most important adage to remember in the management of a fracture is 'Reduce–Hold–Rehabilitate'.

In the context of high-energy injuries, this is precluded by resuscitation following ATLS (Advanced Trauma Life Support) principles.

Immobilization provides the basis for fracture healing. For many complex and unstable fractures, immobilization is achieved by means of internal fixation. However, many stable fractures at low risk of displacement can be immobilized effectively with casting, which can be performed by orthopedists or knowledgeable primary care clinicians.

Casting is standard treatment for many closed, nondisplaced, or reduced fractures. The optimal time to place a cast is after post-traumatic swelling has resolved. This usually takes 5 to 7 days following an injury but varies

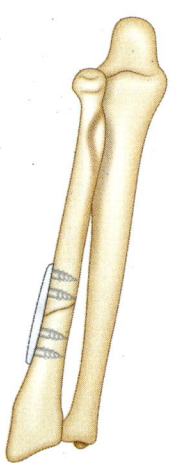

Type of fixation: Compression plate and screws	
Biomechanics	Stress shielding
Type of bone healing	Primary
Speed of recovery	Slow
Advantages	Allows perfect alignment of the fracture. Holds bone in compression allowing for primary healing
Disadvantanges	Stress shielding at the site of the plate. Some periosteal stripping inevitable
Other information	May initially need secondary support such as a splint or cast
Applications	Tibial plateau fracture. Displaced distal radial fracture

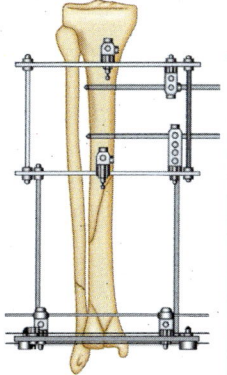

Type of fixation: External fixator devices	
Biomechanics	Stress shielding
Type of bone healing	Secondary
Speed of recovery	Fast
Advantages	Allows access to soft tissue, if wounds are open
Disadvantanges	Pin tract infections cumbersome
Other information	Mainly used if patients have associated soft tissue injuries that prevent ORIF, or if patient is too sick to undergo lengthy surgery
Applications	Open tibial fracture. Severely communited distal radial fractures

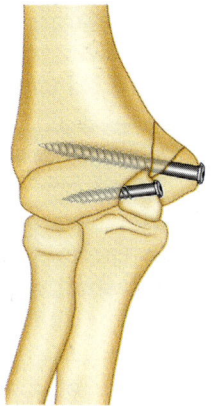

Type of fixation: Screws, pins, or wires

Biomechanics	Stress shielding
Type of bone healing	Secondary
Speed of recovery	Fast
Advantages	Minimal incision size often needed. Less chance of growth plate damage with the use of smooth wires (Kirschner wires/K-wires)
Disadvantanges	Difficult to get perfect alignment. Hardware may need to be removed after healing is achieved
Other information	Reamed rods are most commonly used
Applications	Midshaft tibial and femoral fractures

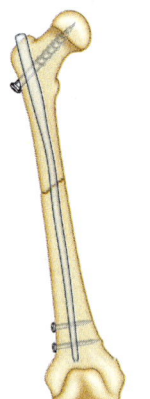

Type of fixation: Rods/nails

Biomechanics	Stress shielding
Type of bone healing	Secondary
Speed of recovery	Fast
Advantages	Smaller incision than plates so often less soft tissue damage caused by surgery. Early weight bearing possible
Disadvantanges	Disruption of endosteal blood supply. Reaming may cause fat emboli
Other information	Reamed rods are most commonly used
Applications	Midshaft tibial and femoral fractures

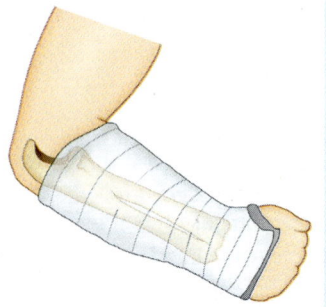

Type of fixation: Short or long cast of plaster or fiberglass' brace

Biomechanics	Stress shielding
Type of bone healing	Secondary
Speed of recovery	Fast
Advantages	Noninvasive. Easy to apply. Inexpensive
Disadvantanges	Skin breakdown or maceration. Reduction of fracture may be lost, if cast becomes loose. Potential for harmful pressure on nerve/blood vessels
Other information	Most commonly used means of fracture support
Applications	Torus fracture of the wrist. Nondisplaced later malleolar fracture

depending upon the location and type of fracture.

Implants Types

- Pin and wire fixation
- Screw fixation
- Plate and screw fixation
- Intramedullary nail fixation
- External fixation

Complications of Fractures

Early
- Visceral injury
- Vascular injury
- Nerve injury
- Compartment syndrome
- Hemarthrosis
- Infection
- Gas gangrene
- Fracture blisters
- Plaster and pressure sores

Late
- Delayed union
- Non-union
- Avascular necrosis
- Malunion (Fig. 57.10)
- Bedsores
- Myositis ossificans
- Tendon lesion
- Nerve compression
- Muscle contracture

- Joint instability—joint stiffness—algody-strophy RSD—osteoarthritis

COMPLICATIONS OF FRACTURE (Detailed)

Acute complications
- Neurologic and vascular injury (e.g. bleeding, hematoma, seroma)
- Compartment syndrome
- Wound infection, osteomyelitis

Long-term complications
- Avascular necrosis
- Complex regional pain syndrome
- Post-traumatic osteoarthritis
- Joint stiffness/contracture
- Joint instability
- Heterotopic ossification
- *Children:* Growth disturbances after growth plate injury (→ Salter-Harris fracture)
- *Nonunion:* Incomplete healing of a fracture which results in the creation of a false joint (pseudarthrosis)
- *Clinical features:* Pain, swelling, limited weight-bearing capacity, and reduced range of motion persisting after the normal duration of healing (usually 6–9 months)
- *Treatment:* Debridement and resection, osteosynthesis (fixation), antibiotics in the case of infected nonunion

Complications due to immobilization
- Thrombosis, pulmonary embolism
- Infections (e.g. pneumonia, urinary tract infection)

BIBLIOGRAPHY

- https://www.amboss.com/us/knowledge/General_principles_of_fractures
- https://www.uptodate.com/contents/general-principles-of-fracture-management
- https://metronorth.health.qld.gov.au/
- https://gmch.gov.in/e-study/e%20lectures/Surgery
- https://www.sciencedirect.com/topics/medicine-and-dentistry/fracture-management
- https://medrevise.co.uk/index.php?title
- https://www.youtube.com › watch
- https://orthopaedicprinciples.com › 2017/07

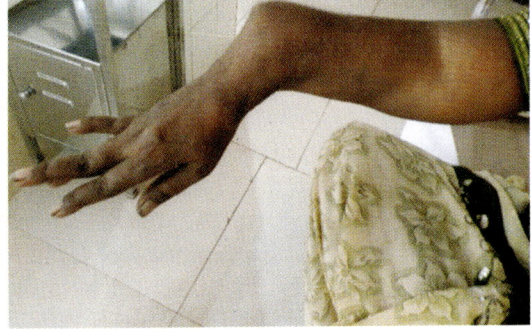

Fig. 57.10: Malunion of forearm bone fracture

Chapter
58

Injuries of Thoracic Cage

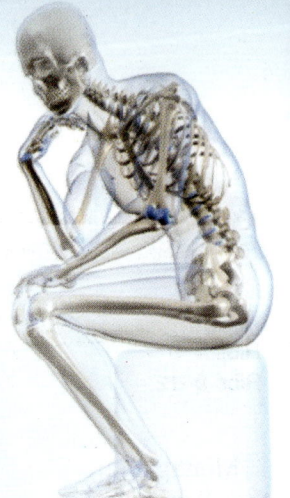

Rib fractures are the most common form of blunt thoracic injury. The ribs are frequently affected by blunt or penetrating injury to the thorax. Rib fractures are the most common form of significant chest injury, resulting from more than half of cases of blunt trauma. Rib fractures are very common and are detected in at least 10% of all injured patients, the majority of which are as a consequence of blunt thoracic trauma (75%) with road traffic collisions being the main cause. The remaining 25% are due to penetrating injuries. The issue with a rib fracture is not in the fracture itself; an isolated rib fracture is painful but not life-threatening. The danger with rib fractures lies with the potential for underlying injury such as pneumothorax, hemothorax, cardiac injury, and liver and spleen lacerations. Multiple rib fractures are an important indicator of trauma severity, with increased morbidity and mortality occurring with increasing numbers of rib fractures, especially in the elderly. Four or more fractured ribs are associated with higher mortality rates and seven or more have a mortality rate of 29%.

Fractures to the first three ribs are uncommon, as they are short and stiff and protected by the clavicle, scapula and muscles of the upper chest wall. A fracture to these ribs suggests significant force was transmitted into the thorax, and the risk of intrathoracic injury is high. The presence of two or more rib fractures at any level on the thoracic cage is associated with a higher incidence of internal injuries. Ribs 4–9 are the most commonly injured because of their exposed position and relative immobility, as they are attached to the sternum anteriorly and the spine posteriorly. Fractures to ribs 9–11 are associated with increased risk of intra-abdominal injury, specifically to the liver and spleen.

A standard posteroanterior chest radiograph usually suffices for evaluation of suspected rib fractures after minor trauma.

For isolated injuries (i.e. single rib fracture), clinicians generally begin treatment with nonsteroidal anti-inflammatory drugs (NSAIDs) with or without opioids. For more severe injuries, particularly if ventilation is compromised, admission and invasive treatments, such as intercostal nerve blocks may be needed.

Patients with one or two nondisplaced rib fractures found on imaging studies, or focal tenderness over one or two ribs but no evidence of fracture on CXR and who are assumed to have a rib fracture, may be treated with analgesics and discharged without a period of observation, assuming there are no other injuries of concern.

Thoracic cage injuries may be associated with concomitant and potentially life-threating injuries. In the acute setting, correct recognition of the pattern, extent and severity of thoracic cage injuries, may aid in more accurate delineation of concomitant injuries (Table 58.1 and Flowchart 58.1).

Table 58.1: Rib location and associated injury sites

Rib location	Associated injury sites
Rib 1	Subclavian vessel
Ribs 1–3	Vascular, brachial plexus
Ribs 4–9	Pulmonary, cardiovascular
Ribs 9–12	Liver (right ribs), spleen (left ribs)

Management of rib fractures by stabilizing the chest has been around for centuries, but has gone in and out of fashion. However, more recently, rib fracture fixation has made a resurgence with evidence suggesting it is beneficial for a certain group of patients. Intubated patients with a flail chest, respiratory failure, and prolonged ventilation, or non-intubated patients with a flail with deteriorating pulmonary function, are now considered for operative fixation. Once accessed, the fracture is reduced and a plate of appropriate length, usually 6–10 holes, is applied. The majority of plates are pre-contoured for different rib levels, although sometimes additional moulding is required.

Surgical fixation may be of benefit with some types of rib fractures, particularly those associated with chest wall deformity, flail chest, or symptomatic nonunion (Fig. 58.1).

HEMOTHORAX (Fig. 58.2)

A hemothorax occurs when blood collects in the pleural cavity. It can occur with both blunt and penetrating chest trauma. Large injuries to the lung parenchyma and to arteries and/or veins can bleed considerably (more than 1 liter) and lead to hypovolemic shock.

The usual cause of hemothorax is laceration of the lung, intercostal vessel, or an internal mammary artery. It can result from penetrating or blunt trauma. Hemothorax is often accompanied by pneumothorax (hemopneumothorax). Massive hemothorax is most

Flowchart 58.1: A simple, rapid assessment of patients with thoracic trauma and respiratory distress during the primary survey

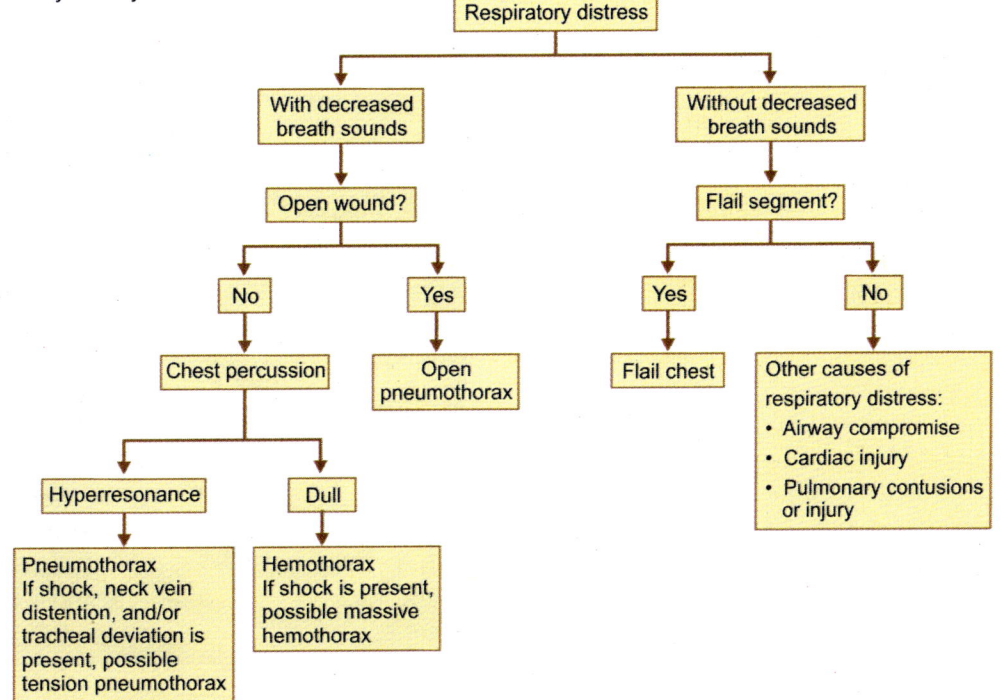

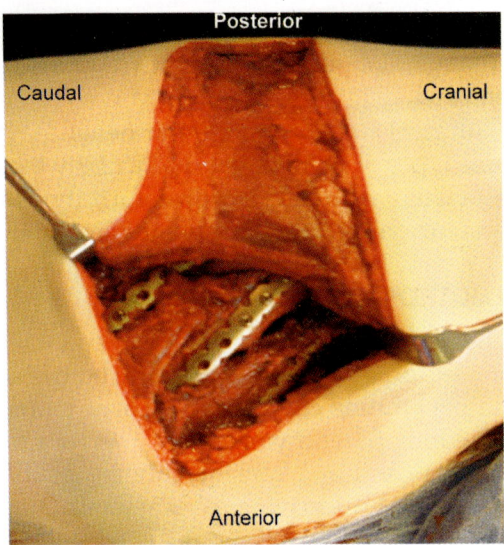

Fig. 58.1: Plating of rib fractures

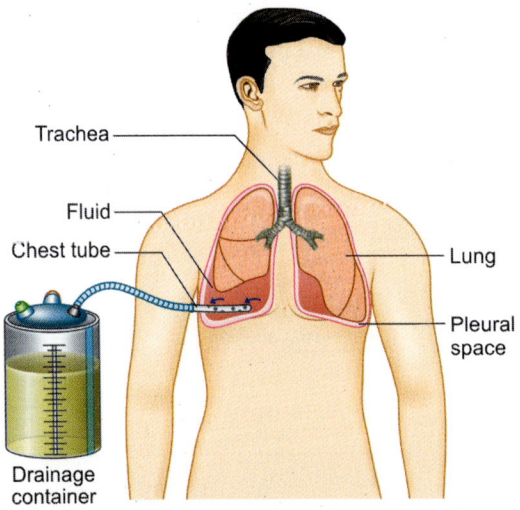

Fig. 58.2: Intercostal chest drainage tube

often defined as rapid accumulation of ≥1000 mL of blood. Hypovolemic shock is common.

Patients with large hemorrhage volume are often dyspneic and have decreased breath sounds and dullness to percussion (often difficult to appreciate during initial evaluation of patients with multiple injuries).

If allowed to progress, an uncommon complication termed a tension hemothorax can develop that will present similarly to a tension pneumothorax.

FLAIL CHEST (Fig. 58.3)

Flail chest is multiple fractures in ≥3 adjacent ribs that result in a segment of the chest wall separating from the rest of the thoracic cage; it is a marker for injury to the underlying lung. A single rib may fracture in more than one place. A flail chest is created when three or more ribs are fractured at two or more places each, creating a freely moving segment of chest wall that moves paradoxically to the rest of the chest. Flail segments can be located anteriorly, laterally or posteriorly, and a flail sternum can result from anterior blunt force trauma that disarticulates the sternum from all the ribs (costochondral separation). If multiple (3 or more) adjacent ribs fracture in ≥2 places, the breaks in each rib result in a segment of chest wall that is not mechanically connected to the rest of the thoracic cage (flail segment). This flail segment moves paradoxically (i.e. outward during expiration and inward during inspiration). Paradoxical chest wall motion is the classic sign of flail chest, but may not initially be present, if muscular

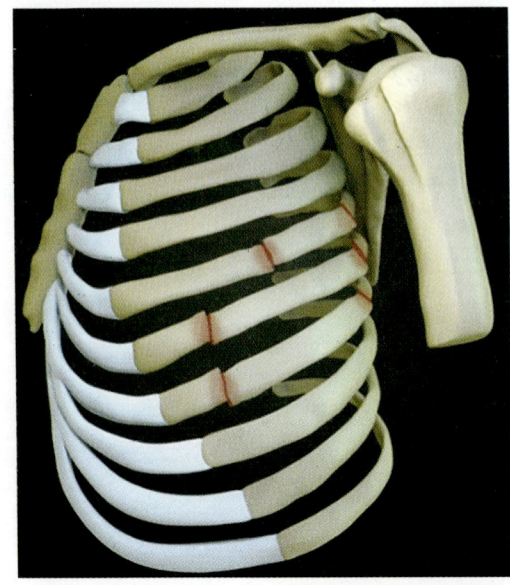

Fig. 58.3: Flail chest

splinting of the chest wall stabilizes the segment in place.

Flail chest is usually managed supportively, with adequate analgesia and chest physiotherapy to assist with volume expansion, and secretion management to prevent secondary complications of atelectasis and pneumonia. 'Internal splinting' with positive pressure ventilation can help and select cases can be treated surgically by internal fixation.

TENSION PNEUMOTHORAX (Fig. 58.4)

Tension pneumothorax develops when a lung or chest wall injury is such that it allows air into the pleural space but not out of it (a one-way valve). As a result, air accumulates and compresses the lung, eventually shifting the mediastinum, compressing the contralateral lung, and increasing intrathoracic pressure enough to decrease venous return to the heart, causing shock.

Treatment

Needle decompression followed by tube thoracostomy: Treatment is immediate needle decompression by inserting a large-bore (e.g. 14- or 16 gauge) needle into the 2nd intercostal space in the midclavicular line. Air will usually gush out. Because needle decompression causes a simple pneumothorax, tube thoracostomy should be done immediately thereafter.

In patients with thoracic trauma and impaired circulation (signs of shock), severe injuries to consider during the primary survey include the following:
- Massive hemothorax
- Tension pneumothorax
- Cardiac tamponade

The common symptoms and signs of tension pneumothorax include:
- Respiratory distress
- Agitation with tachypnea
- Hypoxia
- Tachycardia
- Hypotension
- Decreased or absent breath sounds on the affected side
- Hyperexpansion
- Decreased movement of the affected hemithorax
- Subcutaneous emphysema.

Management

If tension pneumothorax is suspected, or cannot be excluded in the hypotensive multi-

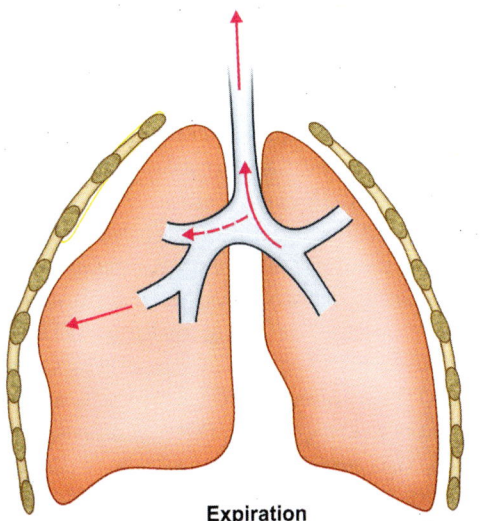
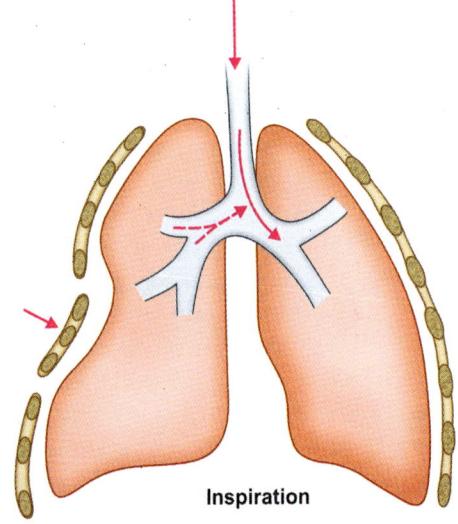

Expiration   Inspiration

Fig. 58.4: Tension pneumothorax

trauma patient who is not responding to volume resuscitation, then chest decompression must be performed without delay. Needle decompression is performed preferably at the 5th intercostal space, mid-axillary line (with the arm in the abducted position). This location may not be easily accessible, and in such circumstances the 2nd intercostal space, mid-axillary line is used. A large bore IV cannula (14 or 16G) with a 10 mL syringe attached is inserted, and air is drawn. Alternatively a pneumocath can be used. Needle decompression will allow time to transport the patient to a medical facility for definitive decompression and intercostal catheter insertion.

If the patient is conscious, and equipment for finger thoracostomy is not immediately at hand, then a needle decompression should be performed at the 5th intercostal space, mid-axillary line.

Chest Tube Insertion

Re-expanding the lung may tamponade any bleeding vessels, as well as draining a pneumothorax. Once the chest is decompressed via finger thoracostomy under aseptic technique, an ICC is inserted, and is directed posterior and apical. Tube size is important and should be a large bore (28–32 Fr) in order to facilitate rapid drainage, prevent air leaks and to allow large blood clots to be removed. Once advanced, ensure fogging of the tube with expiration and suture in place. Placement should be confirmed with CXR. Auto-transfusion could be considered in some circumstances, if capabilities exist.

Sternal fracture and costochondral separation (separation of the sternum from the ribs) are most often caused by anterior blunt force trauma, the most frequent mechanism being collision of the chest with a steering wheel. Contrary to intuition, a restrained passenger is more likely than an unrestrained passenger to suffer sternal fracture. An isolated sternal fracture has extremely low mortality risk, but this rises rapidly with the presence of associated injuries. Associated injuries that contribute to this high mortality include flail chest, aortic injury, pulmonary and myocardial contusions, intra-abdominal injuries and head injury.

PNEUMOTHORAX

A pneumothorax occurs when air collects in the pleural space between the lung and inside of the chest wall. It is a common complication of blunt and penetrating chest trauma and is present by default in every patient with penetrating injuries that pass through the parietal and visceral pleura. Pneumothoraces are classified as simple, open or tension.

A simple pneumothorax occurs when a hole in the visceral pleura allows air to escape the lung and collect in the pleural space. A simple pneumothorax is most often caused when a fractured rib lacerates the pleura. It may also occur without a fracture when blunt trauma is delivered at full inspiration with the glottis closed.

An open pneumothorax occurs when a hole in the chest wall and pleura allows air to collect in the pleural space. The violation of the pleural space eliminates the normally negative intrapleural pressure that exists between the lung and chest wall, causing the affected lung to collapse. Air may move in and out of the hole in the chest wall with inspiration, resulting in a sucking chest wound.

A tension pneumothorax occurs when the initial defect in the chest wall or lung acts as a one-way valve, allowing air to enter the thorax with inspiration but not escape with exhalation. With each breath, pressure within the hemithorax increases, further deflating the lung. As pressure continues to increase, the mediastinum is pushed toward the unaffected side. This shift causes the vena cava to kink, resulting in decreased venous return. This creates a chain reaction of decreased preload, decreased stroke volume, decreased cardiac output and, ultimately, decreased blood pressure.

BIBLIOGRAPHY

- pubs.rsna.org>doi> full Flail chest-Injuries; Poisoning-MSD Manual Professional; Traumatic Rib Injury: Patterns, Imaging Pitfalls, Complications.
- radiologykey.com>traumatic-chest-wall-injuries; Traumatic Chest Wall Injuries. Radiology Key
- www.msdmanuals.com; Flail Chest-Injuries; Poisoning–MSD Manual Professional
- www.msdmanuals.com; Thoracic Trauma
- accessurgery.mhmedical.com; Thoracic Injuries. Quick Answers Surgery. Access Surgery

Index

303